Henry B. M. Murphy

Comparative Psychiatry

The International and Intercultural Distribution of Mental Illness

With 28 Figures

Springer-Verlag
Berlin Heidelberg New York 1982

Professor Dr. H. B. M. Murphy
McGill University, Department of Psychiatry,
1025 Pine Avenue West, Montreal, PQ/Canada H3A 1A1

ISBN-13:978-3-642-81716-8 e-ISBN-13:978-3-642-81714-4
DOI: 10.1007978-3-642-81714-4

Library of Congress Cataloging in Publication Data. Murphy, H. B. M. (Henry Brian Megget), 1915– Comparative psychiatry. (Monographien aus dem Gesamtgebiete der Psychiatrie ; 28) Bibliography: p. Includes index. 1. Psychiatry, Transcultural. I. Title. II. Title: The International and intercultural distribution of mental illness. III. Series. [DNLM: 1. Mental disorders — Occurrence. 2. Cross-cultural comparison. W1 MO561B v. 28 / MW 100 M978c] RC454.4.M87 362.2'0422 81-16638 ISBN-13:978-3-642-81716-8 (U.S.) AACR2

Softcover reprint of the hardcover 1st edition 1982

Typesetting: Fa. B. Steiner, Heidelberg

2125 / 3130-54321 0

Preface

The history of this book dates back to 1946, when I was put in charge of the medical services for a group of refugee camps in Germany. Each camp tended to be occupied by people of a particular cultural origin – Estonian, Jewish, Latvian, Lithuanian, Polish – and as I sat with the camp doctors seeing patients or discussing cases it became apparent that some syndromes, particularly the more psychiatric, could be common across the camps of one cultural group while uncommon in the camps of another. My clinical teachers had said nothing about such variance, and when I sought to learn more about it I found that very little had been written. In due course that led me to search out employment in some location where I would be able to investigate the phenomenon systematically, and this has become my prime interest ever since, encouraged by my wife, who not only tolerated the discomforts which it sometimes led to but also assisted in the work in numerous ways.

Over much of the time during which I have been engaged in this pursuit, it has been McGill University, with its Section for Transcultural Psychiatric Studies established by my colleague Eric Wittkower, that sheltered and encouraged me. Nevertheless, until relatively recently the two main reasons why I had found it difficult in 1946 to learn about national and cultural differences in mental disorders have persisted, and they deserve mention here as a warning to those who are tempted to embark on similar enquiries. The first of these reasons is that societies can feel uncomfortable when their mental health is compared with that of their neighbors – except perhaps when the comparison is in their favor – since the results may appear to cast doubt on their efficiency and values, more specifically on what the Swedish philosopher Harald Ofstad * has called their "value-myths"; consequently they prefer that such comparisons be avoided. The second reason is that they, and their representatives, see little purpose in funding investigations in other societies when the results are unlikely to have a concrete application in their own; unless the investigation is requested by the other society as a form of aid, something which rarely occurs. The force of these problems is weakening, and the number of people engaged in such studies has grown greatly in recent years, so that the subject has become part of mainstream psychiatric teaching. Nevertheless, it continues to be difficult to persuade psychiatrists to examine the mental health of their own society as compared with that of others at the same developmental stage, although it is now much easier to interest them in examining the mental health of societies with which they are less personally identified.

This book attempts to bring together the main lessons which we can infer from such examinations. I apologize if I sometimes appear to make too much use of my own researches and not enough use of those of other people, but one's own work is always what comes easiest to mind when one is searching for an illustration. I apologize also for the fact that some of the illustrations draw on findings – my own and those of others – which have never been properly published and therefore cannot be verified by the critical reader, my excuse being that in this book the principles being illustrated are of more importance than the facts which illustrate them. These principles do not come from any one tradition or school; rather they are the crystallization of the ideas of many prior authorities and current colleagues in the social sciences as well as in medicine, and to these I gladly express my debt, although they are too many to mention. Regarding the preparation of the book itself, however, there are three sources of aid which I would like specifically to acknowledge. First, that of Dr. Fred Fenton, to whom I turned, as someone not so well acquainted with the field that his own knowledge would unconsciously bridge my omissions, for criticisms of successive chapter drafts, and who has pointed out numerous errors in my thinking, ones which I hope I have been able to correct. Secondly, that of the librarians at the McGill Medical and Osler libraries, who undertook the tracking down of a host of difficult-to-find texts. Without their help I would have often had to rely on not-always-accurate secondary sources, and sometimes would have been misled. Thirdly, that of my secretary, Mrs. Vibeke Teller, without whose criticisms my English would be much more tortuous and difficult to follow. To these in particular, but also to the many others who know themselves to have helped me at particular stages, I extend my thanks.

Montreal, November 1981 — Henry B.M. Murphy

---

* Ofstad H (1981) Identity and minority; value conflicts and conflicts of identity. In: Eitinger L, Schwarz D (eds) Strangers in the world. Huber, Berne, pp 42–69

Contents

Chapter 1 Introduction

It is to Emil Kraepelin that we are indebted for the term Comparative Psychiatry in the particular meaning which it customarily carries today, and the meaning which inspires this book. In a 1904 paper under this title, he pointed out that while comparisons of mental disorders in groups of different age, sex, and occupation are quite familiar and would not seem to need putting into any special category, these had almost entirely "been confined to groups of the same nationality so that it is virtually unknown whether the psychiatric morbidity of the French, English, or Italians differs from that of ourselves (i.e., the Germans), and if so in what respects" [317]. He thus implicitly proposed that the term Comparative Psychiatry be applied to international and cross-cultural studies, and immediately illustrated what he had in mind by reporting impressions which he had obtained from visits to Java and Singapore, comparing samples of patients there with samples in Europe. Since the contrast in that paper is mainly between Asians and Europeans, one may get the impression that it is racial variations that were in his mind, but the subsequent editions of his famous textbook [318] make it clear that he was thinking of comparisons within Europe, even within Germany itself, as well. The purpose of such comparisons was for him self-evident, namely to obtain more information upon which could be built the "scientific" psychiatry which he believed he had so strongly promoted in distinguishing dementia praecox, paranoia, and manic-depressive psychosis from the muddle of ambiguous terms with which psychiatrists had had to work previously. His approach was pragmatic, to break down the barriers to the collection of relevant knowledge, and although racial factors enter into consideration he does not seem to have been biased for or against particular theories, so long as they were "scientific" and not "philosophical."

Subsequent authors, most recently P.M. Yap in his book *Comparative Psychiatry, a Theoretical Framework* [680], have largely shared that position, seeing international comparisons as a means of developing and testing etiological theory and the soundness of our classifications. However, in the three–quarters of a century since Kraepelin wrote, the lines of development in psychiatry have not been entirely what he would have expected, and his assumption that a "scientific" psychiatry would triumph at the expense of what he saw as merely philosophical ramblings has not proved true. We still do not know how to identify with confidence the dementia praecox which he thought he had delimited, and some of the considerations which he called philosophical appear to possess real substance when it comes to assessing the prognosis of that disorder. New doubts regarding the nature of psychiatry have developed since his day, and we no longer view the researcher as a neutral recorder of data which are independent of his presence. Therefore, while Kraeplin's insight into the need for Comparative Psychiatry is still valid and relevant today, it is desirable that the nature and parameters of the field be defined more clearly than he undertook to do.

This chapter is concerned with these definitions, and in the process will attempt to indicate the concepts, assumptions, biases, and limitations which are likely to have influenced the choice of material for the chapters that follow. The reader whose interest is only in research data and their interpretation is advised to pass on to questions of method in the next two chapters or even directly to the presentation of comparative data in Chap. 4. The reader more concerned about the ways in which definitions and viewpoint may affect findings is invited to continue here.

1 Definition, Goals, and Parameters

By Comparative Psychiatry is here meant the study of the relations between mental disorder and the psychological characteristics which differentiate nations, peoples, or cultures. Its main goals are to identify, verify, and explain the links between mental disorder and these broad psychosocial characteristics, and its main tool is explicit comparison rather than the implicit comparison which takes place all the time in any clinical field. What marks it off from psychiatry in general is firstly that it is an academic discipline rather than a healing art. One does not apply it directly to the care of the individual patient, even though its findings may be used on his behalf and though that care may be the subject of its investigations. Secondly, it is not directly concerned with organic factors, whether they be genetic, traumatic, infectious, dietary, or other. All these factors may influence the results which one obtains when comparing one nation or culture with another, but they are not best investigated by this type of comparison since the overlap is too imprecise. Two nations may differ markedly in their predominant racial, i.e., genetic, inheritance, but that does not make this the best way of studying genetic factors. Normally, a nation has quite a mixture of genetic origins, even though this may be something its members prefer to overlook, and in any case genetic comparisons are best made between groups whose psychosocial characteristics are highly similar so that it is only the genetic factor which distinguishes them. Thirdly, it is not concerned with all psychosocial factors or even with those which normally attract the most attention in psychiatry; rather it is concerned with those which, because they are all pervasive in a society, tend to get overlooked by the great majority of researchers who work only within single societies. All good clinicians and many researchers consciously or unconsciously compare the mentally ill with their healthy neighbors and draw clinically relevant inferences from the contrast, but they tend not to draw inferences from what the patients and their neighbors have in common even though some of that which they have in common – and which differentiates them from people in another society – may equally be of clinical relevance.

These are the rough delimitations of the field, but they conceal a host of uncertainties. What do we mean by mental disorder, by nation, by psychosocial characteristic? What theories are being relied on to justify the assumption that mental health can be affected by psychosocial characteristics so general that they are shared by whole societies? How can one pretend to derive sound findings from international comparisons when it is well known that nations tend to have different systems of psychiatric care, use different diagnostic criteria, and have different concepts of normality? Points such as these require separate examination.

2 Concepts of Mental Disorder

In Kraepelin's initial paper, he stated that "A reasonably reliable comparison is only possible, of course, if we contrast real disease entities rather than vague syndromes ..." [317]. The era in which he was writing was one in which bacteriology and micropathology were enabling medical science to differentiate the key features and causes of various diseases much more sharply than had been possible previously. He therefore seemed justified in assuming that the same would happen in psychiatry and that the "real disease entities" to which he refers would soon be as confidently differentiated as syphilis from tuberculosis. This has not occurred, the whole "medical model" of psychiatry has been challenged, and even when that model is retained there are major questions whether the main concern of psychiatry should be with "disease," i.e., what the clinician can objectively identify, or with "illness," i.e., what the patient experiences. So: what concept of mental disorder should underlie international and cross-cultural comparisons?

The answer coming closest to Kraepelin's model is the Schneiderian one [544], which sees mental diseases as analogous to somatic diseases and makes a fairly clear distinction between the former and what are seen as "abnormal psychic reactions." e.g., various forms of neuroticism. With such a view of mental disorder, Comparative Psychiatry can model itself on international epidemiology, seeking to measure the frequency and character of specific diseases in different societies. It is a view which yields good results, both practical and theoretical, when one has diseases for which there is an objective indicator, as is the case with general paresis, or whose features are so distinctive that their presence or absence can easily be ascertained in any individual, as is the case with *koro* and some other "culture-bound" syndromes. However, the disorders that fit these criteria form only a small minority of those with which psychiatry deals, and this "medical model" of mental disorder does not correspond as well to the modern concerns of psychiatry as some would like to believe.

The reason for this is twofold. In the first place, although we have reasonably clear, typical or core pictures of what this school of thought considers to be the mental diseases, and although authorities in most countries would agree with these pictures, patients stubbornly refuse to group themselves neatly in the same fashion. In all societies one can find abundant patients with some of the features of the typical syndromes just mentioned, but whose general clinical picture is mixed or atypical, and there are no agreed criteria for placing them into one or other of the standard catagories in the diagnostic manuals. Of course, for statistical purposes most of these atypical patients do get conventionally labeled eventually, thanks to bureaucratic pressure, but there are abundant studies indicating that different psychiatrists would label them in different ways. Relatively few psychiatrists believe that we know sufficient about psychopathology to be able to say just what symptoms are basic or diagnostic for each disease, and the history of the diagnosis of depression in Africa provides a warning against deciding prematurely on the subject. Prior to the mid-1950s it was generally agreed that endogenous depression was a rare condition in non-Westernized Africans; since then it has come to be seen as one of the commonest mental diseases among them, the shift in opinion arising from the realization that excessive guilt feelings, a common symptom in European endogenous depressions, were not essential to the disorder and were usually absent in African cases.

The second reason why this concept of mental disorder does not correspond well with modern thinking is that it follows a tradition of making a sharp distinction between illness and health (with the latter covering a wide range of states), whereas current opinion tends much more towards the idea of a continuum between the two, and sees everything which is not perfect mental health as being of psychiatric concern. At times this latter attitude appears too broad – little more than the expression of empire-building on the part of the mental health professions – and inappropriate for a scientific text. However, it must be remembered that there are social sciences as well as biological ones, so that a psychiatric concept which makes use of sociological principles can be almost as scientific as one making use of biological principles. Empirically, the well-known ability of one psychiatric syndrome to substitute for another, and the fact that under certain conditions of social stress it is not just a single mental disease that is increased but several, both suggest that handling the concept of mental disorder in terms of discrete diseases may be inadequate. But the question now becomes whether any broader concept of mental disorder has received sufficient international consensus and has sufficient clarity for international comparisons employing it to be satisfactory.

A concept of mental disorder not clearly differentiated into diseases existed long before Kraepelin, and it was to some extent that tradition that he and his predecessor Kahlbaum saw themselves fighting against. However, it was a tradition based not just on an inability to distinguish syndromes but on the idea, so familiar today, that certain types of social stress can increase psychiatric risk, with the particular type of mental disorder that ensues depending on personal factors but being less important than the stress or trauma which precipitated it. Furthermore, in this tradition, the possibility of different peoples having different rates of mental disturbance by reason of social experiences or cultural orientations was widely accepted. In 1794, Benjamin Rush claimed that participation in the American Revolution cured women of hysteria whereas traditional loyalty to the British Crown was encouraging mental illness [527]. In the 1820s, in a survey of British mental hospitals and asylums, Halliday was claiming with almost equal exaggeration that "not one of our African travellers remark their having seen a single madman" [243]. Ten years later, Esquirol, much more relying on his own observations, stated regarding the Paris of 1830–1831 that "the disturbances of that period exercised an influence on the occurrence of insanity, not just through fear and political exaltation but through the social transpositions (*boulversements*) of so many people" [173]. Later in the same century it was widely believed by people like Jarvis, Maudsley, and even Griesinger that insanity was more frequent in modern urban societies than in traditional rural ones, both within the Western world and beyond it, this being "a part of the price we pay for civilization" [278]. And it was insanity in general that these authors were thinking about, mainly the psychoses but extending to hysteria (as Rush's claim indicates) and sometimes to alcoholism as well, so long as the condition was producing a clear interference with social functioning.

Today very similar concerns are voiced, even though civilization and rapid social change are now less often implicated as etiological factors than social disorganization, social exploitation, and the operation of certain social norms. However, where there has been a change for many researchers concerns the point at which mental health and mental ill-health divide. In the earlier studies, regardless of whether official records or survey data were employed, a diagnosis of mental disorder implied an intrapsychic interference with the ability to satisfy basic needs (food, shelter, companionship) and fulfill normal social roles, so that the division between ill-health and health was in practice quite close to what Schneiderians would consider to be the division between psychopathology and "abnormal psychic reactions," even though the underlying theory was very different. Since the 1950s one might say that mental ill-health is seen by a number of authorities as starting at the point where there appears to be an interference with the individual's ability to satisfy his higher needs [in Maslow's sense (384)]; regardless of whether basic needs and social functioning are affected or not.

The shift of the dividing point in the direction of better relative health is in harmony with the trend in medicine generally and the desire to pick up illness at an earlier stage; but whereas in other branches of medicine this can be done objectively with the aid of more refined laboratory techniques, etc., it is a change that poses problems in psychiatry. When disturbances of role playing and inability to meet basic needs are the criteria, psychiatrists and other observers can attempt to apply uniform methods of measuring them. When inability to meet the higher, intrapsychic, needs is the criterion, outsiders cannot directly judge the matter but must infer this from what the individual says regarding his state of mind and psychophysiological symptoms. In a sense this makes each person his own judge, something which is probably welcomed by those who regard psychiatric diagnosis as a social imposition but which makes comparative studies only really valid when all these persons are employing the same definitions and criteria, and are speaking the truth regarding themselves in as far as they know it. Moreover, for such comparisons one faces not just the practical problem of persuading these self-assessors to use the same concepts of need, distress, and symptom, but the theoretical problem of deciding whether certain mental states are normal or not. It is easy enough to say that certain neuroses are true disorders rather than normal psychic variants, but there is no agreement regarding the points at which examination anxiety, separation grief, the low selfesteem of the mental defective, and the memory loss of a septuagenarian should be considered as disorders and cease to be considered as normal experiences.

It is possible that in the future there will be broad agreement on where health ends and ill-health begins, and possible also that a technique will be devised for comparing the self-assessments of different people, but the degree to which different ways of assessing mental health agree with each other at present is low. Table 1.1 presents data from an Austrian survey of patients found in general medical consulting rooms [597], and one sees that if the patients had been assessed according to

Table 1. Disharmony in psychiatric indicators [597]

		Class of patient's main presenting complaint		
		Somatic	Psychiatric	
Class of diagnosis assigned by attending physician	Somatic	289 (34.6%)	192 (20.5%)	481 (55.1%)
	Psychiatric	165 (19.7%)	220 (26.2%)	385 (44.9%)
		454 (54.3%)	412 (46.7%)	836 (100%)

Data derive from adult patients seen in 11 Austrian general practices. Patient's presenting complaints were recorded in a questionnaire administered in the waiting room, and diagnostic class was assigned on the same day by the physician immediately after seeing the patient

the psychiatric content of their presenting complaint there would have been very little agreement with the assessments made by their physicians. Naturally, the problem gets worse when one attempts to compare several cultural groups using more than one measure, as I have done [431]; but even in a single society studied by the same researcher, assessments of neurosis can vary greatly. When Lin repeated in 1962 his well-known 1947 survey of mental disorder in Taiwanese communities, the assessed rate of neurosis jumped from 1.2 to 7.8 per 1000, whereas the rate for all other mental disorders changed only from 8.2 to 9.4 [355].

There are other less widely accepted concepts of mental disorder which could be discussed, some based on structural (e.g., psychoanalytic) and some on functional grounds. All of them, like the forgeoing, can appear sound enough given some premise, but each of them fails when pushed to its logical limits. Hence we appear to have only two alternatives. We can reject the concept of mental disorder as a social fiction, as do some antipsychiatrists, and say that there are only people in need of help, people who should not be labeled any more precisely than this. Or we can accept a compromise between different labeling systems, knowing that this compromise cannnot be defended on sound theoretical grounds, but may still yield empirically useful results.

The first of these is impractical even for the purpose for which it is usually proposed, namely the prevention of stigmatization of patients, since that is going to continue whether there is psychiatric labeling or not, should the society be so inclined. Neither is it going to prevent therapists from consciously or unconsciously putting their patients into categories; and any categorizing tendency is better organized than left to run wild. The second alternative, in contrast, is capable of yielding quite fruitful results under most circumstances, particularly if one remembers that different levels of judgment deserve different degrees of confidence, and also that all compromises tend to be theoretically unsound. For comparative purposes, and particularly for assessing the degree of confidence that data should receive, the level of manifest disfunction which a disorder produces probably offers the best basis on which the compromise should rest, but this is a matter of opinion. The reasons for my preference and the meaning of "degree of confidence" in this context are as follows.

Confidence in data is highest when judgements of mental disorder meet little disagreement, and this is commonest where there is marked interference with social functioning and when only a broad classification of the type of disorder is required. When that marked disfunction is present, distinction between what is mainly a psychic, mainly a somatic, and mainly a social disorder can usually be agreed on, as can the broad distinctions between exogenous psychoses, functional psychoses, neuroses, and psychopathy. However, the specific diagnosis that might be attached to such a case merits less confidence, since there are quite wide differences between psychiatric schools and practitioners regarding, for instance, the differentiation of senile psychosis from the reactive disorders of old age. Where interference with functioning is moderate but still externally observable, there can also be quite high agreement on whether the condition is principally psychic, somatic or social, provided the patients and the professionals come from the same uniform society; and the resultant data are also such as invite much confidence. If the people come from different societies or from one which has marked social variation, however, the confidence that can be placed in such comparative judgements is considerably lower, and it becomes lower still if detailed diagnoses are looked for. To take a concrete example, a Canadian Indian patient who exhibits disturbed behavior while under the influence of alcohol is quite likely to be seen as acting within social norms according to one authority, as suffering from a social disorder according to another, as suffering from alcoholism (a supposedly organic disorder) according to a third, as suffering from depression according to a fourth, and as suffering from a narcissistic neurosis according to a fifth. Finally, if interference with functioning is not externally observable, one's ability to make satisfactory comparisons is very limited unless special means have been used to explore motives and meanings. There is no doubt that we can compare one psychoanalytically investigated patient with another, when the records of the investigations are full enough, but with lesser degrees of investigation the equivalence of meanings becomes uncertain, as I found when I practiced psychotherapy with Chinese and East Indian patients in Singapore. With the information being still more elementary, as from a single brief interview, therefore, confidence in the comparability of judgements must be low.

In practice, this means that when one is dealing with judgments in which confidence can be high, one can take seriously quite limited differences and similarities, so long as they are statistically significant. Where the level of confidence in the comparability of individual or group judgments is low, on the other hand, similarities or differences in rates must be much more marked before one is justified in building hypotheses on them. This is an elementary point, but surprisingly often ignored when international comparisons are made, perhaps because the levels of confidence referred to have never received quantification in a way that, for instance, levels of confidence in anthropological texts have been assessed by Naroll [454].

3 Nations and Cultures

Having attempted to define mental disorder for the purpose of Comparative Psychiatry and having been forced to settle for an imprecise, operational definition, it is now necessary to see whether anything better can be achieved with the concepts of "nation," "people," "race," and perhaps "ethnic group." The assumption implicit in my definition of Comparative Psychiatry is that nations and cultures differ in their broad psychosocial "climates," and the same assumption appears to have been implicit in Kraepelin's desire to compare mental disorder among the French, British, Italians, and Germans. However, terms such as these – nation, culture, British, French – carry very different meanings for different people, and it might be complained that my term "psychosocial climate" is so vague as to be useless. So: why did Kraepelin choose this type of social division, and what can we assume such terms to mean for psychiatry?

Long before Kraepelin, the psychiatric literature had contained two types of either real or implied international comparison. One is that between stable, traditional, preindustrial societies and unstable, industrial, and supposedly more civilized ones. For most of the nineteenth century authors of these ideas, neither nation nor culture was really important, and they were as happy to choose examples from within a single country as from contrasting countries, since they aimed mainly at comparing simple and complex life styles. References to Africa, therefore, were implicitly to a place where life was simpler than in European cities, not to a place where the people were of a different race or had different styles of childrearing. Also, most of these comparisons were in very vague terms, by authors who had not made direct observations for themselves. The second type did involve direct comparisons, initially of a very elementary nature but by the end of the century quite specific and pointed, although relating to legislation and administration rather than psychopathology. The early papers, such as Pinel's reports on visits to Norway and Naples, Morel's on Holland, Belgium, Germany and Italy, and Brigham's on Britain and France, were little more than an indication of where one might meet active psychiatrists and be able to refer foreign patients. Sometimes one meets comments such as that of Morel to the effect that Dutch patients with a condition similar to one seen in France got better without the radical treatment that was thought necessary by Morel himself in the latter country and probably would have succumbed if that treatment had been given them [412]; but that is uncommon. However, the disturbing increase in the chronicity of the average mental hospital patient in the second half of the century, an increase which has never been adequately explained, led to much more serious comparisons regarding whether other countries were having as many problems as one's own, whether the legislation in any of these other countries (or regions within a single country) was more effective in protecting the mental patient, whether there was as administrative structure elsewhere that permitted the overburdened asylum doctors to give their patients better care, and whether there was a model whereby the status of these doctors could be improved. A good example of such a set of comparisons is that undertaken by an official French commsission under the chairmanship of Serieux [552]. What these practicing psychiatrists were clearly comparing when they went abroad were administrative units, i.e., countries or provinces over which particular laws and regulations operated. Their goal was to improve methods of care in the most direct manner possible. It was not to further their understanding of psychopathology, explore whether different peoples responded differently to the same treatment, or assess whether there was anything in their own society (other than the legal system) which might be contributing to mental disorder. This viewpoint does not clash with that which related the increase of mental disorder to civilization, since it was essentially only between "civilized" countries that the comprisons were made, i.e., countries which shared the same problems of trying to handle an excess of mental disorder which earlier in the century had not been apparent.

Towards the end of the nineteenth century, however, a third type of international comparison was being made in psychiatry which did implicitly clash with the "civilization" theory. This was the comparison between Germanic and Latin peoples which had at its roots the "degeneracy" or "decadence" theory first proposed by Morel but achieving its main expression in the writings of the Italian criminologist Lombroso. During the first half of the century, French ideas dominated Western Europe, even in those countries that were opposed to France, but as the German States grew stronger national rivalries increased, fed by the racial theories of Gobineau and Schallmayer; and after the 1870 war German popular writers came increasingly to refer to "Latin decadence," something which unfortunately found an echo in psychiatry. German psychiatrists visiting France had been struck by the abundant cases of hysteria which Janet and Charcot were demonstrating and which had apparently so few equivalents in Germany itself. One theory which existed even within France itself was that hysteria arose in "degenerate" families, and an apparently common opinion among German physicians was that "among the French... there are just more hereditarily tainted individuals than among the German races" [170]. In consequence, a new reason for making international comparisons appeared, one related to theories of racial superiority and the genetic origin of mental disorders.

Kraepelin neither accepted nor rejected these ideas (although he suspected that some of the cases of hysteria demonstrated by Janet and Charcot might be iatrogenic), but they were almost certainly one of the reasons why he called for comparisons within Europe and collected the data in Java. Handled correctly, they were quite legitimate grounds for carrying out comparative studies, but those of his successors who were attracted to these concepts did not have Kraepelin's dispassionate interest in facts for their own sake. From 1900 until World War II, a steady flow of usually poor quality papers based on this theory were published, most often having the Jews and the United States Blacks as their examples and making no allowance for the social factors which could affect the hospitalization rates of these groups. Unfortunately, this section of the literature has stamped Comparative Psychiatry in many European minds as being racist, so that there is still a reluctance to make certain types of comparison, for that reason.

Until the Second World War, therefore, if the terms nation, culture, and people were used by psychiatrists in more than a casual or operational fashion, they tended to refer sometimes to particular levels of social complexity, sometimes to alleged degrees of inherited degeneracy, and sometimes to the populations over which particular sets of laws and medical administration practices held sway. Today the same may apply, or there may be a deliberate vagueness of definition as was true of Kraepelin's use of the term *Volksart* (people); but it is much more likely that attention has been paid to the definitions used by social scientists for describing large social groups. It is desirable that we are aware of what these definitions are, and the

UNESCO-sponsored *Dictionary of the Social Sciences* [230] is as good as source as any.

Of the terms referred to at the beginning of this section, a *people* in Kraepelin's sense is not defined, having by now been replaced for scientific purposes by more precise terms. *Race* is given purely biological definitions, e.g., "a subgroup of people possessing a definite combination of physical characters, of genetic origin." *Nation* is relatively easily defined as "a considerable group of people, united by common culture, values, standards, and political aspirations, usually occupying a definite territory," but the dictionary recognized that the French usage (and perhaps the German) is more ideational or even idealizing than this. A *culture* in the demographic sense is simply a group that shares the same "culture" in the ideational sense, but regarding the latter this dictionary states that "it is difficult to settle on a single definition for this extremely important term," and those definitions which it does quote are certainly complex. Simplifying somewhat, it can be said that *culture* for the social scientist comprises the ideas, values, habits, and other patterns of behavior which a human group consciously or unconsciously transmits from one generation to another and hence usually treats as traditional or worthy of reproduction. A culture (demographic) may comprise a single society or be dispersed as in a diaspora, and although a nation is supposed to be "united by a common culture," it is recognized that it may contain within it various *subcultures*, groups which share some of the national traits but for historical or situational reasons do not share others. A particular social class within a national society can sometimes be called a subculture insofar as certain traditions exist within it which do not exist elsewhere, but the term is more commonly applied to situations where groups of different backgrounds have come together to form a nation, thus developing some traits or features in common but maintaining limited differences.

The final term which calls for definition at this point is *ethnic group*, one which I have not used until now and which I will try to avoid. According to the dictionary being quoted, it "denotes a social group which, within a larger cultural or social system, claims or is accorded a special status in terms of a complex of traits which it exhibits or is believed to exhibit." This appears very similar to the definition of subculture, and in fact "ethnic group" is often used where subculture is intended; but since the traits of an ethnic group can be physical or mental, individual or social, political or religious, and since they need only be claimed or attributed rather than demonstrated, it is clear that this latter term is a catchall. The researcher may be forced by popular or political practice to use it – census classifications may employ it, for instance – but the very popularity of the term arises from the fact that it is ambiguous and avoids specifications, whereas it is a scientist's task to reduce ambiguity and to be precise in what he means.

The purpose of my going into these definitions in some detail is to show that when one refers to international or cross-cultural comparisons, the properties most fundamentally underlying the groups being compared are shared mental states, not political divisions or, except secondarily, social structures, and certainly not biological traits. It is to these shared mental states that I have applied the term "psychosocial climate," since the average member of a nation or culture is surrounded and affected by them since infancy, and since he tends to take their major features for granted just as, in a temperate zone, he takes the rain for granted. However, they are more than just surrounding him, and here the climatic metaphor breaks down. They usually have an imperative quality and hence become internalized, affecting his thoughts and behavior from within as well as from without. Central to the definitions of "nation" and "a culture" is culture in the ideational sense of a transmitted tradition, but both in popular usage and in the sense employed here is left space for change and for social elements not deriving from tradition. After the Bourbon restoration the French were found to differ from the Germans and British in much the same ways as they had differed before the Revolution, but during the Revolution there were many more differences, and after the Restoration some of these remained. It can be argued that for medical (and hence psychiatric) purposes, such genetic differences as exist between nations are of considerably greater importance than the psychosocial ones, and hence that when international differences in morbidity are found, these should first be attributed to some genetic factor, with the psychosocial dimension only being given serious consideration when the genetic and other biological aspects have been proven irrelevant. Genetics are certainly relevant to psychiatry, but whether these or psychosocial factors are more important in a given situation is a matter for exploration, not for presumption. Comparisons of nations are in my opinion no more suited for the testing of genetic hypotheses than comparison of races are for testing of psychosocial ones. Nationhood and culture are mental states, and genetic research is better done within a single culture rather than between cultures, since there are then fewer complicating variables to handle.

Definitions, as always, tend to deal with typical cases, not boundaries. A point which neither the cited definitions nor any others, to my knowledge, solve is how wide a difference in transmitted ideas, values, habits, etc., needs to be present before it is proper to say that one is dealing with different cultures, and how similar these features must be between two groups before one can say that they belong to the same culture. In theory the matter can be determined by measuring through opinion surveys whether the within-group variance is as great as the between-group variance on a number of key cultural features. It would be difficult to reach agreement regarding which features are the key ones differentiating cultures, however, and in any case one is rarely going to be in the position of having such data. In practice, therefore, operational definitions have to be used, usually those which are employed in some population census, and if the researcher feels that the groupings he is using are not customary, it is up to him to justify them. One can treat all Europeans as a single cultural group when compared with, say, Japanese, insofar as to someone from a third region the former will have certain common cultural (as distinct from racial) traits which make their behavior and thought patterns different from those of the average Japanese, and which derive from shared historic forces such as that of Christianity. However, one must guard against lumping together in this fashion groups whose only common feature is that they are different from one's own reference group, e.g., in the way that the "colored immigrants" to Britain appear alien to the average Briton.

Another question concerning nations and cultures is the extent to which a part can be taken to represent the whole. If one has country-wide statistics on mental disorder then their national representativeness is rarely at issue, but if one has information only from or about a limited section of the nation or cultural group, how far can one generalize regarding the whole? A notable illustration of this problem can be found, for the social sciences, in the attempt to compare semantic differential responses internationally [477]. For that, information was collected in 26 cultures regarding the connotations of a range of common substantives (nouns) including, incidentally, many of interest to psychiatry. Numerous inferences regarding both universality and differences in meaning have been made from these comparisons, but when one learns that all the data were collected from male highschool students aged 14 - 18, the question immediately arises whether they could be taken to represent their cultures or whether samples of older persons of both sexes might have yielded substantially different connotations.

In the mental health field the problem of representativity particularly arises with respect to migrants. To what extent can international migrants be taken to represent the dominant culture of the country from which they came, particularly when they have had years of acculturation to their new society? Migrants are usually not a random sampling of their originating society; they are self-selected, sometimes chosen from the brightest individuals in their communities and sometimes from the dullest. Also, if a country contains minority subcultures that feel disadvantaged,

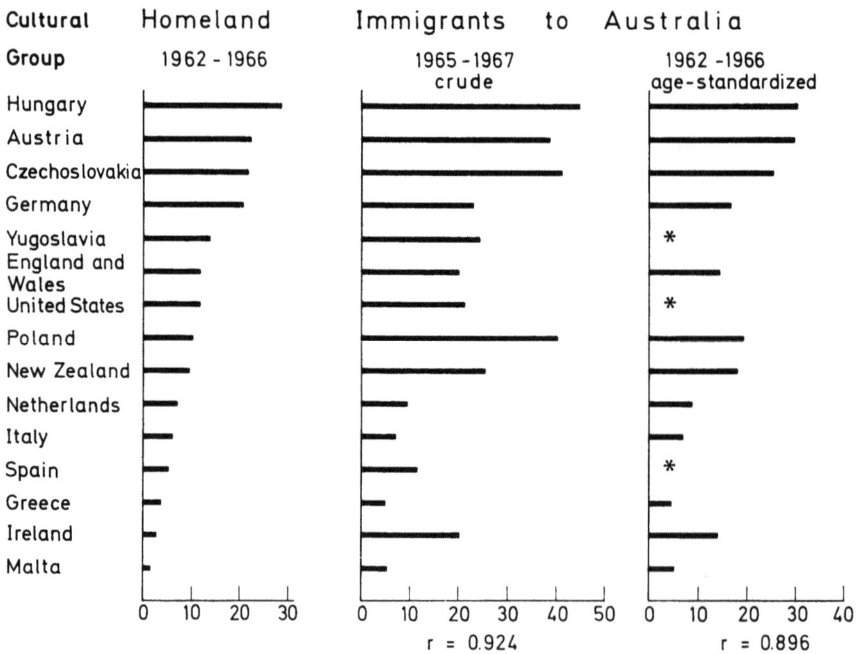

Fig. 1.1. Culture-specific suicide rates in Australia as compared with rates in countries of origin. Rate per 100 000 per annum. 1965–1967 data from Whitlock [65b]; 1962–1966 data from Burvill [83]. Pearsonian correlations are between the Australian rates and those in the countries of origin. All sets are standardized for sex, but only those from Burvill by age. * indicates that rates are not available

these are more likely to migrate than groups that do not feel disadvantaged. Yet these migrating individuals have usually been brought up within the culture that they are leaving, and willingly or unwillingly have absorbed most of the habits, value orientations, and ways of thinking of that culture.

The most concrete answer to that question has been given by comparing suicide rates among European immigrants to Australia with those in their homelands. Such a comparison has the advantage of dealing with a reasonably clear measure, and even if suicide may not always be the result of a mental disturbance, it certainly reflects an attitude towards death which culture is likely to have influenced. As can be seen in Fig. 1.1, independent studies of this question have demonstrated a high correlation between the rates which the different Australian subcultures exhibit and the rates which their parent cultural groups exhibit at home. Moreover, according to Whitlock [656] the numbers of suicides to be expected in these Australian subcultures are closer to what is actually observed when the expectations are based on the natal country's mean rate than when they are based on the mean rate for Australians as a whole. From this it seems reasonable to conclude that subgroups from a culture do reflect the influence of that culture on their mental health even though they may now be separated from it and though other pertinent factors affecting the mental health of the subgroup may complicate the issue.

One such complicating factor occurs when the chosen sample is in a situation which one culture can handle much easier than another. For instance, during World War II Indian army soldiers from the Tamil-speaking south developed considerably more serious mental disorders than those from the Punjab and neighboring northern parts [659]. That could have been taken to indicate a general psychiatric difference, but for cultural reasons the Punjabi accepted the hierarchical army structure easily while the southerners had great difficulty in accepting it. It would therefore not be correct to extrapolate from the army findings and expect southern villages to produce more serious mental disorder than northern ones. A similar error would be to take a single village study in France to represent the whole rural society there.

Two final points concerning culture and nationality require slight amplification: complexity and change over time. Earlier generations of social anthropologists tended to think of culture as static, and since they also tended to focus on small and relatively isolated communities they usually felt it possible to identify the key elements in the local culture, perhaps even to cover everything of importance in it. Culture is not static, however, and with large and complex societies it may appear almost impossible to identify all the features which can be said to distinguish each culture.

Culture change is the easier aspect to tackle, and can even be turned to the researcher's advantage, since it may enable him to undertake the equivalent of cross-cultural studies within a single society, by comparing one period with another [437]. The problem which such changes create in Comparative Psychiatry is that one often possesses psychiatric data from one period and sociocultural data from another, and one may make a big mistake by assuming that the culture has been static in the meantime. For instance, given the shift in public attitudes toward divorce throughout the Western world during the past 20 years, it is almost certainly a mistake (although one which is still made) to assume that mental disorder rates for the divorced and

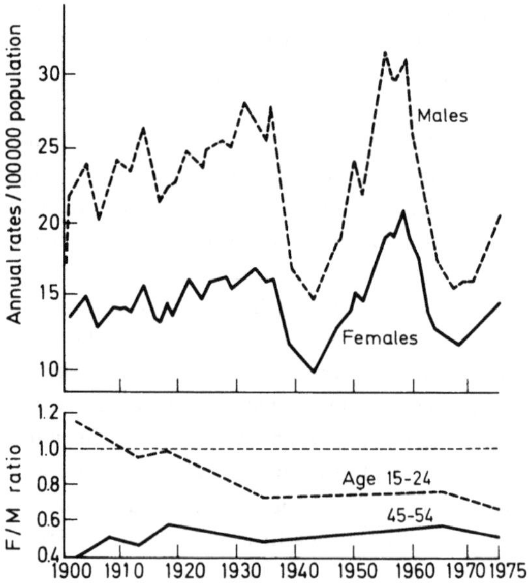

Fig. 1.2. Sex-specific suicide rates in Japan, 1900 to 1975, with sex ratios for two age groups. From Kato [295]

separated are as much above those of the currently married today as was the case in the 1950s and earlier. Rather than reciting earlier statistics in such a situation one should be according it special study, since it is particularly when attitudes toward something like divorce change that one can test the different hypotheses which relate it to mental disorder.

Naturally, if one does attempt to analyze changes in morbidity and link them to cultural trends, either contemporaneously or historically, one has to allow for changes in the processes and people through which the information is being collected. In most countries one cannot compare mental hospitalization rates today with those in the 1950s, since the perceived function of the mental hospital has changed and psychiatric outpatient clinics exist much more abundantly than they did then. However, ways are often available for getting round such difficulties or (still better) for incorporating the changes in medical services or concepts into one's design. Alterations in suicide rates, such as shown in the upper part of Fig. 1.2, are largely independent of medical services, and although affected by clinical trends are almost certainly influenced by culture change as well, particularly with the Japanese. The shifts illustrated in the lower part of this figure are definitely not due only to something like a business cycle.

The problem of cultural complexity is more difficult to tackle, so much more difficult in fact that in Comparative Psychiatry one usually has to abandon comprehending it and to be satisfied with exploring a few of the more obvious possible relationships with the aid of theories which we know are still largely unproven. At the stage which we have reached, some researchers are even satisfied to draw attention to some difference in morbidity and leave to others the task of looking for related sociocultural variables. However, in considering ideal approaches to the problem, it is appropriate to mention here two conflicting schools of thought which have developed in the social sciences, entitled the "emic" and the "etic" approaches after terms used in linguistics.

4 The "Emic" and "Etic" Viewpoints

The "emic" approach focuses on the cultural gestalt and seeks to understand the relationships between its elements (psychiatric disorder sometimes being included in the latter), while allowing the culture to impose itself on one's own thinking about it. Thus, if patients in a given society show a marked concern for household cleanliness, as Ellenberger described in 1950 respecting the German Swiss [166], the proper task of the researcher would be seen as establishing links between this and other features of the culture in terms of the culture's own value system, but not comparing such obsessions with those in another culture. This is because the character of the obsessions in the former group cannot, in theory, be precisely the same as in the latter, owing to the cultural difference, and hence precise comparison cannot be possible. Such a point of view is valuable for reminding us how we tend to incorrectly assume that a term in one language or culture has the same connotations as it has in another, and for stressing the interrelatedness of different aspects of life. Probably the best illustration of the force of such a viewpoint for psychiatry lies in Doi's elegant discussions of the psychopathological and nonpathological aspects of certain Japanese terms or concepts which are extremely difficult to translate into a Western language [153] (see p 263ff). However, when carried to its logical extreme the "emic" position becomes untenable, since all knowledge is acquired through a process of comparisons, and to say that one must stop comparing is neither sound nor practicable.

The "etic" position rejects the idea of allowing the studied culture (or perhaps any culture, at the extreme) to impose its values or other ideas on one's way of looking at it, and calls instead for the researcher to develop an analytic structure from the outside, employing concepts and criteria which are assumed to be universal [53]. A little consideration will lead the medical reader to realize that this is in somewhat unfamiliar terms the standard medical viewpoint, one which most other branches of medicine take for granted and which dominates much psychiatric teaching. With biology it works, universal concepts and criteria being satisfactorily applied not just across nations but across races and often species, the neurochemistry of the rat being in many respects identical to that of the human. With not just culture but much else relating to mental disorder it is less satisfactory, since these have to do with thought patterns and it is much more questionable how many true universals relating to these have yet been discovered. To take an elementary example, classic psychological texts on perception assumed that men not having a physiological defect all see three primary colors in the same way and combine these in standard fashion. But linguistics then demonstrated that the spectrum is divided very differently in one language as compared with another; it was found that culture as well as environmental experience affects these differences; and today it is accepted that there is as much psychology as physiology in the way that colors are perceived. If that can occur such such a relatively simple, apparently objective matter, it is bound to happen much more with supposedly universal but more complex concepts like achievement motivation, mourning, the psychodynamics of dreaming, and sex-linked roles. Comparative Psychiatry must lean to the etic rather than to the emic position, since with the emic no comparisons are usually possible. However, when pushed to its logical extreme of requiring that the researcher employ only concepts of proven universality, the etic position is no more tenable than the emic. As with the definition of mental disorder, therefore, it is necessary to compromise, assuming a position which is easy to attack in the light of pure theory.

5 Varieties of Approach

Emic and etic do not represent only viewpoints; they also represent styles of approach. In what has been presented so far, emphasis has been placed on the logic of different positions, concepts, and definitions. However, in much research, particularly in the human sciences, what is undertaken is determined quite as much by personal inclination as by logic. Guided strictly by logic, research in Comparative Psychiatry would probably follow the path of identifying a problem, formulating hypotheses concerning it, and then selecting from among the world's vast variety of societies those best suited for the testing of these hypotheses. This is almost never done. In part it is not done because of practical difficulties, because working in particular societies may be much more expensive than working in others, or because the information on which to base a logical choice of test site for a given problem or hypothesis is very hard to come by. However, the cause is also to a great extent personal inclination – a reluctance to make the effort of learning a new language; a desire to work in one society rather than in another; or a reluctance to tackle questions which would necessitate too close an examination of one's own value system, or which might be politically embarrassing. (I have twice been refused permission to undertake research for the latter reason, and I have felt it necessary to delay publication of findings once on similar grounds.) As well as grasping the logic behind Comparative Psychiatry, therefore, it is desirable that one grasps the broad lines along which the field has developed, and the gaps which have been left in it for one or another reason.

One of the clearest and most long-lasting lines of development has been the adapting of psychoanalytic theory to the life-styles of non-Eurpoean peoples, or alternatively the devising of ways of describing these life-styles which would fit that theory. Through a thin succession of distinguished workers – Malinowski, Roheim, Devereux, and Parin, among others – there is over 50 years of research into peoples with cultures extremely different from those in which psychoanalytic theory developed, much of this work being consciously or unconsciously directed to demonstrating that the theory has universality and will work anywhere. The researchers made their own field observations, sometimes giving us only their theoretical interpretations and sometimes as full detail as one would get in a psychoanalytic study anywhere. The main difficulty with this line of work, as with psychoanalysis in general, is to marry it to other approaches and to achieve more objectivity; but progress in these directions is being achieved. Another problem with it is that it has tentended to focus on relatively little-known peoples – Trobrianders, Pitjentara, Navaho, and Dogon, for instance – and has shunned the obvious chance of comparing the psychodynamics in different European cultures. It is only relatively recently that I was able to persuade followers of that tradition to undertake a limited comparison of patients from two European groups [484], although the application of psychoanalytic theory to the task of explaining differences in suicide rates in three European countries [256] had earlier offered what seemed to be a promising model. This line of work has been a little disadvantaged by premature attempts to use psychoanalytic theory for explaining broad cultural differences, as for instance in the book by Gorer and Rickman [229]. Also, the unwary reader is liable to confuse the serious work of this type, work which involves field investigations or a thorough knowledge of primary sources, with the facile psychologizing around historical or international topics which one also meets.

At the other pole of Comparative Psychiatry, but covering almost the same time span, is the analysis of mental hospitalization data in terms of subculture, a tradition dominated by Malzberg in New York from the 1930s [373] to the 1960s, but with contributions from Australia, Canada, and Great Britain. The main characteristics of this line of studies were the employment of state-wide or country-wide data on thousands of cases, the differentiation within this mass of cases of numerous categories of first generation and second-generation immigrants all treated in the same hospitals by the same body of physicians, and the analysis of this large body of data in terms of official diagnosis. A further characteristic, important in view of the abnormal structure of most immigrant populations, was an effort to standardize for age and sex, and eventually for more complex variables such as occupation, education, and district of residence. The value of these analyses lay in their demonstration of marked differences in morbidity rates between groups of different European cultural origins. Their weaknesses were that they tended to put excessive reliance on official statistics, not investigating how accurately hospitals were reporting on their patients or how far the patients represented the mass of hospitalizable mental disorder in their different subcultures; and that they usually avoided any theory which might link mental illness to culture or national origin. Today these large-scale studies have almost died out, in part because mental hospitalization does not carry the same meaning as it did previously, in part because population censuses have tended to shift away from recording subcultural differences, and in part because the weaknesses just mentioned have become more widely recognized. However, when combined with parallel approaches which compensate for these weaknesses they are still capable of yielding valuable data, as the work of Cochrane [112, 115] in Britain has shown.

The nearest approach to bridging the psychoanalytic and statistical approches just mentioned has been the comparative study within North America of relatively small samples of hopitalized patients from two or more subcultures, something which has focused on the distribution of symptoms among patients rather than the distribution of diseases among populations, and has employed psychodynamic theory not on whole tribes or subcultures but on the mentally disordered persons from among them. The pioneer study of this type was that by Opler and Singer [471] comparing Irish Americans with Italian Americans, and since then the general approach has been used to cover persons of Chinese, French, German, Polish, and Polynesian background, among others. The advantages of this are that one gets a clinical picture of the patients whom the statistical studies of the Malzberg school had quantified, and that numerous psychodynamic hypotheses were generated which appeared open to testing. The disadvantages are that (usually) the observations tend to be slanted by the researchers' own theoretical biases; that it is usually unclear how far the observed differences relate to the mental disorder or are characteristics of members of the compared subcultures whether mentally healthy or not; and that one is left uncertain whether the discussion and hypotheses offered relate only to the types of symptom exhibited by persons who fall ill, or to the risk of developing the studied illness (usually schizophrenia) in that particular people. The same spirit, and much the same strengths and weaknesses, is found in studies in which only patients of a single culture are investigated but where a comparison is implied, as in the book *Oedipe Africain* [471]. This whole family of research is undoubtedly the most central to the field of Comparative Psychiatry in general, since the researchers deliberately seek to establish links between cultural or national characteristics and important aspects of psychopathology. However, because their results are insufficiently objective in the eyes of many other researchers and because it is usually unclear whether one is dealing with the basic disorder itself or only with the superficial characteristics which it assumes in different settings, these studies have not received the attention which they might have deserved.

One way of improving on the approaches so far mentioned is to develop more standardized methods of clinical description and assessment for use internationally and crossculturally, and the 1960s saw a promising surge of activity in this direction. Interview schedules and rating scales focusing on different levels or categories of mental disorder were developed and then used in a wide variety of societies. International committees were set up for the purpose of reducing the amount of unacknowledged variation in the ways in which national schools of psychiatry approached the task of diagnosis, and also to obtain agreements on nosology, where possible, while videotapes of patient interviews were distributed internationally with the idea of training psychiatrists in different countries to use the agreed criteria.

This work has been valuable, but the spirit inspiring it has too often been a negative one, i.e., to circumvent or nullify national and cross-cultural differences in psychopathology rather than to exploit these differences for the purpose of understanding psychopathology better. (Much of this research was linked to the task of using chemotherapy more effectively, and it is easier to issue guides to chemotherapy if one treats all mankind as equal than if one has to accomodate the fact that some drugs are more effective in some races or cultures than in others.) As a result, a study like the US/UK Diagnostic Project [123] tells us in detail to what degree certain diagnostic criteria differ in the two countries and how to get round this difference, but it offers very little in the way of discussion or explanation of the numerous clinical differences that remained between the two national samples after a standard method of assessment had been applied, and none of the eight psychiatrists involved in this project has (to my knowledge) gone any deeper into the matter.

Similarly, the international conferences and committee work which took place around the problem of bringing national diagnostic concepts and criteria closer together yielded information on their agreements and a little on their disagreements, but virtually nothing on the ways in which national schools of psychiatry and national approaches to nosology are linked to, or maybe even determined by, other aspects of the national culture. To get an adequate discussion of the latter, potentially important, subject one has to leave European and North American cultures out of consideration and take a safely distant example such as China [313]!

As the last remark indicates, the objective of comparing the effects of therapies linked to particular cultures, and of understanding the philosophy behind such therapies, has been less enthusiastically pursued by medical men than other objectives we have been considering; but it is a subject which is of considerable interest in the field of medical anthropology which has burgeoned during the 1970s, and psychiatrists themselves are becoming increasingly involved in this type of study as a result. When the Milbank Memorial Fund sent a high status group of American psychiatrists to study the open ward system in some British mental hospitals in 1957, it was agreed that something of that system derived from British tradition but that it was exportable, and the event sparked what was for a time called the "third psychiatric revolution." When other commissions and investigators crossed the Atlantic to look into Querido's community psychiatry services in Amsterdam and the British system of registered treatment for drug addicts, the general conclusions were that these were not reproducible in the United States; but there was no serious discussion of why one type of program should be exportable and another not, a major reason for this being that it was felt that such discussion would inevitably hurt the sensibilities on one side or the other. (Dutch doctors were seen as too authoritarian and as being according too much authority by their patients for their model to suit the United States, while the American public was thought to be too irresponsible to accept the type of rationing of drugs which at that time was working in Britain.) When it became apparent that modern medicine, although technically superior, was going to be unable to meet the needs of the large mass of people in Africa and Asia, however, attention was drawn to the need for evaluating what the various "folk" medicine traditions were offering, and it appeared that their results were best in the fields of psychotherapy and sociotherapy. During the 1970s, therefore, this became quite an active although rather unscientific subfield (the methods of evaluation still being very vague) extending from Zaire to the heart of New York with investigations into the methods and results obtained by unofficial healers in the different locations.

There are numerous other less popular approaches to be found in the field, and probably still further ones fully appropriate to it which have not yet been taken up. How much effort and time it takes to pursue any approach properly, however, can be seen in the World Health Association Mental Health Division's series of international collaborative studies on schizophrenia and related functional psychoses. Starting in 1965, the first steps in this series had to be agreement on definitions, the development of instruments whereby the criteria attached to these definitions could be uniformly applied in different countries, and an assessment of how far psychiatrists from different schools could agree on the meaning of the information thus obtained.

This was followed by a study of some 1200 patients in nine countries, with the initial focus being on how far the disorders in the different countries resembled each other, but also with some indication of the ways in which those from one country differed from those of another [674]. Since the latter differences could have been due to differences in case selection and the channels whereby patients come to official attention in each field center, they were not such as could be given much weight, but by arranging for follow-up of the same patients at a 2- and a 5-year interval it was possible to assess whether nationality was linked to the course of illness in patients who initially presented with very similar pictures. This has been done [677]; marked differences have been uncovered which may not be explainable in terms of case selection; hypotheses have been developed to account for these differences in other, culture-linked, ways; and new studies have been launched both to test these hypotheses and to explore variations in treated incidence. The whole series is expected to last at least 20 years, has been very costly, and for the first half of that time appeared to be yielding very little.

To follow the same careful process with each other aspect of Comparative Psychiatry is not possible. What one has mainly to do instead is to draw inferences from comparisons with the mass of data which already exist or are easily available, while accepting the limitations which their heterogenous origins impose. In pursuing clues in this mass of material, one can be looking mainly for similarities, i.e., for indications of universal states or processes, or one can be looking mainly for differences, i.e., for evidence that local factors have had an influence. I must declare here a frank bias towards investigating differences rather than similarities, and I can legitimately be reproached for discussing certain differences in a given body of data while ignoring the more obvious similarities. My reasons for this bias are as follows. Firstly, there is to my mind too great a tendency in psychiatry to assume that findings derived from one set of patients can be applied to all other sets despite the fact that there may be marked differences between these sets in what they have been taught regarding coping styles, symbols, social relationships, and thinking processes. Secondly, it is a general principle in all science that when attempting to develop a universal law, an early and essential step is to look for apparent exceptions to it, since it is in this way that laws are not merely tested but improved. In psychiatry the great variation in symptomatology and in course of illness has led us to grasp at what similarities we think we can detect, while setting aside the differences which accompany these. This is the correct first step in developing any universal law; but we ought now to be beyond that step with respect to many disorders and ready to ask ourselves how our theories would explain this or that apparent exception. In this book I am mainly concerned with presenting instances where the data show a greater degree of difference (or, occasionally, of similarity) than would be expected by chance or by the influence of the data-collecting process, and not with discussing theory. However, I would think myself remiss if I did not also point out the possible significance of the findings for certain theories, and suggestions regarding directions in which these theories might be modified are sometimes given.

Earlier, mention was made of the levels of confidence which can be entrusted to different types of data, and these levels of confidence become highly important when it comes to assessing how far a given finding should be regarded as supporting or as challenging existing theory. To judge how much confidence can be placed in data one must know something about how it is likely to have been collected. Therefore, before passing to specific observations, the next two chapters will discuss the scope and limitations of the data on which international and cross-cultural comparisons depend.

Chapter 2 Comparability of Official Sources of Data

International comparisons of health and disease customarily derive from a relatively small range of national data regarding which there has been some effort made to achieve international uniformity. Death certificates, hospitalization records, and infectious disease notifications are the major sources, with clinic attendances, autopsy reports, and community surveys of pathogens and antibodies playing a lesser role. In psychiatry it has been customary to think of hospitalizations as providing a good reflection of the level and variety of major mental disorders in a society, while the other conventional sources tell us little, apart from death certification for suicides. However, mortality statistics and autopsy reports can be of use when comparing certain psychosomatic disorders and perhaps drug abuse, while infectious disease notifications and immunological surveys provide the basis on which one can begin to assess the significance of national or cultural differences in general paresis. Some countries have maintained registers of the chronic insane, the mentally defective, and alcoholics, whether ever hospitalized or not; and although psychiatric outpatient clinics are still of little value as a basis from which to measure incidence or prevalence, they are able to yield interesting comparisons with respect to symptomatology provided one knows something about the sources and conditions of referral. Moreover, since mental disorder overlaps social disorder and in children often comes first to official attention in the form of juvenile delinquency, police and court records can be relevant to psychiatry in ways which are not true for other branches of medicine.

With all official sources of data, medical or nonmedical, we know that clinical detail and local variation have had to be sacrificed to the need to fit each case into a single pigeonhole for statistical purposes. However, the uniformity of these pigeonholes and the large numbers of cases which are brought together in this way may enable us to recognize broad patterns which are imperceptible when only parts of the total picture are taken. Therefore, an effort must be made to see what inferences can be drawn from them after various biasing factors are allowed for, even though such inferences only deal with superficial variables and need to be checked by in-depth studies.

This chapter will consider the broad factors affecting the representativity of different categories of official data, i.e., of data which are routinely collected and lie within the public domain for researchers to work on. Having considered such factors, it will then go on to assess what sorts of inferences might legitimately be drawn from comparing these data internationally or crossculturally.

1 Hospitalizations

a) International Comparisons

In much psychiatric writing during the twentieth century, it has been assumed that mental hospital patients are representative of, and even constitute the great majority of, persons suffering from major mental disorders in the society, the term "major" referring to the psychoses and to a less clearly defined group of nonpsychotic disorders causing serious social disability. Ødegaard, for instance, argued in 1952 that community surveys (what he calls census investigations) do not yield results which are importantly different from the results obtained from hospital admission statistics, since although the former detect many not-yet-hospitalized patients, these patients tend to appear in the hospital statistics at a later date [467]. This assumption is based on the still more fundamental ones that a psychotic is someone who cannot look after his own affairs, and that a special setting with medical services, i.e., a mental hospital, must be provided in which he can be looked after. However, there are situations in which this assumption is patently untrue, namely where mental hospitals do not exist; and even where they do exist they may be much too small to look after all the psychotics. Prior to the 1870s, only a minority of psychotics in even the most advanced countries were in mental hospital, and a century later an overview of psychiatric services around the globe shows it to be extremely unlikely that a majority of countries possess sufficient mental hospital beds to take care of all their psychotics.

Figure 2.1 illustrates the range of ratios of psychiatric beds to population which existed around 1970 in countries providing such data to the WHO, and one sees that this range is so great that a log scale has had to be used in place of the customary arithmetic one. Moreover, the figure indicates that over this range there is a highly significant correlation between the bed ratio and an elementary measure of national economic level, the per capita Gross National Product (GNP). If one holds to the assumption that mental hospitalizations reflect the level of major mental disorders in a society, one must conclude that national economic status is positively associated with risk of mental disorder, but the obvious alternative is that countries provide mental hospital beds not in relation to what they see as the need but in relation to what they feel they can afford.

The first of these alternatives cannot be rejected out of hand. It was one which was seriously discussed by leading psychiatrists during the nineteenth century, and later in this book we will have to examine the possible truth of the statement by one of America's leading psychiatrists, Jarvis, at that time, to the effect that "Insanity is a part of the price which we pay for civilisation" [278]. As Rosen's admirable review of the topic documents [520], international leaders like Griesinger, Maudsley, and Tuke were much concerned by the apparent increase in insanity during their lifetimes in countries which thought themselves to be at the forefront of civilization. However, what becomes apparent in retrospect is that they were allowing themselves at least in part to be overimpressed by the increase in mental hospital populations, and that they were misinterpreting their own history. A review of the nineteenth century debate on the establishment of public mental asylums reveals that it was not the psychotic's incompetence which had led to these being

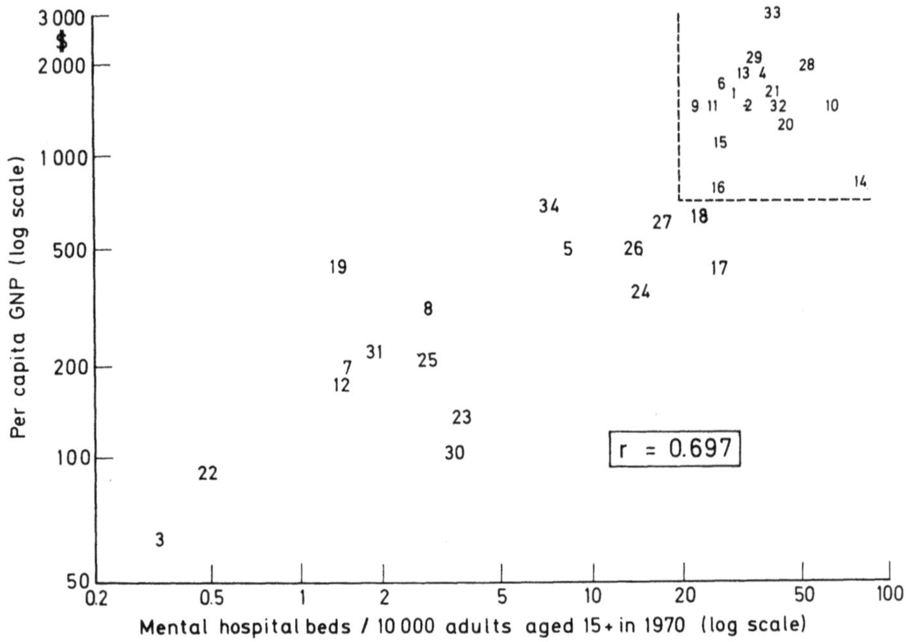

Fig. 2.1. Ratios of psychiatric beds per 10 000 adult population in 34 countries as related to per capita Gross National Product. 1, Australia; 2, Belgium; 3, Burma; 4, Canada; 5, Chile; 6, Denmark; 7, Ghana; 8, Guatamala; 9, France; 10, Finland; 11, Germany, West; 12, Honduras; 13, Iceland; 14, Ireland; 15, Israel; 16, Italy; 17, Jamaica; 18, Japan; 19, Mexico; 20, Netherlands; 21, New Zealand; 22, Pakistan; 23, Phillipines; 24, Portugal; 25, Rhodesia; 26, South Africa; 27, Spain; 28, Sweden; 29, Switzerland; 30, Thailand; 31, Turkey; 32, United Kingdom; 33, United States; 34, Venezuela. Bed ratios are for 1970 [676]; GNP data [71] are from 5 years earlier to allow for development lag

seen as necessary, but the fact that other people were abusing that incompetence in ways which were becoming unacceptable. In Britain, it was not the disturbance created by the masses of unhospitalized insanes in the general population but the plight of the relatively few insanes in private hospitals [notably the infamous White House in Bethnal Green near London (288)] which prompted the drive first to control the private mental hospitals and later to build public ones. Despite what some social scientists have argued regarding mental hospitals being created out of a desire to limit yet another form of social deviance, history indicates that these places were mainly developed to protect patients against social injustice, and if the reader is puzzled why these massive asylums were established rather than open colonies after the model of Gheel in Belgium, he should read how the latter impressed the Australian psychiatrist Tucker in 1880. At the conclusion of a tightly packed nine-page report, Tucker states: "I have visited some hundreds of Lunatic Asylums in four out of the five geographic divisions of the globe, and in the worst of them I have seen some cheerful faces. At Gheel I did not see a single one ... Gheel is an abode of desolation – a lingering survival of remote and barbarous ages – a monstrosity in this nineteenth century, and a humiliating reproach to our modern civilization" [622, pp

754–795]. (His report contributed to conditions improving there, after numerous recriminations.)

It would therefore be wrong to interpret the increase in psychiatric bed ratios in the more developed countries during the nineteenth century as a response to an increase in the prevalence of psychosis in the general population at that time, and in returning to the present day it would equally be wrong to interpret the fall in psychiatric bed ratios in some countries during the last decades as indicating a decline in prevalence. Between 1955 and 1968, the mental hospital bed ratio in California dropped from 29 to 10 per 10 000 general population, but the number of patients in protective living arrangements outside hospital in that state increased from less than 1000 to over 12 000 [26], and has further increased since. Mental hospitals and their bed ratios depend on the attitudes of governments much more than on the supposed need of all psychotics to be hospitalized.

From this it follows that across the range of countries included in Fig. 2.1, hospitalized prevalence, hospitalized incidence, and the clinical features of hospitalized patients cannot be assumed to reflect the level and character of major psychopathology in society. Given the correlation with GNP, it is much sounder to interpret these as a reflection of what each country sees itself as able to afford, and this makes any further comparison of hospitalizations on such a scale largely useless for most psychiatric purposes. We are not here dealing with something comparable to international mortality statistics.

But Comparative Psychiatry fortunately does not need to depend on such wide comparisons at its present stage; it is enough to be able to compare a few countries at a time, and in Fig. 2.1 there are some surprisingly different psychiatric bed ratios in countries having similar GNPs per capita. Moreover, at the upper right corner of the chart, in the part delineated by dotted lines, one can see that the correlation between psychiatric bed ratio and GNP becomes insignificant ($r = -0.12$). To compare the bed ratios of countries which are in the process of rapid development, such as Mexico (19), Chile (5), and Jamaica (17), can still be of doubtful value even though they possess relatively similar GNPs per capita at the chosen date, since their health services can change quite rapidly. To compare countries which are relatively rich and have not become so only recently, however, would seem more justifiable, since even if we accept that they may not all follow the same rules regarding which psychiatric patients to provide with hospital space, we may still learn much from enquiring what leads them to have different bed ratios.

For this comparison we could simply take the upper part of Fig. 2.1 as it stands and ask, for instance, why the Republic of Ireland (14) needs almost three times the bed ratio which Italy (16) has. However, although mental hospital bed ratios are the easiest indices of psychiatric care to obtain from a large number of countries, they are not the best indices of the numbers of patients being cared for, since some societies may prefer to use relatively few psychiatric beds very actively, either with the aid of supplementary services as in California, or on what has been called the "revolving door" principle (discharging patients rapidly in the expectation that they will need readmission but in the meantime will have avoided some of the dangers of institutionalization), while other societies may possess psychiatric beds in excess of needs. Also, although GNP gives an indication of the ability of a society to pay for

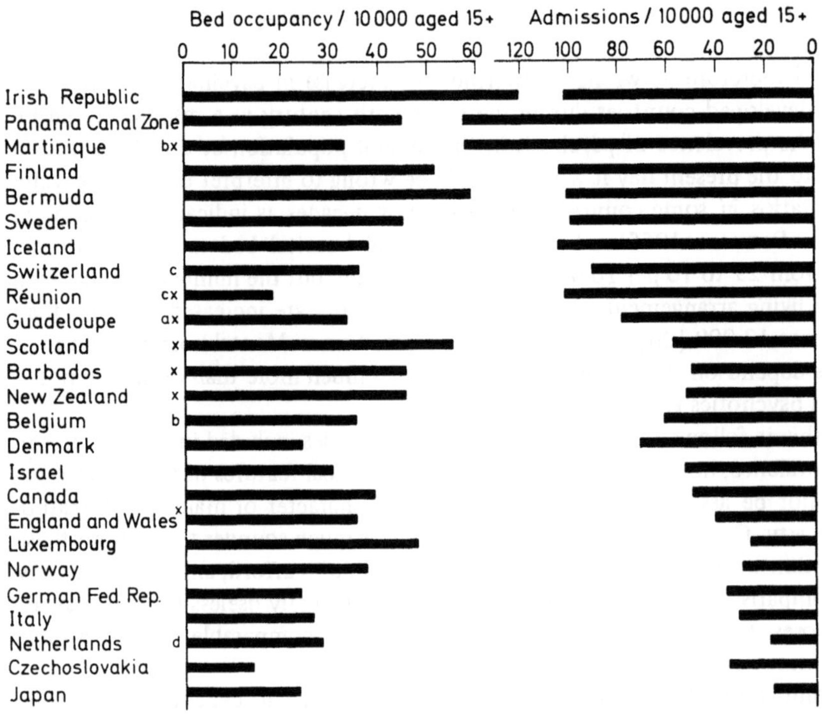

Fig. 2.2. Mental hospitalization in 25 countries and territories. Comparative mental hospital bed occupancy and admission rates per 10 000 aged 15+; countries and territories with more than eight hospital beds (all types) per 1000 total population; averages of 1965, 1970, and 1975. Bed occupancy = psychiatric beds per 10 000 adult population × percentage occupancy during year. Letters alongside names of countries indicate: **a**, 1970 and 1975 only; **b**, 1970 only; **c**, 1965 and 1970 only; **d**, 1965 and 1975 only; **x**, Government hospitals only. From WHO Health Statistics Annual, Vol. III, 1965, 1970, 1975, supplemented in a few instances by national and annual reports and the UN Demographic Yearbook

psychiatric services, it does not give any indication of the priority which health services have in comparison with competing needs such as industrial development, fuel or entertainment. For these reasons I have thought it better to see how much difference exists between one society and another when all have quite rich health services, when hospital admission rates as well as bed ratios are used as psychiatric indicators, and when these bed ratios relate to the average numbers occupied rather than to the numbers officially provided. It is possible that when such modifications are made, the hospitalization pictures in different countries become very similar.

Fig. 2.2 gives the results of that second comparison, and one can see that although it is now possible to use arithmetic scales rather than logarithmic ones to indicate the differences, the latter are still marked. For this chart, the readiness of a society to give reasonably high priority to health services (or, more pertinently, to hospitals) was judged on the basis of it possessing at least eight hospital beds (all types) per 1000 population, something which the United States was not providing that year. All countries and dependent territories included in the *World Health*

Statistics Annual's tables [676] and reaching that ratio of beds to population have been included if they were reporting admission rates to the WHO, but it has unfortunately not been possible to use first admission rates only, as would have been preferable, since the Health Statistics Annual only reports total admissions for psychiatric services. At the top of the figure are those societies which had not just high admission rates but high bed ratios as well, and at the bottom are those societies with the lowest of both rates. Since large numbers of patients have been combined for each society, the standard errors of these rates are very small, almost never exceeding 5 cases per 10 000, something which means that significant differences exist not just between those at the top and at the bottom of the figure, but often between societies whose rates lie quite close to each other.

To find explanations for the very marked differences which one finds in Fig. 2.2, it is necessary to go beyond the official data sources and thus beyond the scope of this chapter. However, while remaining dependent on these sources and on what is common knowledge regarding to societies featured there, it is possible to say a little more. The main question which most psychiatrists would ask when faced with such differences in rates is whether they seem likely to derive mainly from differences in frequency of mental illness of a certain degree of severity, or mainly from other factors such as criteria of admission to hospital. One way of beginning the pursuit of these matters is to compare the rank order of the societies in this figure with their rank order with respect to some other mental health indicator. Another way is to ask whether there are some known features of these societies which might be expected to lead to an above average or below average use of mental hospitals.

Taking the latter question first, one point which springs to mind when these societies are considered is that the Panama Canal Zone has a very large transient population in relation to its residential one (on which these rates are based) and that its hospitalizations could easily be inflated by sailors and others from the thousands of ships which pass through it each year, particularly if its hospital had a reputation for giving responsible care. Hence the position of that territory at the top of the figure need not mean that its residential population has much mental illness. A similar though less obvious factor may help account for the fact that there are four Caribbean territories in the upper half of the figure and none in the lower. Such territories depend much on tourism, and I found when I did a mental health survey of another Caribbean island (H.B.M. Murphy, H. M. Sampath, 1967, Mental illness in a Caribbean Community. A mental health survey of St. Thomas, V.I.; report to the government of the Virgin Islands; unpublished work) that the police were very quick to remove from the streets anyone whose behavior might make the tourists uncomfortable, one place to put such people being the psychiatric ward. Moreover, during the tourist season the population can be inflated by temporary workers from other islands, people who do not feature in the population census but may require hospital admission. Accordingly, while it is quite possible that the residential population of the featured Caribbean territories has a high rate of major mental disorder, this is not something which it would be wise to assess only on the basis of total mental hospital admissions.

Regarding comparing international levels of mental hospitalization with levels of some other measure of mental health, there are two main possibilities involving official statistics open to us. Comparison with suicide rates is easy, and although it is well known that some societies with high levels of of suicide can have low levels of other mental disorder indicators and vice versa, this is still worth undertaking. Secondly, as was discussed in the previous chapter (p 13), it may be possible to compare the hospitalization rates in such societies with those of peoples from the same national origins who have settled overseas. In Fig. 1.1 it was shown that a quite high correlation existed between the suicide rates of Australian minorities and those of the national populations from which they stemmed, and such a comparison is potentially of greater value with respect to mental hospitalization rates. Italy and Sweden, for instance, may differ greatly regarding their mental hospitalization policies, and this difference may conceal whether there is any difference in "true" prevalence or not; but if Italians and Swedes both migrate to the same overseas country having a uniform hospitalization policy, their relative vulnerabilities to major mental disorder may become clearer.

Table 2.1 provides the results of the two types of comparison just mentioned for European countries sending migrants overseas. As expected, there is no significant correlation between the ranks of the different countries with respect to suicide and mental hospitalization. If we had reason to believe that suicide was a good indicator of national mental health, we would therefore have to conclude that mental hospitalizations, even in countries with rich health services, are a wholly unsatisfactory measure of nonfatal mental disorder. However, we know that suicide forms only a small part of the spectrum of mental disorder and may also occur in the absence of this disorder, so that such a conclusion is not justifiable. Passing to the second part of the table, we see that there is a surpisingly high correlation between the mental hospitalization ranks of European-derived groups in Canada and the corresponding ranks of the societies from which they derived. Both comparisons are quite crude, insofar as most of the data are not age standardized and the European mental hospitalization ranks were based on the averages of 3 years while those of the other two measures were each based on single years. However, the rank order correlations are so clear that it is unlikely that in this type of population either age standardizations or the use of data from other years would have made much difference.

To conclude this section of the chapter, therefore, it can be said that comparisons of mental hospitalization rates are able to reveal quite striking differences which seem unattributable to economics or to hospitalization policies, provided enough care is taken to exclude instances where the latter are obviously playing a part, and provided one makes some allowance for such factors as the ratio of adults to children in the population. Official data by themselves cannot usually offer any explanations for these differences, although clues might be forthcoming if one used national reports with diagnostic distributions rather than merely the WHO compilations on which I have relied at this point. (For instance, one might find that one country treats its alcoholics in mental hospital while another treats them in a different type of service.) But the idea that it is impossible to make international comparisons of this sort does not appear to be valid, and the time appears overdue for an investigation into the reasons why countries like Ireland and Finland make so much more use of mental hospitals than others with similar per capita GNPs, while countries like Italy and the Netherlands seem to need such facilities so much less than average.

Table 2.1. Rank ordering of European peoples in terms of (a) suicide rates in 1970; (b) mental hospital admission rates in homeland (from Fig. 2.1); and (c) mental hospital admission rates of their descendants living in Canada, 1961

National group	Comparison A		Comparison B	
	Suicides in homeland (676)	Mental hospitalizations in homeland		Mental hospitalizations in Canada[a]
Irish (Southern)	15	1	1	1
Finns	4=	2	2	2
Swedes	3	3	3	3
Icelanders	14	4	4	5
Swiss	6	5		n.s.a.
Scots	12	6		n.s.a.
Belgians	7	7		n.s.a.
Danes	2	8	5	11
Other British	11	9	6	4
Luxembourgers	8	10		n.s.a.
Norwegians	9	11	7	6
Germans (Fed. Rep.)	4=	12	8	8
Italians	13	13	9	7
Dutch	10	14	10	9
Czechoslovaks	1	15	11	10
r_s	-0.18		0.83	
t	N.S.		4.49	

Rank order correlations by Pearson's method. In Comparison B, Canadians regarded as of Irish descent had to be estimated indirectly by taking Roman Catholics whose families originated from the British Isles, and those regarded as of "Other British" descent by taking all others deriving from the British Isles, Scots included. n.s.a., "not separately available."

[a]H.B.M. Murphy, 1968, Mental hospitalisation patterns in twelve Canadian subcultures, unpublished work

b) Within-Country Comparisons

In comparison with the problems which confront one in attempting to compare mental hospitalization rates and other data between countries, a comparison of ethnic groups within the same country would seem to be quite easy. That is sometimes the case, most obviously where racial and genetic influences are important and sociocultural factors can be ignored. However, if the influence of culture and social circumstances is accepted as relevant, as it is for the conditions being discussed in this book, then problems of comparability arise also within countries, and these may loom all the larger if we expect more detail from within-country comparisons than from international ones.

One such problem is inequality of access to services, something which can conveniently be illustrated by reference to a study which was ahead of its time and deserves to be remembered, but which is difficult to interpret for this reason. In the 1920s, Skliar and Starikowa undertook an analysis of almost 2000 patients admitted to the psychiatric unit at Astrakhan (U.S.S.R.) [571], and this remains one of the very few studies in psychiatric epidemiology to be published from that part of the

Table 2.2. Diagnostic distributions and comparative incidence rates of male patients admitted to the Astrakhan Psychiatric Unit, U.S.S.R., in the 1920s; by ethnic group [571]

	Persians %	Russians %	Armenians %	Jews %	Tatars %	Kalmuks %	Kirgis %
Schizophrenia, paranoia	3.0	6.0	18.5	13.5	4.8	5.6	4.5
Reactive psychoses	25.7	23.4	10.7	23.1	27.4	10.4	11.4
Manic-depressive psychoses	34.4	13.0	15.4	13.5	25.2	58.3	68.2
Alcoholic psychoses	5.7	35.9	15.4	3.8	8.5	10.4	2.3
General paresis	20.0	8.3	21.5	9.6	4.5	–	–
Other diagnoses	11.2	13.4	18.5	36.5	29.6	15.3	13.6
	100.0	100.0	100.0	100.0	100.0	100.0	100.0
Number of cases	35	580	65	52	270	249	44
Estimated rate per 100 000 population	350	180	150	80	29	9	0.8

Notes:

1. It is not completely clear over what period the data were accumulated, or whether all ethnic groups were covered for the same period, but the latter seems probable.
2. Many more diagnostic categories are given by the authors than indicated here, and their combination into the above six is done on my own responsibility.
3. There are a number of probable errors in the authors' original calculations; where sufficient clues exist, these have been corrected.
4. Female data are available in the original, but their inclusion would have made the table too complicated for present purposes.

world. Table 2.2 presents a reworking of some of their data, and there are features in the body of the table which either challenge expectation (the comparatively low proportion of affective psychoses in a Jewish patient population at that time, for instance) or invite speculation, as is the case with the high ratio of schizophrenic to reactive psychoses among the Armenians as compared with the rest. However, when one looks to the foot of the table where the estimated rates of admission are given, it becomes clear that some of the ethnic groups were scarcely using the hospital while others were using it quite heavily, most probably because of geographic access. If the authors had prepared separate tables for the patients and population stemming from the area immediately surrounding the hospital, their material would have been much more instructive, but that was not done, even for the patients alone, and as a result these unique historical data become less useful, since when only a very small percentage of psychotics are hospitalized, it cannot be assumed that the factors determining their selection are the same as when a much larger percentage are admitted.

Even in countries which are quite well supplied with medical services, geographic factors may result in some subcultures being much less well served than others, or there may be regional differences in hospitalization policy which would affect any comparison of unevenly distributed subcultures even though all regions were well served. Given enough detail on both patients and population, standardization can be undertaken for geographic distribution just as one standardizes for age or social class. (This was done with reasonably satisfactory results for most of the Canadian groups included in Table 2.1.) However, such standardization may not always be possible, or may be unable to allow for some key factor. For instance, New Caledonia is rich in medical services, being a French overseas territory, but these services are concentrated in Noumea at one end of a mountainous island 400 km long with few roads and poor public transport. Mental hospitalization rates from Noumea itself are considerably higher than from the rest of the island, this urban-rural difference affecting all ethnic groups but being much more marked for the Melanesians than for the Europeans [153]. If one wished to compare the mental health of the Melanesians and Europeans using hospitalization data, standardization for distance from the hospitals would be necessary since the two groups are not evenly distributed, but it is doubtful whether that would be sufficient, in the first place because it is much easier for the rural Europeans to get into Noumea than for the poorer Melanesians, and in the second place because traditional healers in the more rural districts may be competing with the hospitals for the Melanesian patients but not for the European ones. Hence it may be impossible to compare these two peoples on the basis of admissions to psychiatric care, no matter how much standardization one does and how abundant the psychiatric services are.

The New Caledonian case illustrates a second problem which can arise when attempting to compare subcultures within the same society, namely differences of class or status. If one is comparing data from two complete societies, such as Sweden and Italy, one knows that any differentiating effect of social drift or social stress is only likely to have occurred within each group, but not between them. If in a single society one subculture has started off at a considerable social disadvantage in relation to another, however, both social drift and differential social stress must be allowed for when they are compared, and it may be impossible to do this adequately. Social *drift*, whereby the most mentally healthy and competent families rise in social status while the least healthy decline, is liable to lead to the "passing" of the more aspiring families from the lower-status to the higher-status subculture, so that the more healthy members of the lower-status one hide their membership of it. Social *stresses* are liable to lead to the disadvantaged subculture having more mental disorder than the other subculture, not because of anything inherent to the culture or race but because the former's members have more difficult lives. The obvious example of such a confusion of culture and class relates to the Blacks and Chicanos in the United States, but many others exist, for instance the Gypsies in eastern Europe, Arabs in Israel, and Indians in Peru.

In general, crosscultural comparisons of mental health are best undertaken in societies where one has ascertained that each of the groups to be compared has free vertical mobility and is not debarred from any social stratum (something which need not imply that they must have equal proportions in each stratum). Such societies are quite possible to find, but they tend to be small, insular, and to have a relatively short history in their present form, suggesting that multiculturialism tends over time either toward cultural fusion or to the dominance of one group by another. Where they are to be found, as in Hawaii, Singapore, Switzerland, and Mauritius, they invite psychiatric study.

2 Clinic Attendance and Combined Case Registers

Until the mid-1960s, mental hospitals provided a relatively consistent and reliable source of epidemiological data in most developed societies, since there was usually no other form of care that was socially approved and available for the major mental disorders. With the expansion of psychopharmacology and the attack on institutionalizing during that decade, however, the question of who would and who would not be hospitalized became increasingly unclear, not just between societies but within them. Whether a given psychotic is hospitalized or treated as an outpatient has come to be determined less by his clinical features or by the society's attitudes than by the therapeutic orientation of his clinician and the attitude of his family. Accordingly, it can be argued that the act of mental hospitalization no longer carries any stable meaning and the official data should now represent both inpatient and outpatient populations. (For this reason, the mental hospital data to be cited in later chapters will usually derive from earlier decades rather than be the most recent available.)

Unfortunately, despite the help which the computer now offers, it is still difficult to obtain such combined data, or even to get good outpatient data alone. When a patient comes into hospital it is known that he is being taken in charge for a certain period and it is therefore relatively easily accepted by both patient and staff that standard information be collected and stored about him. In many mental health clinics, a substantial number of the patients or clients are seen once only, so that there is understandable reluctance to record as much clinical and demographic information as one would at a hospital. Moreover, with only a single visit, the reliability of whatever is recorded is more in question. One can argue that if a patient comes only once to a clinic, then his condition cannot be serious and he can be ignored; but the problem then arises of agreeing on the point at which cases do become serious enough to merit full registration. If all patients are required to obtain referral from a general medical practitioner or an agency then they can all probably be fully registered, and if such data can then be linked to data from other sources we have a very powerful tool. However, one of the unsolved problems of such linked case registers is to persuade therapists to cooperate.

At the time of writing, the best source of crosscultural comparisons of treated mental illness including more than simply hospitalizations is the Camberwell Psychiatric Case Register [662] maintained by the Institute of Psychiatry in London. Although a specially funded research project, this is a type of register which is being taken as a model by health service administrations and could therefore represent what a number of official data sources are likely to be able to provide in the future. Other linked case registers exist, but Camberwell has a relatively high proportion of immigrants in its approximately quarter million population and its Register was started in 1964, so that by 1970 it was possible to compare a number of cultural minorities, for instance West African [530], West Indian, and Irish [30]. The papers dealing with culture and based on that Register are not such as one would yet wish to put much weight on, since the clinical information is rather thin and one is not sure how far the figures used for the population base are sufficiently accurate. (In the comparison of West African and West Indian rates there, the patient data derived from a 4-year period, whereas the population estimates were based on a 10 % sample

Table 2.3. Symptomatology of patients attending psychiatric outpatient clinics in New York and the Netherlands [531]

	New York		Netherlands	
Number of clinics	6		5	
	%		%	
A. Percentage of clinic patients given diagnosis of schizophrenia	35.2		2.7	
	%		%	
B. Frequency in all patients of certain symptoms often associated with schizophrenia, regardless of assigned diagnosis				
Inappropriate affect	30		28	
Hallucinations	4		3	
Delusions	9		5	
Incoherence	4		5	
Autistic thinking	10		3	
Other thought disorder	14		13	
	M	F	M	F
C. Problems of social adjustment	%	%	%	%
Unemployed (as % of those in labor market)	28	25	14	26
Problems in marital role (of those married)	34	50	11	31
Problems in interpersonal relationships	56	54	45	47
Feeling of isolation	50	57	17	31
Feeling of inadequacy	64	59	15	23
Number of patients	194	340	145	144

from only one of these years [530], and one does not know how much the population changes from year to year in that part of London.) Nevertheless, it can be expected that better means of comparison will develop out of this and other case registers as time passes, and persons thinking of doing such comparative research should pay attention to the care which needs to be taken to ensure that all clinics and agencies continue to cooperate.

From the limited results which have just been cited, it might be inferred that international comparisons involving outpatient data are still far from being possible. However, that is not entirely true. Even if one cannot be sure that the criteria determining consultation at a mental health clinic in two or more countries are similiar, or that the diagnostic criteria are comparable, one may still learn something from a comparison of clinical pictures. Table 2.3 reproduces certain data collected during a comparison of psychiatric clinics in New York and in the Netherlands [531]. Judging by the percentages given a diagnosis of schizophrenia by the clinic psychiatrists, as shown first, it would seem that the groups are not at all comparable. Judging by the frequency of certain schizophrenia-like symptoms in the total patient samples (part B), the two groups look much more similiar and one might be tempted to think that it is only the perceptions of their clinicians which distinguish them. Judging by the complaints in part C, however, the two groups look very different again, or at least seem beset by different problems. It is not my purpose in this chapter to discuss the possible meaning of such differences, and if I were to do so I would first have to examine how far they might have derived from some of the New York clinics being in a large metropolis while the Dutch ones were all in smaller university centers rather than in Amsterdam or Rotterdam. But the table indicates that comparisons of this type can provoke thought and are worth repeating.

Another category of outpatient data which is occasionally to be found comprises the registers which are sometimes maintained by nurses, temperance boards (in Scandinavia), and other bodies in parishes or districts. These are too few today to offer new possibilities of comparison, but they have been used thus in the past.

3 Mortality from Suicide and Other Causes

With respect to mental illness in the strict sense of the term, death certificates yield very little epidemiological information. Even with such a condition as general paresis before the discovery of penicillin, mortality data proved of less value than hospitalization data, since if the condition escaped mental hospitalization it was likely to escape diagnosis entirely. At one time the mortality rates of patients in mental hospitals, regardless of cause of death, attracted considerable attention, since they showed how far the staff had managed to keep out such conditions as typhoid; but since the First World War the main influence on such rates has been administrative policy. If the mental hospital was regarded as the appropriate dumping ground for elderly patients with multiple disorders, then its mortality rate was inevitably high; if it was regarded as having to care only for patients who were free of serious somatic illness, then its mortality rate was low. A question which is more pertinent today but has been relatively little researched is the period of survival of mental patients from the time at which their illness is recognized, since if the mortality among such patients is excessive in relation to age this may call for special preventive measures; and that mortality rate may vary with culture. For instance, when 112 Indian and 107 non-Indian patients first admitted to mental hospital in Mauritius in 1955 were followed up 12 years later [444], 14 Indians but only one non-Indian were found to have died in the interval ($P < 0.005$), although the average ages of the two groups on admission were similar. (Further data from this Mauritian study are referred to in Chaps. 4, 6.) However, for such work individual follow-up rather than recourse to official sources will often be necessary.

Where mortality rates become considerably more interesting for psychiatrists is when the latter look beyond the question of frank mental illness and consider how far death might be delayed by paying attention to contributory psychological factors. The obvious cause of death being referred to here is suicide, but death from psychosomatic disorders is also pertinent, as well as homicide, accidental death, and some purely statistical correlations. For instance, a highly significant correlation has been shown between score on the Cornell Medical Index and risk of dying within the following decade, even after allowing for age, blood pressure, serum cholesterol, and some other variables [137]. In attempting international or crosscultural comparisons of such mortality rates the problems are the same as are encountered in international epidemiology generally [4], and they will therefore not be discussed here. However, the over- and under-reporting of suicide involve problems specific to this cause of death and therefore demand separate consideration. The overreporting of suicide is not a subject on which I can remember having seen a single scientific paper, but it may have to be borne in mind in particular international comparisons even though it is irrelevant to the majority of such. It occurs mostly in societies where the police have excessive power and where prisoners who die from ill-treatment or neglect are said on the death certificate to have committed suicide, since such a statement avoids embarrassment to the authorities. The reports of Amnesty International give many alleged instances of this happening, but the countries cited are not usually ones in which serious studies of suicide are undertaken. Other instances of overreporting are said to occur among women in societies where they are very much under the thumb of their husbands' families and may be murdered or killed by neglect under circumstances which permit the death to be labeled suicide, particularly if the husband's family want him to take a more financially rewarding marriage. In a part of India, I once came across a situation where almost 10 % of recorded suicides were in children under the age of 10, and enquiry revealed that some of these cases were where the mother had killed herself and her children.

Underreporting is commoner and has attracted much more attention, but we need to distinguish between the form which exists in nearly all societies and that which is much commoner in some than in others. In most societies, the death of a family member or friend by suicide causes more distress to the survivors than his death by other causes, and if the person committing suicide desires to avoid causing that extra distress he will usually try to make the cause of death seem uncertain. Drowning, highway deaths, the incorrect use of medical drugs, and deaths from exposure may all therefore conceal a suicidal intent but the authorities will rarely attach the suicide label to them and we will rarely be able to assign them confidently to that category either. It is for this reason, most probably, that what Durkheim called altruistic suicide is so rarely reported and discussed in most societies, since if altruistic feelings are acted on then the effort will be made to protect family and friends against the self-reproach which frank suicide would occasion. It is only in the few societies where altruistic suicide can be a cause for pride in the family that it is likely to be undisguised. Elsewhere, official statistics are likely to reflect merely the types of suicide which are accompanied by feelings of resentment towards – or disinterest in – family and friends.

Even where there is resentment, however, other factors may lead the actor to make the suicidal nature of his act ambiguous, and his survivors may then seize on whatever ambiguity exists to avoid having to use the suicide label. If the culture despises or condemns suicide and at the same time encourages individuals to hope that they will be well remembered by their acquaintances after death, then the act is unlikely to be blatant and the actor may balance his feelings of resentment by telling himself that if his survivors manage to obtain a "good burial" for him they will have made up for their earlier neglect. One country in which the question of underreporting has been relatively fully investigated is the Republic of Ireland, since its recorded suicide rate has for long been one of the lowest in the world. Irish Catholicism still condemns suicide strongly; the act is still nominally a criminal offence; and the physicians or other authorities called upon to certify the cause of death will often know the family quite intimately and hence desire to save its members pain. A study by McCarthy and Walsh in Dublin [392] concludes that the actual rate of suicide is between two and four times higher than the official figure, a range which at its lowest still leaves Ireland with one of the lowest suicide rates in the world but which at its highest brings the level up closer to that of neighboring England. In making such a comparison it must be remembered that the English rate would also be pushed up if the same type of reexamination of coroners' verdicts were undertaken, so that it is probable that Ireland does possess a genuinely low rate by international standards. However, that does not mean that suicidal thoughts are rare, since the rate of parasuicide (attempts not leading to death) has become quite high during the 1970s [640].

In general, neither underreporting nor overreporting is going to make much difference to most discussions of international variations in suicide rates, since these variations are much wider than could be accounted for on this basis; but they should be kept in mind. What is much more important than misreporting is the fact that most information routinely recorded on suicide – method used, time of day, etc. – has little psychiatric relevance, while what would be of relevance is usually not recorded. Suicide can be undertaken on logical grounds and with clear sensorium, and although it must usually signal distress, that distress can be somatic or social rather than primarily psychological. Comparative studies of suicide can contribute substantially to psychiatry when sufficient detail is available to permit a differentiation of psychological states, but this detail must be sought in police or coroner's records (which are also official sources of data) rather than in death registers. Accordingly, although it is temptingly easy to make wide-ranging international comparisons using official statistics, it is much better to undertake more limited comparisons using fuller information.

4 Delinquency and Crime

What has just been stated regarding suicide applies equally to juvenile delinquency and in lesser degree to certain types of adult crime. Criminal behavior can be undertaken for logical reasons and with a clear sensorium, but there is a certain percentage of cases in which that is not true and with which psychiatrists should concern themselves. For the study of this minority of cases, national statistics are of still more limited value than was the case with suicide, but comparisons of two or more societies on the basis of police or court records hold more promise, even though the lack of uniformity respecting what gets recorded will sometimes make such a comparison fruitless. I have found it profitable to compare case records in Madras and Singapore, and the presence of distinct cultural groups in the latter city enabled findings of the

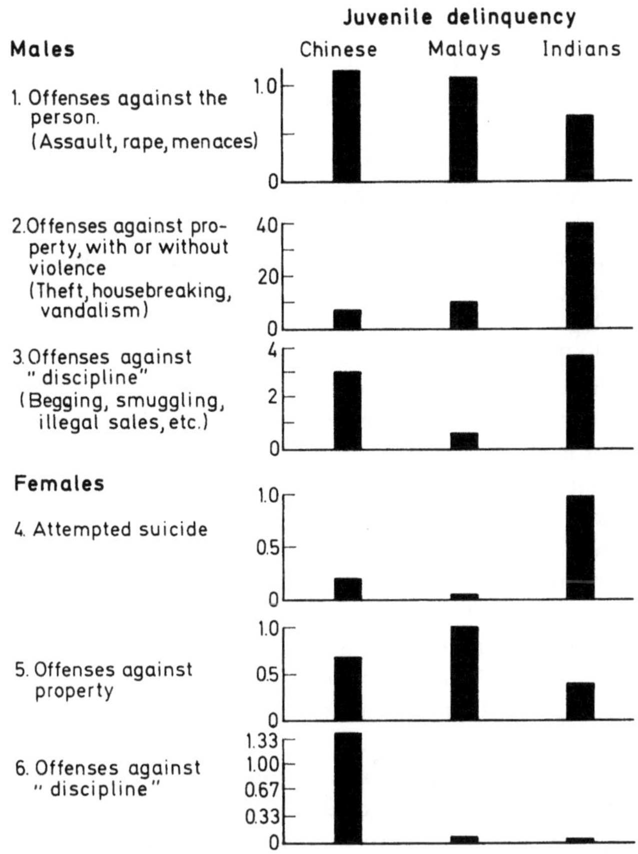

Fig. 2.3. Rates of juvenile delinquency per 1000 aged 10–15 in three Singapore cultures, 1948–1955, by type of offence and sex [422]. (Note that each section of this figure has its own scale.)

type illustrated in Fig. 2.3 to be obtained. Even as broad categories of offense as those used in this figure yield sgnificant differences, and when the more precise nature of the offenses is noted the cultures are quite distinctive. Broadly speaking, the Chinese juvenile delinquents tended to be acting on behalf of their parents or other adults, usually in directions of which – although technically illegal – their own community approved. The Malays tended to be acting individually, impulsively and out of direct material need. The Indian boys, however, were most often apprehended for stealing objects which they got little or no profit from, so that their thefts have to be interpreted as an indirect form of aggression, and one can infer that the attempted suicides of their more closely supervised sisters were also an expression of aggressive feelings which dared not be ventilated more directly.

It is frequently argued that delinquency data have no value, since the number of persons breaking the law is very much larger than the number recorded; but from the psychiatric as opposed to the strictly legal or sociological angles the very fact of getting caught is significant. In the examples just cited, the Chinese probably have a higher rate of actual law infringement by juveniles than the Indians do, but the former only rarely reflect any psychological or intrafamilial disorder while the delinquency of the Indian juveniles probably did often reflect such disorder, and the impulsive, irrational character of the latters' acts contributed to them being caught. Where the police are allowed some latitude regarding what actions to take concerning law-breaking juveniles, they tend to recognize distinctions of this sort, so that the relative numbers of juveniles brought to court may have greater significance for psychiatrists than the relative numbers admitting to illegal acts on an anonymous questionnaire.

Regarding adult crime somewhat similar comments can be made, but variations in the laws and their enforcement from one society to another make comparisons useful only for the most distinctive and universally recognized crimes. It is certainly not possible to use national statistics as a basis from which to discuss possible differences in the prevalence of psychopathy or personality disorders. Homicide statistics are more comparable, and they are sometimes taken as an index of the degree to which aggression is allowed free expression in a culture, something which could be relevant not just to the suicide rate (a matter quite often discussed) but to the rate of mental disorder deriving from ego-superego conflict. What needs to be said in this chapter is that in contrast to suicide, rates of homicide are recorded in more than one way in many countries, and the different sets of statistics often disagree in any one year. With suicide, the labeling is completed once a death certificate is provided, at latest after a coroner's inquest, which takes place soon after the discovery of the body. With homicide it is not on the basis of death certificates that national statistics are usually published, but on the basis of police returns, and to label a death homicide before someone has been tried and found guilty can be conceived as prejudging the case, so that in some administrations the reporting is delayed until a court trial has taken place or it is decided that any such trial is unlikely. Averaged data over a number of years are much more necessary here than with suicide, therefore, and if one seeks to distinguish between "rational" and "irrational" homicide for psychiatric purposes, it must be remembered that, in contrast to suicide, the identity of the person causing the death is often unknown, particularly where psychological disturbance is absent.

5 Populations-at-Risk

In contrast to all that has just been noted regarding the problems of obtaining satisfactory data about the cases from offical sources, the problems of obtaining satisfactory data regarding the populations-at-risk are usually simple. Either the data exist or they do not. There are instances when the official census is reporting on a population different from that from which one's cases are being drawn, as when there is much illegal migration or a large transient population; but these are uncommon. There can also be problems of cultural definitions (most obvious with the Jews) or of shifting frontiers (most obvious in Central Europe); but these can usually be allowed for. Occasionally, the way in which a group is defined in the census is quite different from the way it is defined for other official purposes, but the common situation is for the same definition to be used throughout, with the same range of error. The major problem for the researcher is when the population census fails to enquire into the variable the researcher is interested in. Sometimes it will be possible to derive an adequate estimate from a prior census or from immigration data (if emigration is slight). Sometimes the semiofficial records of a religious group or a cultural association will be sufficiently complete. But in most instances where the population census does not give the relevant data one has to be content with clinical descriptions of small case samples, perhaps compared with local population estimates obtained from nonofficial sources.

6 Conclusions

A Canadian criminologist has suggested that in his field it might be best to "treat the official statistics as guilty until proven innocent. With such an approach, when a difference in rates is found, the initial assumption is that the statistics are at fault, and attention is directed to discovering differences in the faithfulness of reporting or in the methods of classification which could account for it" (215). That approach, like all others in which guilt is assumed until innocence can be proven, is dangerous insofar as it tempts the judges to announce their verdicts before the case for the defence has been heard; but it is useful nevertheless. In international or crosscultural comparisons of official data having psychiatric significance, the first step should be to examine how far the methods of data collection are likely to have been the main cause of the observed differences in the results or – and this is no less important, although the criminologist just cited forgot it – of the observed similarities. Many apparent similarities and differences stem from the methods of data collection and classification rather than from any deeper cause. But the case for the defense must be heard, and if the defendant has no spokesman the judges must arrange for his case to be stated. It is not necessary for the methods of data collection to be perfect in order for them to be found innocent of producing the particular difference or similarity which is at issue; it is only necessary that the weaknesses in the data gathering are not such as would be likely to produce the particular degree of difference or similarity which is under discussion. In all comparisons of official data, one is going to find features which derive mainly from the recording method employed, but that does not mean that *all* features share that characteristic. Problems of comparability will always exist, but this does not mean that they are insurmountable.

In seeking to surmount these problems, an important step which has been illustrated repeatedly in this chapter is to set aside much of the data and focus on a limited part of it. With any type of research data whatever, there are going to be weak or faulty elements, but even with the poorest material, the researcher should ask himself: What can we salvage from this? When one is dealing with official data, one must always remember that although other sources are likely to be more accurate or more detailed, none are likely to yield the same *quantity* of usable information. It will often be necessary to reach the Scottish verdict of "not proven" rather than one of guilt or innocence when the data-gathering system is accused of producing a spurious similarity or difference. But the next step should not be to abandon working with the suspect source; rather, one should see whether other sources of information support or refute the impression obtained. These other sources may also be official, as was illustrated in Table 2.1, but the greatest help is when they derive from methods of enquiry more specific to one's particular objective, such as those to be discussed in the next chapter.

Chapter 3 Comparability of Special Survey Technique Findings

Given the frequent occasions on which official sources of data do not provide the means of making the comparisons one wishes, it is natural to think of collecting one's own data or at least of drawing on those from other field studies. Making use of such supplementary data greatly widens the range of comparisons possible, but it is not a panacea. Each research method tends to be good for answering particular questions and poor for answering others. In consequence, one needs to know each method's capabilities, and needs to avoid depending completely on results which derive from some special study if that study has not used a technique fully appropriate to the questions which one seeks to answer. Most special study methods provide greater detail and more careful classification than one gets in official sources, but on the other hand they usually cover much smaller numbers of subjects, thus raising questions regarding their representativity and the range of chance variation which they may conceal.

This chapter will review the main sources of nonofficial data that tend to be used in Comparative Psychiatry, and will attempt to indicate their strengths and weaknesses. In theory all types of research findings can be drawn on, including the study of single patients and experiments in a laboratory. Because Comparative Psychiatry is primarily concerned with the effects of broad psychosocial climates and seeks to distinguish these from the effects of idiosyncratic experiences, however, the goal must be to obtain as representative a group of subjects as possible from each of the nations or cultures being compared, and it is thus mainly with survey techniques that I will be concerned, surveys of patients or surveys of total populations. My comments will be addressed to their suitability for comparative work, not to their suitability for other purposes.

1 Case Identification by Practicing Psychiatrists

When hospital records prove unsatisfactory as a source of information on the distribution and character of an illness, the most obvious resources to turn to next are the medical practitioners outside hospital, either those specializing in the particular illness in question or general practitioners, with the resultant information being used either by itself or in combination with that obtained from hospitals and other sources. The enquiry may be by questionnaire, interview, record screening, or any combination of these. It may be aimed at getting precise figures, rough estimates, or even just qualitative impressions if head-counting is inappropriate, depending on what level of knowledge one is seeking to tap and can realistically expect to reach.

The use of *questionnaires* directed to physicians whom the researcher does not know, and without face-to-face contact, is clearly the least satisfactory approach although the easiest to follow internationally. Its use is appropriate when one is attempting to collect full clinical descriptions of cases of some rare disorder such as Gilles de la Tourette's syndrome [2], but seldom for other purposes. Usually, the physicians approached do not answer or answer carelessly, and one can never know how representative the answers are. Unfortunately, this approach is relatively popular with researchers into alcoholism, and it has been shown that the results are quite unsatisfactory [658].

Questionnaires addressed to a limited circle of professional acquaintances whom the researcher knows or who are in his debt invite more consideration, as long as one is seeking only rough impressions. Sir John Megaw, head of the health services in India around 1930, used this approach to survey village health [403] and was able to derive some interesting statistics revealing, among other things, a regional difference in the prevalence of gross insanity, a difference which received some confirmation in later studies. I myself have used this method by addressing questionnaires to correspondants in different countries, not asking them to count cases (which they would be too busy to do) but to give their general impressions regarding possible cultural differences in the symptomatology of schizophrenia [446], symptomatology of psychotic depression [447], and responsiveness to psychotropic drugs [425]. Some results from these enquiries will be indicated later, but it should be emphasized that this approach ought really only to be used for obtaining pointers toward future research, and that one must enquire into such matters as diagnostic orientation and work setting as well as into the clinical impressions which the respondants have acquired.

The *questionnaire-cum-interview* method of collecting information from specialists is capable of yielding much more satisfactory data, whether used alone or combined with hospitalization data, but the selective relationship of most medical specialists to the population which they are presumed to serve must be kept fully in view, since this varies from one country to another and may be quite unbalanced within a single country or society. Thus, when patients have direct access to specialists, as in North America, the disorders which the latter are going to encounter will be considerably different from when access is only attainable through a general practitioner, as in much of Europe, while within Europe still other differences are going to arise depending on whether the general practitioner sees the specialist as a rival (when payment is by consultation) or as a too slowly available help (when the doctor is paid a salary or on the basis of a "panel" of patients as in Britain).

The most serious attempt to tap specialists' records for the purpose of an internal comparison was the Texas mental health survey by Gartly Jaco [275] in the 1950s, one which covered 11298 cases of psychosis entering psychiatric treatment for the first time, 47% receiving that treatment from a public (i.e., hospital) source and 53% from a private one. The Texas population at that time had roughly 13% "Non-Whites," i.e., Blacks; 13% persons with Spanish surnames; and Jaco calls the remaining 74% "Anglo-Americans." Table 3.1 shows the treated incidence rates which he obtained, and it can be seen that although there are substantial and interesting differences between the three groups, the picture is very different when the cases treated

Table 3.1. Case identification through private psychiatrists [275]

	Anglo-Americans			Hispano-Americans			Nonwhites		
	Hosp.	Priv.	Total	Hosp.	Priv.	Total	Hosp.	Priv.	Total
Schizophrenia	14	23	37	17	7	24	28	2	30
Affective psychoses	3	18	21	3	3	6	2	–	2
Organic and other psychoses	15	7	22	11	1	12	22	1	23
Total	32	48	80	31	11	42	52	3	55

Age-adjusted treated incidence rates of psychosis by source of treatment; for major subcultural groups per 100 000 Texas population, 1951 and 1952.

privately are included from that which would have been obtained had only hospitalized cases been covered. Hence, valuable though this study was for showing up the marked class bias in the medical statistics of certain types of society, it is very doubtful whether its data can tell us anything about the "true" relative incidence of psychosis in the three cultural groups. Jaco brought in a whole group of patients who did not feature in the official hospital records, but he did not reach: (a) the Black and Spanish American psychotics whose families wished to avoid the shame of sending them to hospital and yet could not pay for private care; (b) psychotic vagrants considered harmless by the police; and (c) those other psychotics, particularly in the senile and depressive categories, who were able to survive outside hospital with the aid of general practitioners and folk healers and who rejected psychiatric aid, either public or private. In some societies these missed groups constitute so small a percentage of the total that they can be ignored, but only a slight knowledge of rural Texas even into the 1970s suggests that they were substantial there. Accordingly, one does not know what weight to put on Jaco's finding that the "Anglo-Americans" had so much more psychosis than the two minorities, and as far as I am aware no further work was done to explore this finding. It seems that most local psychiatrists took it as reflecting merely the differential access to services, rather than a real difference in vulnerability.

Since that pioneering work, regional case registers drawing on private and general hospital or clinic psychiatrists (and sometimes psychologists or other therapists) have developed in a few locations along lines similar to those of the Camberwell Case Register mentioned in the previous chapter. [663] One such is in Monroe County, New York State. The degree to which local private psychiatrists all collaborate with such registers is still quite a problem, but as an increasing percentage of private psychiatric care becomes covered by state or private insurance schemes the proportion collaborating may grow, and that side of the input should be watched. As noted in the previous chapter, these registers are better for comparison between local subcultures than for international comparisons, but there are certain questions which it would be quite instructive to use an international comparison of their data for. One of these is treatment outcome, i.e., an examination of whether the longer term results of one national system of psychiatric care gives better results than another, with roughly comparable disorders. [28]

Even when regional case registers cover private as well as public treatment, the data which can be obtained from them tends to be very limited. Not just to assess outcomes but to compare the finer details of symptomatology, it is going to be necessary to go beyond the register to the individual case record or to special research. However, before leaving the question of the individual psychiatrist being a source of comparative information, mention needs to be made of the relatively few but interesting reports in which such psychiatrists, working with people of more than one culture or country, have systematically attempted to compare the mean clinical pictures observed in each. (Every clinician who attempts to describe the patients he has met in some foreign country is implicitly making such a comparison, but what is being referred to now is the deliberate comparison of groups of patients individually remembered and well recorded.) The question of the representativity of the patients chosen for such comparison needs once again to be kept in mind, but Japanese psychiatrists trained in the West have made particularly good use if this type of approach, notably Kimura [307] and Doi [153], and there is at least one comparison of patients from contiguous countries in Europe [484]. The results differ from the more formal cross-cultural comparisons by researchers such as Opler and Singer [471], in that the writers have been responsible for their patients' treatment, often over years, and have probably made more effort to understand them fully; but on the other hand, for that very reason they are less likely to be objective.

2 Case Identification by General Practitioners

The problem of patients who reach the hospital and the specialist being unrepresentative can at least in theory be overcome by turning to those seeking *primary medical care*. In most developed countries the great majority of the population sees a physician every 2 or 3 years, and it would therefore seem that if we could get a picture of the frequency and character of mental disorders which physicians see in general practice, the result would be much more comprehensive and satisfactory than anything else we could obtain in the way of a general picture of the mental health of a population.

In a few instances this proves true. We have few better pictures of the mental health of a community and what disadvantages mental illness brings to daily life than the reports of Bremer from northern Norway [68], Primrose from Scotland [501], and Llewellyn-Thomas from eastern Canada [358]. These men all lived in their rural communities for years as the only local physicians and they were all personally interested in psychiatry. They therefore knew not just what patients told them in their offices, but what was seen and talked about in the community and how neighbors handled the sick individual. However, to draw conclusions from their figures regarding the relative distribution of mental disorder in Norway, Scotland, and Canada would be quite wrong, not just because of differences in diagnostic orientation, and because the populations are small, but because they are atypical in a number of ways with respect to the people whom we would like them to represent. The Arctic

Table 3.2. Case identification by general practitioners

	Britain		Germany		Norway
	England and Wales [359]	London [565]	Mannheim [685]	Bavaria [149]	[67]
Date of data collection	1955–1956	1961–1962	1973–1974	1973–1974	1972
Number of practitioners	171	50	13	18	56
Number of patients covered by survey	195 034	8943	1026	1274	12 698
Senile and presenile dementia	4	2	45	17	14
Other psychoses		10	38	32	9
Neuroses and psychosomatic disorders	87	195	210	158	215
Personality disorders and alcoholism	1	9	29	32	20
Oligophrenia	0.5	4	2	6	8
Total	93	220	327	232	266

Active prevalence of psychiatric disorder per 1000 adults consulting general practitioners in three countries. (See text for differences in approach.).

Norwegian community was under special stress due to the 1939–1945 war, was unusually isolated, and had an unusually high percentage of immigrants in it, many of them fugitives. The Canadian one had an abnormal age distribution, with many old people, and was exceptionally individualistic in value orientations even for Canada, as befits a people who make their living in small fishing boats. Only the Scottish community seems fairly representative of its region, despite its "Calvinistic traditions, with tendencies to shotgun marriages and excessive consumption of alcohol" [501, p 15]. To get more reports such as that of Primrose for other reasonably representative communities would obviously be valuable for comparative purposes, but they are likely to be rare.

One obvious way round the problem of unrepresentativity of such reports by individual physicians is to obtain information from a number of them, preferably typical of the medical practitioners in a fairly representative part of the country, and this has been done a number of times, both for small rural groups [214, 390] and for larger urban or national ones. Table 3.2 provides comparative data from the larger studies in three countries, Germany, Great Britain, and Norway. Looking at the bottom line, one sees that three of the surveys yield fairly similar total rates, whereas the first British one gives an unusually low and the first German an unusually high one. How far can we infer that the other three are genuinely similar and that these two are genuinely different?

The first point to note about these surveys is that the two British called on the general practitioners to maintain notes during a whole year, while the other three called on them to do this over much shorter periods. Since the rates concern active prevalence, not incidence, one does not expect the year-long rate to be 26 times the 2-week rate, but Mazer has shown that a 12-month active prevalence rate for mental disorder is 58% higher than that for a 3-month period [389] in a general practice study. Therefore it would not seem unreasonable to expect the first two to yield roughly double the prevalence rates of the other three, other things being equal, whereas we see that they do not. The second point to note is that the 1955 British study called on the physicians to take notes on *every* patient seen, and it was organized as a general medical survey, whereas the 1961 survey called on them to take notes on only approximately every tenth patient and, like the German and Norwegian studies, it was organized with specific focus on psychological disturbances. This means that in the 1955 survey, the physicians were paying no particular attention to the possibility that a patient had a psychological disturbance as well as a presenting somatic one, and they were also working very routinely, while in the others special attention to psychological problems could be expected over the brief survey period, and there might also be a special alertness concerning the diagnosis of the patients whom the research staff would be expected to interview. A third point is that the mean age of the Mannheim patients was significantly older than that for the population from which they were drawn, and that there is some doubt whether they comprised a random or representative sample of the patients consulting these practitioners.

In the face of this lack of uniformity, the easy thing is to say that no comparison is possible; but if such a rule had been applied generally to medicine in the past we would probably not have made any advances at all, since no good clinician examines his patients in a completely uniform fashion. The better reaction is to say that the 1955 British data should probably be disregarded and that the high Mannheim rate for senile and presenile dementia may be unrepresentative of the city itself, but that the other data do invite comparison, allowance being made for the duration of each study. On this basis, probably the most important feature in Table 3.2 is the substantially higher rate of "Other psychoses" in the two German samples as compared with the British and Norwegian ones, such "other psychoses" being the diagnostic group in which one would expect the least disagreement between clinicians either in the same country or in different countries. Previously, Mannheim had appeared to have a very much higher incidence of psychosis than another British town, Salford [7, 240], based on new entries to regional registers of patients coming to the attention of psychiatric services. These general practice prevalence data seem more comparable but still suggest that a difference in the incidence and prevalence of psychosis must exist between England and Germany.

Given the fact that the London survey spanned a year as compared to the briefer German and Norwegian ones, and given also the known fact that neuroses can be quite transitory, the data in Table 3.2 also suggest that London general practices are seeing fewer neuroses than the German and Norwegian ones. However, the London survey tabulates various additional categories of lesser psychological disorders which I have not included in the table and which may or may not be equivalent to what are treated as neuroses and psychosomatic disorders in the other studies, and because definitions are so vague in this diagnostic range it seems better to suspend judgement on the matter.

3 Direct Identification by Research Psychiatrists

Although the general practice data such as cited above appear to be the most comprehensive of the types so far discussed, they still have well-known disadvantages. It has been argued that general practitioners do not have the training to make confident psychiatric diagnoses and that they vary widely in their readiness to recognize a psychiatric disorder or even listen to a patient trying to explain a mental problem. Perhaps more seriously, the time which they customarily must allot to each patient's visit (6 minutes has been a suggested average) is too short in most peoples' view to arrive at a proper psychiatric diagnosis, and this shortage of time also leads in many instances to very sketchy record-keeping. Thirdly, individual physicians in many heavily populated areas acquire a reputation for being good with certain types of illness and poorer with others, regardless of any formal specialization, so that a survey which covers only certain physicians serving a city, and not all, can still get a distorted picture. Finally, where governmental or private sickness insurance is not dominant, patients may not stay with any one physician for primary care but may prefer to go to different hospital clinics or specialists depending on what illness they think they have; and then the primary care physician does not know his patients as persons.

Because of this and because of the limitations which official sources harbor, it has frequently been said that the psychiatric researcher must get away from service settings and look for cases in the community himself, not necessarily ignoring the information which hospitals and doctors can offer, but not remaining dependent on the latter.

The advantages of this are that cases are likely to be picked up which would escape the general practitioner's eye and which would never be brought to a psychiatric clinic or hospital. Also, the study's criteria of "caseness" are more likely to harmonize with those which other psychiatrists would use than is true when general practitioners are doing the diagnosing. However, there are disadvantages also, namely that the research interview may be a one-shot affair with someone whom the psychiatrist has never seen before; the person interviewed lacks the motive to be forthcoming which a patient seeking treatment has; and the psychiatrist's training, being entirely with people who are seeking or otherwise clearly needing help, may initially be quite a handicap when it comes to assessing someone who is not seeking help.

There are three main ways in which such "direct" clinical assessments can be undertaken, namely by the research psychiatrist seeing every adult or every child (but rarely both) in the population under study; by him seeing those subjects whom his assistants have interviewed during a household survey and who are suspected of having some psychiatric disturbance; and by him seeing only those subjects on whom information from key informants, records, etc., appears insufficient to permit a judgement.

With the first type of approach, pioneered by Essen-Moeller [174] in Sweden, both the size of the population covered and the amount of information available from each person are limited by the cost of the psychiatrist's time. Moreover, if only self-reports are being sought much important information may remain concealed, and it may be impossible to pose certain questions for fear of losing the public's cooperation. In practice, therefore, this is usually only worth trying if one either (a) has ample other information as well, as was the case with the Swedish studies, or (b) is searching only for types of disorder that cannot be concealed from the professional eye and that are currently active. However, if the investigator gets to know his communities well, as Hagnell [241] has done, then much indirect information can be gained from neighbors during the casual conversations which take place before or after the formal interviews, and this may constitute the other source of information.

The second "direct" method, namely for the psychiatrist to accompany teams of lesser trained field investigators or at least have cases referred to him by these, retains the advantage of uniformity of diagnostic viewpoint but risks losing cases by reason of the assistants being less trained to recognize psychopathology which the subject does not himself report. This method, pioneered by Rosanoff in New York State in 1916 [519], is of particular value today in countries where psychiatric services are comparatively inadequate, so that records are little guide, and where one wishes to know whether certain types of social stress are being accompanied by an increase in mental disorder. Although employed in the well-known Hutterite survey [161] the most notable use of this technique has been in Taiwan [354, 512] and in India. Theoretically, it can be employed to measure lifetime prevalence and unit-time incidence, by getting subjects to provide sufficiently full psychiatric histories of themselves, but a reanalysis of Lin's otherwise admirable survey of Taiwan Chinese communities shows that his subjects' memories must have faded quite rapidly respecting illnesses which were no longer active. To produce rates in terms of active prevalence is much more satisfactory unless, as Nandi *et al* did [452], the same community is visited at two points in time so that the incidence of new cases can be recorded.

Table 3.3 summarizes the findings of the majority of Indian surveys which have used this technique, and yields a number of points of interest. One is that the shift from traditional village to city life seems accompanied by a decrease in the mean prevalence of schizophrenia and not an increase as might have been expected. The second is that refugee migrants continue to have more mental disturbance than non-refugees, even years after their migration. A third, not so obvious point, is that the prevalence of hysterical neuroses appears to be declining over time (as illustrated in the three reports from Lucknow), and also with the shift from a rural to an urban setting. A negative finding is that there is no convincing difference between the results from Vellore in the Tamil-speaking, more Dravidian, south of India and those from Lucknow in the more Aryan north. The schizophrenia rates are a little suspect, insofar as the surveys were done by household and hence did not cover beggars, religious saddhus, and others living outside a normal household; and there is some evidence that camps af saddhus may contain a disproportionately high percentage of schizophrenics [386]. However, this is a disadvantage which applies to virtually all field surveys of stable populations, whether by household survey or key informant,

Table 3.3. Household interview assessments with research assistants: India

	Populations 15+[a]	Schizophrenia	Organic psychoses Brain syndrome	Endogenous depression	Reactive depression	Anxiety neuroses	Hysterical and other neuroses	Alcoholism and addiction
RURAL								
Punjab [450] 1978	570	12.3	–	7.0		19.3		–
U. Pradesh [556] 1972	1430	2.1				10.5		2.1
W. Bengal [168] 1971	750	8.0		5.3		2.7		24.6
W. Bengal [452] 1976	562	7.1	16.0	72.9	8.9	17.8	23.1	3.6
Karnataka [93] 1976	1233	8.1	4.9		30.8	??		4.0
URBAN AND MIXED								
Agra [155] 1968	16 800	2.6		0.9	5.8		10.6	
Lucknow [554] 1967	1040	3.8		11.5		40.4		
Lucknow [555] 1972	1010	2.0		3.0	7.9	14.8		
Lucknow [557] 1974	3240	3.4	6.2	10.8	12.3	20.5	5.0	0.3
Vellore [633] 1973	1760	2.8	2.8	3.4	35.3	12.0	3.4	5.1
REFUGEES								
Lucknow [555] 1972	1110	4.5		3.6	20.7	41.4		
W. Bengal [453] 1978	490			22.6	41.2		6.2	

Active prevalence of mental disorder per 1000 aged 15+, in 11 Indian household surveys.

[a]Where the report did not give the population aged 15+, but either used other age divisions or only a total figure, this has been estimated on the basis of internal evidence and other data from India. Some of the papers yield data of more than one kind, but only those data giving active prevalence in the indicated population as obtained by household visit are used.

and the results should therefore not be incomparable with results obtained from other countries by roughly equivalent methods.

In Taiwan, interesting differences were obtained between the prevalence of mental disorders in the Chinese [354] and in the aboriginal hill tribes [512], the former suffering more from schizophrenia than the latter, but less from alcoholism and acute transient psychoses. If we assume that the two groups of subjects cooperated equally with the surveys, these differences ought to be valid since the same techniques were used in each, but the actual rates reported should not be compared with rates from elsewhere, since they combine current and former disorders without there having been the means to yield an accurate "lifetime prevalence" estimate. Another potentially very interesting survey using a similar field survey technique was the large-scale survey of Chinese, Iban, and Malay peoples in Sarawak during the 1960s by a team under the direction of K.E. Schmidt; but unfortunately only a very small part of this has been published [105].

When a sound assessment of lifetime prevalence is desired, as it often must for genetic studies, one obviously requires good community records; but in addition to these the third type of "direct" survey is also desirable. Lifetime prevalence, being so dependent on good community records and a stable population, is calculable in only a few societies, principally some parts of Scandinavia and Switzerland. Moreover, even when the records are well maintained, the very fact that they are public property may result in their registrars being reluctant to report mental illness in them until it is both unquestionable and public knowledge. Böök [61] indicates that most parish registrars in northern Sweden waited for news from a hospital or clinic before making the "insanity" entry, and that 60% of his "confirmed schizophrenics" had to wait at least 2 years for their first hospitalization, time for a brief psychosis to have terminated. Accordingly, Fremming found that he had to pay "about 1800 visits to the subjects of my enquiry or their relatives" [204, p 19] although his whole studied population was only a little over 5000.

Table 3.4 summarizes what is probably the most trustworthy international comparison of lifetime prevalence, thanks both to the abundance of records which the two researchers could tap (Helgason had the private files which his father, Helge Tomasson, had collected on 18000 patients during 30 years of psychiatric practice in Iceland) and in part because of the Icelander's deliberate effort to follow Fremming's model. The two populations yield very similar rates in most categories, but manic-depressive psychosis was significantly more frequent in the Icelandic than in the Danish males, thus confirming, with some correction, previous impressions.

4 Household Survey by Questionnaire and Interview

A major disadvantage of the type of approach we have just been considering is that although it may count heads more thoroughly than many other methods, it can tell us very little about the clinical pictures encountered. This is because the research assistants have neither the time nor the training to bring back such pictures. One well-known solution to this problem is to have these assistants ask a series of precisely worded questions, bring back the answers with or without their own com-

Table 3.4. Birth cohort studies with follow-up by psychiatrists. Based on Table 33 in Helgason [253]

	Iceland Helgason [253]		Denmark Fremming [204]	
Sample population at age 10	Males (2729) %	Females (2666) %	Males (2086) %	Females (1979) %
Schizophrenia (confirmed)	0.57	0.90	0.75	1.02
Manic-depressive psychoses (confirmed)	1.80	2.46	1.02	2.24
Other psychoses (including ? schizophrenia and ? manic-depressive psychoses)	1.00	2.19	0.73	1.72
Epilepsy (all types)	0.59	0.52	0.56	0.48

Percentage lifetime expectancy (to age 55) of developing psychoses or epilepsy in Iceland and Denmark, based on cohorts born between 1895–1897 (Iceland) and 1883–1887 (Bornholm, Denmark).

ments, and submit the results to psychiatrists for the latter to assess and classify. As noted earlier, the main disadvantage of this approach is that one is dependent on the subject's willingness and ability to answer truthfully, particularly when, as is often necessary, interviewers are being employed who have no professional training at all. Its main advantage is that within a given research budget one can, with such lesser-trained interviewers, cover a larger population and/or take time to enquire about lesser levels of mental distress than would normally be brought to the attention of any medical practitioner. Where subjects answer truthfully, therefore, one can frequently get a subjective picture of their disorders which is unlikely to be got in any other way from such a population, although there may still be a problem of assessing how this subjective picture relates to psychiatric classifications employed in the same, or more importantly in another, society.

Whereas the techniques which we were previously considering were developed largely in Europe and received further exploitation in Asia, the idea of having the field interviewers ask precise questions and bring back precise answers was developed mainly in North America and has seen further development mainly in West Africa (although one notable Indian study [93] using this technique exists). The classic models of this approach are the Midtown Manhattan [583] and the Stirling County [345] surveys, both of which appeared in several volumes. At the time of publication they were received with some suspicion by both the public and the profession. The public was not too happy to be told that, for instance, "57% of the adult population of the County (Stirling) would be considered 'psychiatric cases' according to the criteria of the Manual" [345, p 121]. (The "manual" referred to was the American Psychiatric Association's *Diagnostic and Statistical Manual, Mental Disorders*, 1952 edition.) Sections of the medical profession were similarly uneasy to learn that in neither study could the psychiatrists entrusted with assessing the mental health of the interviewed subjects agree on conventional diagnostic labels for the inferred disorders, so that the ratings of "impairment" had to be substituted, this meaning "Can this person perform his usual duties? If not, to what extent is he incapacitated?" [345, p 52]. As a result, these studies have not contributed much to conventional, i.e., medically based, psychiatric thought and practice. However, if one's concern is mental health in a different sense, particularly the effect of different social factors on mental stress and distress, then what they and the method they pioneered have to offer is much, due to the fact that the method permits, at least in theory, quite fine gradations between the mental health assessments of a high percentage of the public. The second volume of the Midtown Manhattan Study [336] is crammed with illuminating data on the mental health ratings of groups compared in terms of such rarely studied variables as parents' religion, generation of immigration, interpersonal affiliations, and economic mobility.

The fact that one can have almost exactly the same questions posed to subjects in different societies and cultures, and can then have their answers precisely recorded and assessed by a central team of psychiatrists, has made this method seem to some researchers particularly suitable for international and cross-cultural comparisons. However, quite early in the analysis of the Midtown Manhattan data, results were produced which cast doubt on that assumption. The survey sample had by chance included a small number of Puerto Ricans, and when mental health assessments of this group were separated from the rest it was found that not one had been assessed as "well," while a majority had been assessed as definitely "impaired," a rating assigned to only 23% of other persons in the area. While it was agreed that the Puerto Ricans in New York at that time were under some strain, it seemed highly unlikely that a random sample of them should contain no mentally healthy person, and workers who knew this group were quick to suggest that the poor ratings which they received were the results not so much of pathology as of a "response style" which led them to agree with what they thought the interviewer was suggesting, and also perhaps to dramatize their problems. The impact of this response style was probably exaggerated by the fact that the interview contained very few questions about positive aspects of mental health or enjoyment (e.g., "Do you have a lot of fun when you get together with your friends?") and also paid relatively little attention to how far the reported symptoms were interfering with daily life. However, even if these adjustments had been made, it was recognized that it would probably still have been quite difficult to assess from a reading of the answers alone how much allowance should be made for such cultural factors.

Because of such considerations, it was decided at the first main attempt at carrying this technique to another continent and obtaining international comparisons with it [334], to have the psychiatrists more closely involved in the field work from the start. Table 3.5 shows some results from this attempted comparison and provides a valuable lesson regarding the difficulties which any such attempt must face. As one can see from the main part of the table, the Nigerian sample reported more of almost all symptoms than the Canadian sample did, the exception being sleep disturbance. From a certain angle that might have been expected, since the Canadians had been benefitting so much more from the delights of civilization, including better medical and psychiatric care. However, when one looks at the bottom line of the table, which indicates the percentages thought to be "significantly impaired" by mental disturbances, the Canadian sample appears twice as bad as the Nigerian one. The main explanation for this seems to be that "significant impairment" was judged on

Table 3.5. Symptom comparisons through household interviews

	Nigeria [61]		Canada [633]	
	Town	Country	Town	Country
N	64	262	143	1010
	%	%	%	%
Psychoneurotic symptom groups				
Anxiety	36	27	13	10
Depressive	27	30	8	7
Hypochondriacal	–	–	4	4
Other	61	53	46	41
Psychophysiological symptom groups				
Gastrointestinal	50	42	36	33
Musculoskeletal	52	34	29	22
Cardiovascular	33	20	15	15
Headaches	55	42	9	12
Genitourinary	47	24	8	4
Respiratory	16	8	3	3
Skin	28	18	3	1
Frequent sleep disturbance	2	5	(a)	15
Rated as "significantly impaired"	19	16	38	32

Percentage of respondents in sample communities of the western region of Nigeria and of Nova Scotia in Canada reporting selected categories of symptoms during home interviews, with the percentages of each group rated as "significantly impaired" by the research psychiatrists. Data taken from various locations in each source; questionnaires were not identical for each location. (a) Sleep disturbances were not independently reported for the Canadian town.

the basis of questions regarding behavior as opposed to subjective experience. The Nigerians reported more distress in response to the team's enquiries, and they may have suffered more, but they did not usually allow the matters complained of to interfere with their daily work whereas the Canadians often did do this, or at least allowed themselves to believe that their work was being interfered with thus.

Since that Nigerian study, attempts have been made to improve the technique [45, 93], and improvements have also been made towards making impairment assessments more objective. However, international comparisons by this method still remain problematic, and in developing countries a question of the ethics of such surveys has been raised. In nearly all field health surveys, certain expectations are raised in the minds of those interviewed, whether general public or physician, and it is both dishonest and often harmful if these expectations cannot be met. In an advanced society these expectations can be slight and the abundance of medical services available ensures that any health anxiety aroused by the questions can receive prompt attention. In a developing country, however, that is not usually the case, and there is some evidence that such a survey may turn the minds of the respondents away from traditional styles of complaint and sources of help toward new symptoms and to services which may not be available. Researchers contemplating such studies in developing countries should read Beiser's article [44] on this subject. Where the approach is clearly of value is for comparing different sections of a single society in which response styles and the significance of particular symptoms are likely to be uniform.

5 Direct Case Identification by Questionnaire Alone

When a psychiatrist or physician accompanies the interviewing teams in the foregoing type of survey, it is his presence which particularly arouses expectations. When he is absent, the expectations tend to be less although the level of cooperation may also decline, and if such a professional is not needed to read each protocol there can in addition be considerable economies in time and money. For this reason, an obvious step for researchers to explore has been the elimination of individual case judgements entirely, by having "caseness" depend automatically on the responses to certain questions or the total score on a symptom checklist. This possibility is particularly attractive to social scientists, freeing them from dependence on the clinician, but clinicians have also employed it, getting a secretary or technician to score a self-administered questionnaire and report the score only. Typically, with this approach, the respondent is rated as "normal" if his score of positive answers is less than a predetermined figure, and as a "case" if that score exceeds the same or a higher predetermined figure.

For survey purposes, the strengths of the approach are that it can be applied in strictly uniform fashion to quite large samples of the population; can be combined, thanks to its brevity, with many other types of enquiry; and can focus on subjective feelings of distress or discomfort which may not be reported in clinical interviews. Its weaknesses are that it does not reach those types of mental disturbance which the respondent either cannot or will not report regarding himself but which may be apparent to others; it makes no allowance for differences in response style and motivation (whereas the professional interviewer tends automatically to allow for these); and it is inflexible, unable to pursue additional information touching the respondent's key problem or to give the answers touching that key problem more weight than answers which do not. A further point to note is that whereas the results from the other special methods often seem equivalent, using the same concepts and differing only in the intensity of their search, the results obtained by this method are not really comparable with those obtained by others, since the subject is now his own judge and the opinions of a third party are not brought to bear on the assessment.

As an example of the proper use of this method, one may take Amiel's mental health survey of the French teaching profession and some other control groups in France [15, 16]. Here, the goal was not to count cases of particular disorders but to assess whether certain categories of teachers were more mentally distressed or disturbed than other categories and than socially comparable groups in other occupations. A sample of 776 teachers could relatively easily be covered, allowing quite detailed demographic analysis; data from large control groups could also be quite easily obtained; the professional organizations concerned did not see the enquiry as primarily

Table 3.6. Symptom-checklist responses from general populations [272]

N	India 736 %	Chile 931 %	Israel 1300 %	Nigeria 720 %
Average frequency with which symptoms are reported in each sample	24	29	22	28
Individual symptoms				
Nervousness	48	36	27	9
Heart beating hard without exertion	13	24	13	45
Shortness of breath without exertion	8	15	6	32
Disturbing dreams	21	22	35	48
Correlation between symptoms score and score on dissatisfaction with treatment at work	0.01	0.13	0.04	0.31

Frequency with which certain symptoms are reported by male blue-collar workers aged 18 to 32 in four countries; and correlation of symptoms scores with score of dissatisfaction regarding way treated at work.

psychiatric, i.e., as threatening to label some of their members as crazy or otherwise deviant; and this was a population all likely to be using the same language in the same fashion. The results are instructive, but if one wished to compare them with those from another country there is much that would have to be done first in the way of assessing what representative persons in each culture meant by their answers, and then in the way of assessing whether the particular symptoms employed in the questionnaire had roughly the same significance in each location.

The last point is often overlooked when cross-cultural comparisons are made with such questionnaires, it being assumed not just that symptoms are symptoms all the world over but that answers to such a questionnaire represent a general level of subjective distress rather than the presence of particular syndromes. The latter point seems true, but there are still in each culture ways in which that distress tends to be experienced or expressed and ways in which it does not come forth, so that the choice of questions can be crucial when cross-cultural comparisons are intended. This was shown most dramatically when an attempt was made to add a brief mental health rating scale to a sociological study of 5500 blue-collar workers in six developing societies [272]. It was decided that only about ten questions on mental health could be accepted, since so many other aspects of social adjustment, etc., had to be covered, and when the research group's adviser in mental health questions referred them to standard symptom checklists, it was found that some of the items either did not translate well or were not well accepted in some countries, so that the resultant list of theoretically comparable questions was rather limited.

Table 3.6 shows some of the results from that enquiry in four countries. On the top line one sees that the average percentage frequency with which the symptoms in this mental health scale were reported positively was quite similar in the four countries, suggesting that the scale must have had roughly the same meaning in each. However, when one looks at the frequencies with which certain individual symptoms were reported by each country's sample, it becomes clear that the uniformity just mentioned is accidental. If some of these symptoms had been omitted, and probably if different ones had been added, the average score in each country could have been very different. Moreover, when one looks at how the scores on the mental health scale correlate with a sense of dissatisfaction about treatment in the workplace, something which one expects to be related, one sees on the last row that while that correlation is probably significant in Nigeria, it is negligible in India and Israel. That shows how difficult it is to compare answers from this type of instrument internationally. In fact, the meaning of scores on such a symptom checklist has been shown to differ between one part of a city and another, even within a reasonably homogeneous population [433].

Nevertheless, this type of instrument can be used for international comparisons of a certain type, namely those seeking to assess how far certain associations between mental health and other variables remain constant from one society to another, or vary. An illustration of this type of application is given in a paper by Chance, Rin, and Chu [103], in which symptom checklist material obtained in Taiwan and from Alaskan Eskimos were examined to assess whether under conditions of rapid social change mental health was better in those who changed most rapidly or in those who changed least. For both the Eskimos and the first generation Chinese immigrants to Taiwan, it was discovered that the poorest scores were at neither end of that hypothetical continuum, but rather derived from individuals who either sought to modernize their lives but lacked the means, or sought to remain more traditional but were being denied that choice. However, in a third cultural group, the long-settled traditional inhabitants of Taiwan itself, that relation did not operate, presumably because their greater social security enabled them to accomodate modernizing trends at their own pace. In this comparison, each study had been undertaken separately, with different symptom checklists, and no attempt was made to equate the items in them; but that did not appear to invalidate the later comparison of their results (once roughly comparable measures of orientation to and experience of change had been agreed upon) provided each scale appeared to cover roughly the range of symptoms and behavior thought to be relevant. Where even this limited comparison would not have been legitimate, of course, is if one suspected that the relevant psychopathology was not being tackled by the instrument, as would be the case if alcoholism or schizophrenia were important. (The work just cited has been challenged [191] on technical grounds and requires repeating before its conclusions can be fully accepted; but that does not detract from its value as an example of legitimate international comparisons using symptom checklist scales.)

6 Case Identification by Lay Informants

The identification of cases by self-report, either through interviewer or through questionnaire, has the disadvantage of not getting satisfactory information out of a variety of respondents. There are those whose illness interferes with their ability to interpret and communicate clearly, those who may be motivated to conceal facts about themselves, and those not mature enough to be able to communicate their symptoms properly. Moreover, if the researched condition is quite rare, self-report approaches become quite uneconomical, 100 or 1000 persons having to be contacted for every case recorded.

One potential answer to these problems is to have third parties provide the desired information. We have already seen an example of this approach through the use of general practitioners, but for some conditions they also may seem less than satisfactory, for instance if they treat diseases rather than treat people, or if the researched condition is one that is not usually brought to them. A further, attempted solution has been to use *lay* third party informants, i.e., people who can claim no medical knowledge and thus provide no reliable diagnoses, but who can testify to what they have observed and have been told. With such informants one can only reliably enquire into behavior, not sensations; signs, not symptoms in the conventional modern sense. If the informant is intimately associated with the potential "case," then he may be able to report on the latter's feelings, but that very intimacy may color his perception and reporting. (Wives cannot be trusted to report accurately on the spouse's alcohol abuse.) If the informant is not close to the potential "case" then greater objectivity can be expected, but the chances of direct observation are correspondingly less and what the informant can offer may be mainly hearsay.

The disturbances on which third party reporting is not merely accepted but virtually routine are those of childhood, many clinicians interrogating the mother and asking the child almost nothing. Langner's mental health rating scales for children [337] exploit this fact, being addressed to the mothers, and the care with which they are designed to differentiate between various syndromes is a great advance over the 22-item scale for adults which bears his name. However, the degree to which the answers are affected by the mental health and other characteristics of the mother still remains to be explored, and we are given no information regarding the degree to which such ratings agree with ratings effected by other means. Rutter's questionnaire for teachers [529] seems in some respects more promising, since such teachers are less intimately involved with the children than mothers are and if the one teacher rates several children it should be easier to make corrections for rater bias. However, when the British team compared the ratings obtained from the teachers' questionnaires with ratings obtained through psychiatric interviews of mothers, as shown in Table 3.7 (lower half), the degree of agreement is low. Accordingly, although the overall differences found by this team in its three samples are convincing, it is difficult to know how far these results could be compared with results from another country even though the same questionnaire was used, and we are further warned by the authors that "as used here, psychiatric disorder is not equivalent to the presence of an 'illness' or a 'disease' " [529, p 501]. A United States study comparing the ratings obtained from teachers with ratings obtained by direct psychiatric interview concluded that the two agreed in only 11% of girls, although for a higher percentage of boys [225].

Another relatively common use of third party information is when household surveys rely on a single person in each household to report on the other members. This has proved quite satisfactory in surveys relating to diet, somatic health, smoking, and other nonstigmatizing variables, but it has not proved satisfactory either with respect to alcohol abuse [413] or with respect to sociopathy, and has not to my knowledge been evaluated respecting childhood disorders. It seems probable that with this type

Table 3.7. Behavioral ratings by third parties (teachers)

	Isle of Wight [529]		London Local [529]		London Immigrant [528]	
N	1279		1689		354	
	M (%)	F	M (%)	F	M (%)	F
A. From teachers' questionnaires only						
Emotional disturbance	3.9	3.3	7.7	6.5	6.4	6.6
Conduct disorder	9.0	3.0	14.2	5.1	40.1	25.8
Mixed and other	0.9	0.8	2.6	1.6	2.3	1.7
Total disorder	13.8	7.1	24.5	13.2	48.8	34.1
B. Based on psychiatric interview with mother as well as TQ						
(1) TQ + Psy. Int. +	5.9	2.4	11.5	4.8	11.6%	
(2) TQ + Psy. Int. -	7.9	4.7	13.0	7.9	30.0	
(3) TQ - Psy. Int. +	8.2	9.1	9.1	36.1	5.7	

Comparison of mental health ratings of 10-year olds in Britain; three samples studied by two methods, with two categories of disturbance. Figures represent percentages assessed to be mentally disturbed according to predetermined criteria. The upper half of the table represents diagnostic distribution based on teachers' questionnaires (TQ) only, and for children attributed with nine or more abnormalities. The lower half of the table indicates what percentage of children would be rated as mentally disturbed (1) on the basis of both the teacher's questionnaires and a psychiatric interview with the mother; (2) on the TQ but not the interview; and (3) on the interview but not the TQ. Immigrants are all from the West Indies.

of household survey, the respondent's ideas regarding the possible purpose and confidentiality of the survey may weigh still more heavily than when each individual is interviewed separately, and cultural traits (e.g., suspiciousness) will also play a part here. In the south of India there is evidence [289, 598] that it is difficult to overcome suspiciousness whereas in the north this does not seem to be such a problem.

Even interviewing only one person per household, however, can still be an expensive way of tracking down conditions whose prevalence is below 1%, unless the research is taking place in a society where the average household is very large, as was true in Taiwan at the time of Lin's survey [354]. A more economic approach of the same type which is now being tried is to get the household informant to report not just on the houshold members but on a circle of acquaintances [449], something which proves feasible if a method of assuring anonymity is incorporated but which poses problems regarding the representativity of the acquaintance network. (The method was chosen for the purpose of assessing the prevalence of certain types of alcohol-associated behavior unlikely to be revealed by self-report, and one of the problems in interpreting the results is to know whether alcohol abusers have smaller networks of acquaintances than other adults.) Much more widely used for assessing the prevalence of infrequent disorders such as the psychoses is the use of key community informants.

Key informants are people whose position within their communities is assumed to give them special knowledge about the problems encountered and problems created by the community members. Family physicians are obvious candidates for this title, as are the police, clergy, teachers (for certain types of problem only), traditional heads of families or clans in some societies, and local government administrators or representatives in others. Many of the surveys mentioned in this chapter have used such people as auxiliary sources of information, and I suspect that if these had not been used, the number of "cases" identified by direct interview, etc., would have been significantly lower. However, key informants have also been used as the prime source of information, and although this does not receive much support from epidemiologists it is both useful and economical for certain purposes.

The first specifically psychiatric survey depending mainly on key informants (plus official records) was probably that by Brugger in Austria in 1929 [76], and a couple of the errors which he made in that pioneer effort have branded the technique ever since. Brugger correctly understood that key informants can only be used successfully for epidemiological purposes if one can identify with some precision the populations on whom they are reporting, and if these populations are small enough for the informants to know about all the marked deviations in behavior within them. The method therefore cannot usually be employed in urban settings (socialist societies with urban block and sector health representatives are the main exception) and Brugger wisely excluded the city of Jena from his population sample, choosing rural administrative units with 1000 inhabitants or less. However, for eliciting the cooperation of his informants, he relied on State authority, quite forgetting Austrian attitudes toward such authority, and it is immediately apparent that he did not get that cooperation from those informants who should have been most useful. He received only 28 notifications from doctors and 36 from members of the clergy whereas the *bürgermeisters* who should have known least about the mentally ill but whose jobs were most dependent on the authority supporting his survey supplied 165 names. He attempted to compensate for that doubtful result by collecting names from the patients whom he interviewed, and his two later surveys in Germany yield significantly higher rates of psychosis, perhaps because of improved technique, perhaps because of a different public attitude towards authority, and perhaps because of a genuine difference in psychosis prevalence; but one cannot safely cite his data as illustrative of international differences in prevalence.

As that study illustrated, the first point to note regarding the use of key informant surveys is that they can only properly be undertaken in locations where one is reasonably sure of obtaining the cooperation of persons in key positions. For this reason it is an error to launch such a survey in any community without having explored the matter thoroughly, and an error to assume that the cooperation will be forthcoming since there is no obvious reason why it should not. (This is really no different from the rule which says that one does not undertake an epidemiological analysis of admissions to a given hospital before assuring oneself that the records have been adequately kept, or the rule which says that one must test public receptivity before carrying out a household survey; but the reluctance of key informants to cooperate fully may be more hidden and hence needs to be more thoroughly explored.) The second point to note is that this cooperation must be actively wooed and maintained after the initial acceptance of one's research has been obtained, for one is demanding work of people, one's research can in their eyes have unknown

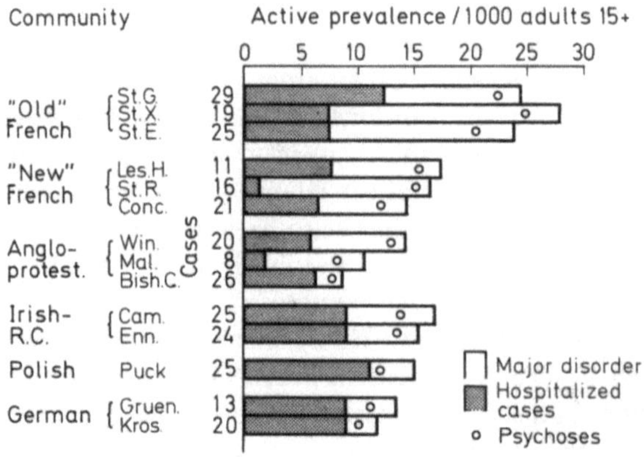

Fig. 3.1. Differences between prevalence rates derived from official sources and from local key informant inquiry in Canadian villages of various cultural origins. "Prevalence" means 1-year active prevalence, not lifetime prevalence. "Major mental disorder" means a disorder producing marked disturbance in social functioning, i.e., mainly psychosis but with a few cases of severe neuroses. Alcoholism was not included

political consequences, and therefore the informants must get sufficient reward for their cooperation to persuade them to search their memories and reveal potentially embarrassing information. (With self-report enquiries, the custom has been to abandon questions that might be perceived as embarrassing, something which can introduce obvious bias.) The third point is that all information needs to be checked, both the positive and the negative, since the apparently unified community may be split into factions which do not speak to each other; the apparently willing informant may have a strong subjective bias on a particular subject; and the most balanced informant can have lapses of memory. These checks should take place both contemporaneously, employing informants from different walks of life, and across time, by returning to the same informants a second or third time, to allow them to have searched their memories and to have verified that the researcher is harmless.

Figure 3.1 illustrates the results obtained by combining a field enquiry of this type [441] with a search of hospital records, for rural communities of different cultural background in the same country, Canada. The adult population covered was slightly under 20 000. Hatched bars represent the active prevalence rates which would have been obtained if only patients known to psychiatric hospitals and services had been considered, empty bars to the right of these indicate the active prevalence of patients with a psychosis or other severely disabling mental disorder who had never been known to the psychiatric services of the region. By taking only the former group one gets the impression that there are no cultural differences in prevalence here, but by adding the latter a statistically significant difference is revealed and the fact that two or three communities (geographically distant) had been taken to represent each of the main cultural groups enables one to assess how likely it is that the differences are culture-linked.

In a survey of this type it is desirable, as goes without saying, that the diagnostic impressions which one gets from the key informants (who are not themselves asked, even the doctors, to make diagnoses but simply to describe people who have shown certain types of abnormality) are confirmed by a psychiatric interview with the named subject himself. However, in societies which stress privacy and disapprove of "gossip," one may find that the informants cooperate much better when assured that the subjects they report about will not be approached, than when they have to fear that such a professional visit would lead to accusations of gossiping. That was the case in these Canadian villages, and hence a majority of patients were not directly assessed, the extra diagnostic difficulty being compensated for to some extent by obtaining additional key informants and additional descriptions of the subject's behavior or talk on specific occasions. The average number of informants in this survey was eight per community, but in societies where people enjoy talking about their neighbors and are not under any disapproval for doing this the required number may be less. Key informant approaches are of little use for comparing symptomatology but, since one can easily combine enquiries about patients with enquiries about the community, they are particularly suitable for studies of the interaction between psychopathology and community structure, or of the ways in which different types of communities treat different types of deviant as was the main goal of the Canadian village survey.

7 Conclusions

For the purpose of clarity, each of the special survey techniques mentioned in this chapter has been treated in relative isolation, as if when one is chosen others are not. In practice, however, the best mental health surveys are those which have combined two or more approaches and have used them, as far as possible, to check on each other. When general medical practitioners have been the prime source of cases, their diagnoses have sometimes been compared with those assigned by a research psychiatrist [149], or a sample of their cases have been given a follow-up interview in order to assess how transient the complaint has been [296]. When household interviews have been undertaken, either by a research psychiatrist or by assistants, it has frequently been the case that these have been checked against what can be learnt from official records or key informants. Symptom checklist scores can be compared with what the subject himself says regarding the degree to which normal functioning has been upset, as one saw in Table 3.5, or with subsequent information regarding need for psychiatric care [431]. However, when more than one approach has been used there are often discrepancies, perhaps quite large ones as one saw in Table 3.7, and then the question arises which of the various measures, if any, to trust. Moreover, if multiple approaches have not been used, so that obvious and maybe embarrassing discrepancies are avoided, is there any reason to think that the one chosen approach is yielding results that are more "true" than another approach which almost certainly would produce different figure?

The answers to these problems depend on the purpose of one's research and, more particularly, on the clarity of the concepts which have guided it. If the purpose of this has been to "measure the mental health of population X," without any particular idea about what use this measurement is going to be put to or which definition of "mental health" is being employed, then it is impossible to choose between one approach and another and there is not much need to worry about that choice either, since such research will be of little use in practice or theory. If on the other hand one is aiming to test a particular theory – genetic, psychoanalytic, social, etc. – concerning a particular clinical entity, then there may be only one approach which yields all the required information efficiently; and if there is a practical goal – expansion of psychiatric services, for instance – then certain types of survey information may be beside the point. Genetic (medical) theory normally concerns itself with the risk of ever getting a particular disease, i.e., with something close to "lifetime prevalence," and for this no "point-of-time" study is going to be adequate; one needs both historical records and informants with long memories such as Helgason was able to tap. Theories concerned with social stress usually (but not always) are more in need of information on minor variations in symptom level and functioning than of information on specific psychoses, whether treated or untreated. To improve the character of consultative services to general practitioners, one needs to know about the types of psychiatric patient who consult these practitioners, but not about patients not consulting them. To develop services that will reach the types of disorder that are currently not being reached, neither general practice nor clinic data are likely to give good guidance and either a self-report or third-party survey will be preferable, regardless of whether such a survey yields satisfactory precision on diagnosis or not.

Because the value of a research approach depends on the question being asked, and because the readers of this book will differ in the questions which they want to ask, it is often impossible to state categorically that the data from one research approach are better than those from another. However, that does not mean that I should then treat all equally and combine results from many different approaches in the one statement or table, such as one finds in some epidemiological texts that have attempted to cover the subject in a short space. One purpose of this chapter has been to show that it is usually not at all legitimate to combine data from different types of approach and (as it were) average the results. In attempting any comparison, whether international or on a much narrower scale, the reader must continually be asking himself how probable it is that in a given society or section of society, someone suffering from a particular type of mental disorder would be identified by a particular type of survey method. Moreover, he should also be asking himself whether some other type of disorder might be substituting for the target one in this given situation, and whether a state that is nonpathological might be assuming the guise of pathology.

Chapter 4 Schizophrenia

Psychiatric textbooks have tended to take a surprisingly narrow or simplistic view when it comes to examining how far this disorder varies between different peoples. Around 1970 one was still meeting statements to the effect that "within rough limits rates are similar in all those cultures that have been carefully studied"[203, p 221], or that "the universal incidence of the disease weighs heavily against any arguments that environmental and psychological factors of any specific kind play an important part in causing the disease" [387]. Such statements are surprising because there has for long been evidence suggesting that the disease is more frequent in one people than in another, and because one would expect some variation of this type regardless of the etiology. Quite marked differences in the hospitalization rates for schizophrenia were reported soon after the term came into use, for instance among North American immigrant groups and between Jews and non-Jews in Europe. By 1953 Böök [61] had reported a prevalence rate in north Sweden which was significantly higher than those reported by other Scandinavian investigators employing the same type of measure. To imply that rates do not vary significantly from one society to another has for a long time, therefore, been incorrect, even though it might be true that the variations do not follow any recognizable pattern, or in some instances could be attributable to factors which are peripheral to psychiatry's true interests.

The main excuse for ignoring these variations has been the lack of agreed diagnostic criteria, and the marked differences between one clinician and another in their use of the term, not just internationally but sometimes within a single hospital. The US/UK Diagnostic Project [123] demonstrated the differences between national schools regarding where to draw the line between schizophrenia and the affective psychoses, while the literature on pseudoneurotic schizophrenia has documented the confusion on a second boundary and some of the African literature [127] has shown that the same exists along the border between schizophrenia and the acute reactive psychoses. Because of this, it has been relatively easy to assume that findings which deviate from the average or which conflict with a pet theory arise from failure to apply standard criteria or from the studied population having undergone adverse and atypical selection. Böök's report was largely ignored in some circles because it was thought that the studied population might be too inbred, but that opinion is having to be revised now that the Lapps, who partly comprised that population, have been shown to have an excess vulnerability in northern Norway as well [18]. In a book such as the present one, it is impossible for the writer to impose his own criteria on the material and assure the reader that only cases meeting these criteria are being discussed. However, as far as possible my intention here is to treat schizophrenia as a unitary condition (not "the schizophrenias") which (a) involves thought disorder; (b) disturbs social functioning; (c) is not predominantly affective in symp-

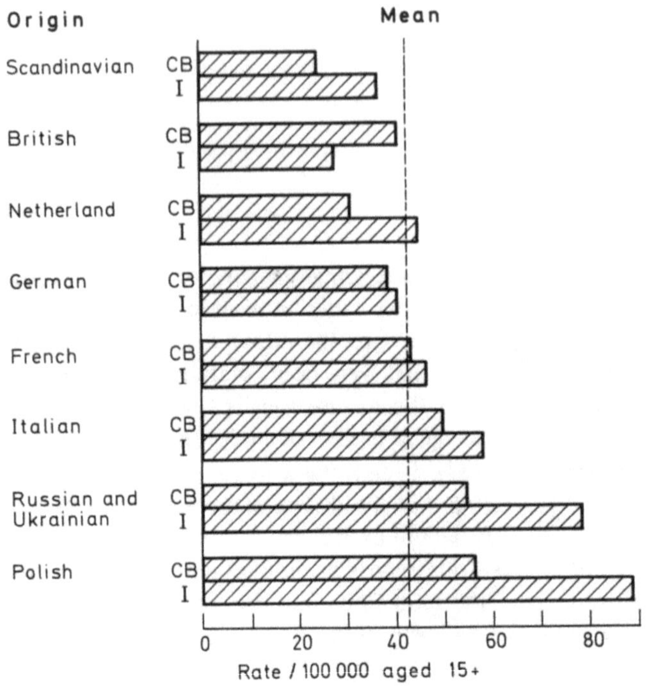

Fig. 4.1. Schizophrenia in Canadian subcultures. Culture-specific rates of first admission for schizophrenia; seven provinces of Canada, 1961, by nativity. Rates standardized for age, sex, and provincial distribution, separately for Canadian born (CB) and for Immigrants (I)

tomatology; (d) has not developed subsequent to mental retardation or some organic brain syndrome (alcohol dependency not being regarded as sufficient evidence of such a syndrome); and (e) has not developed suddenly after some psychic or somatic trauma. This is not to say that I believe that schizophrenia should be diagnosed only when all these criteria are met, but only that they make international and cross-cultural comparisons easier, through eliminating some important areas of potential disagreement.

Because of the variation in diagnostic criteria between and within national schools of psychiatry, there is little point in attempting to rank countries in terms of their schizophrenia hospitalization rates or in terms of prevalence as discovered by different field survey teams. Care even needs to be taken in comparing data obtained for two or more cultural groups attending the same psychiatric services or seen by the same investigator, if there is a reason to suspect that the criteria applied may not have been ones commonly employed internationally. If these criteria are too broad and one of contrasted groups has much less education than the other, then it may appear to have an excess of schizophrenia when a more internationally agreed assessment would probably say that it had merely an excess of affective and reactive psychoses. If the criteria are too narrow, then in the same comparison the less educated group may appear to have unusually few cases of schizophrenia, the reason being that the limited criteria being employed have been developed in a relatively educated population. However, where the criteria appear to be ones often used in other countries, and where peoples of different cultural or national background have all been sharing the same services, there may be some justification for comparing rates as is done in Fig. 4.1.

This figure shows the range of first admisssion rates to hospitals in seven Canadian provinces, for eight groups of European origin, the rates being standardized for age and for provincial distribution, and the "origin" groups being divided into immigrant and Canadian-born. (The Canadian-born are quite likely to have had parents born in Canada also, but administrative tradition called on such people, both at admission to hospital and at the population census, to state their cultural origin on the male side.) The range of rates is not wide, but it goes beyond chance expectation even when the sexes are considered separately, and we also see that there is considerable agreement between the rates for the present generation of immigrants and those for the Canadian-born of the same cultural origins (Pearsonian r = 0.72). It would be possible to discuss these variations here, taking into account such matters as level of education and socioeconomic status as has been done elsewhere [435, 440]; but one would always come back to the question of whether the hospitalized incidence was an adequate reflection of the "true" incidence in the community, and there are not the field survey data to answer this for each of the eight groups. Accordingly, it seems better to consider a few examples of unusually high and usually low schizophrenia incidence, particularly ones on which there is also some background information which might cast light on the phenomenon.

1 Peoples with High Incidence Rates: Irish and Southwestern Croatians

The people on whom we have the most abundant evidence indicating an excess of schizophrenia are the *Irish*. Evidence of them having a higher rate of psychosis than their neighbors dates from the nineteenth century, when the proportion of the population in mental asylums was higher than that in England, despite the fact that the latter had a much higher percentage of the population in urban centers where psychotics would usually have been less tolerated. By 1911 the proportion of the population in asylums was 50% higher than in England [429], and in the United States the Irish immigrants had a psychiatric admission rate four times that of the United States-born and double that of other immigrant groups [498]. Naturally, this excess of psychosis need not have represented an excess of schizophrenia, but when Pollock came to turn his attention to this category of disorder, using data from the year 1920 [499] he found that the Irish-born had the highest age-standardized rate in 11 immigrant subcultures. Since then, the gap between the first admission rates of the overseas Irish and other North American subcultures has narrowed, but that between the rates of the homeland Irish and English has widened. In 1930, the Irish-born had still the highest female rate of various immigrant groups in New York, but their males were only the third highest and the United States-born children of Irish immigrants had rates still closer to the local average [373]. In 1950, rates for the Irish-born and the children of Irish-born in New York were still above average but

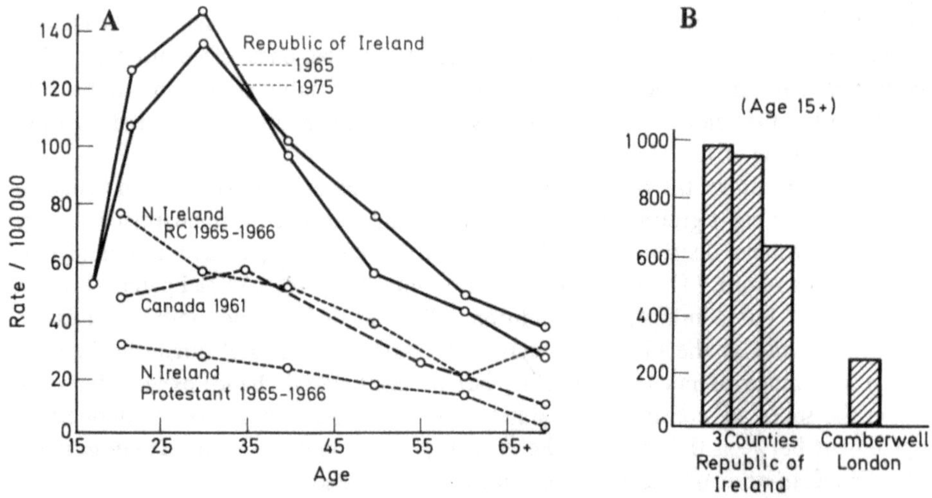

Fig. 4.2 A,B. Incidence and prevalence of schizophrenia in Ireland as compared with selected other populations. **A** Age-specific first admission rates from the Republic of Ireland, Northern Ireland, and Canada at various times during the 1960s and 1970s, standardized for sex [429, 469]. The different sources use different age groupings. **B** One-day active prevalence in three counties of the Republic of Ireland compared with Camberwell, London, based on medical informants and case registers [639]

probably not markedly so (Malzberg [376] does not give precise figures to this year, probably because of difficulties in achieving an accurate age standardization). In 1961 it can be inferred that although Canadian women of Irish origin (mostly third generation) had probably a schizophrenia rate which was significantly above the average for all Canadians, the Irish-origin men did not. (Direct calculation of Irish-Canadian rates was not possible, which is why they had to be combined with the other British-origin in Fig. 4.1; but indirect calculation via religious affiliation was possible [435].)

Returning to the Irish homeland, the first precisely calculated rates for schizophrenia in the Republic of Ireland were produced for 1963 [637], and shortly after that it was possible to compare first admission data from there with similar data from Northern Ireland. Figure 4.2a provides age curves for these two territories at that time, plus the Canadian curve derived from the same source as Figure 4.1 and one for the Republic in 1975. The two Republican curves are clearly much higher than those of the other populations illustrated, and if one calculates age-standardized rates from these they prove to be between three and five times as high as those for most Western countries on which I have data for around the year 1970. From the Figure one also sees that there are much greater age differences in the Republic of Ireland distribution than in the other populations and also that in Northern Ireland the Roman Catholics are significantly more vulnerable than the Protestants.

All that has been written above regarding the Irish refers to hospitalizations, and as such is not above suspicion. Such high official rates could derive either from the treating psychiatrists having used the schizophrenic diagnosis excessively or from the public being abnormally ready to hospitalize their mildly schizophrenic members, without the "true" incidence being significantly different from the world average. Regarding diagnosis, it is true that some of the data derive from New York where psychiatrists are more inclined to use this label than in Europe [123], but the groups against which the Irish-origin rates are being compared there were all being seen by the same clinicians. In Ireland itself, research has been specifically directed at the possibility of the local psychiatrists employing a different set of criteria from those which English psychiatrists do and the conclusion was that the criteria are virtually the same in the two countries [298]. Also, where one diagnosis has been used too freely, it is usual to find a relative dearth of cases carrying other diagnoses, and the opposite proves true here. Although the picture is most dramatic with respect to schizophrenia, the Irish tended to have some excess of other mental disorders as well, both at home and in the early days overseas. However, all these comments provide only an indirect approach to the problem, and what one seeks is a comparative measure of prevalence in the community.

No household survey comparable to some of those cited in the previous chapter has taken place in Ireland, up to the time of writing, but what might be called a modified key informant survey took place through district nurses and physicians of three counties [639], the results being fed into a comprehensive case register comparable to the registers maintained in different parts of England and Scotland. In Figure 4.2 are compared the results obtained in this fashion with those obtained by the Camberwell Psychiatric Case Register, which has been mentioned previously, and one sees that the Irish rates are many times higher than the London ones. The comparison may exaggerate the difference, since it is possible to obtain more detailed knowledge about community members from nurses in a rural area than from the various medical services in a metropolitan district such as Camberwell (for which reason the Camberwell rate cannot be directly compared with ones obtained by household survey), and also because it has been suggested to me by an Irish professor of psychiatry that his colleagues use the schizophrenia label more loosely in practice than was apparent when their diagnostic orientations [298] were being formally investigated. On the latter point a medical anthropologist has written regarding so-called schizophrenic patients in an Irish mental hospital that there "seemed nothing to compel a diagnosis of 'schizophrenia' as opposed to one of 'ontological insecurity' or 'problems of living' " [538]. But the tendency to use a diagnosis more casually in daily practice than during an investigation into diagnostic practices is not confined to the psychiatrists of any one country, and the anthropologist who doubted the diagnosis of some of the hospitalized patients has also provided us with descriptions of untreated individuals in the west of Ireland to whom the average psychiatrist would readily assign a schizophrenic label [538]. On the balance, therefore, the evidence still points to schizophrenia being unusually common in this people.

Why this should be can only be conjectured, and most of the easy guesses are equally easily proved wrong. There is no evidence of an association between the Celtic race and schizophrenia, when one looks beyond Ireland to such people as the Welsh and Bretons, and in any case geneticists indicate the Irish to be a mixture of many racial strains. The idea that the people's mental health might have suffered from an excessive drawing away of its healthier members overseas is apparently disproven by the fact that there is no correlation between the schizophrenia and emigration rates across the country. That the people have suffered for centuries from British domination might seem pertinent, but the more concrete fact is that the schizophrenia rate is now much higher in the south, which has been free of that domination for half a century, than in Northern Ireland where some would say that the domination continues. Adjustment to the modern world came relatively late for many Irish, and one might argue that they are suffering from adaptational strains, but the surprising fact is that the highest schizophrenia rates are not in the more industrialized and anglicized parts of the country, but in the western parts where the effort at maintaining the traditional culture is the strongest. These western parts are also the ones with the poorest soil, and hence direct material poverty might seem a likely factor, but there are other parts of Europe with just as poor soil in which schizophrenia does not appear to be high, and in any case the state provides considerable support.

What remain to be considered are more intangible and debatable factors deriving from culture, from the family and from community life. It has been suggested that this community life traps the less verbally capable members in a type of "double bind" [429]; or that favoritism and maternal ambivalence within the family condems unfavored siblings to constant defeat [538]; or that sexual attitudes in the more traditional communities are exceedingly unhealthy [407]. Yet another feature often alluded to, although not specially in connection with schizophrenia, is the tension between generations which formerly arose from the son having to wait until middle age to inherit the family land, and being subordinate to his father until then. These hypotheses have not been really tested yet, however, and it thus seems better here to pass on to the more concrete facts regarding another highly vulnerable people and see if there are any parallels.

The belief that the *Croatians* of Istria and the neighboring Dalmatian coast have an excess vulnerability to psychosis is said to go back to the end of the nineteenth century, although that might have arisen from the fact that the region happened to be much better supplied with mental hospitals than the rest of Croatia. In the 1920s, when much of the region was under Italian rule, the impression was that it had more schizophrenia than equivalent Italian regions [132], and in the 1930s a first statistical analysis of mental hospital patients appeared to confirm that [328], although it was not possible to allow for age structure. From 1960 to 1971, a series of studies [347] were undertaken to test and explore the matter, with a large team and large population samples, and their results are summarized in Table 4.1. Comparing the population of the "study" area, that of Istria and the neighboring littoral, with a control population residing in representative communities in the rest of Croatia, one sees that the rates for schizophrenia and for other psychoses are roughly twice as high in the former as in the latter, regardless of whether the hospital or the community survey data are used. By themselves these figures do not indicate that the study area rates are unusually high, and comparison with hospitalization rates in other countries is not trustworthy, for the reasons given in Chap. 2. However, when the household survey rates are compared with those from other community surveys, including the three Irish counties shown on the right of Fig. 4.2, it can be inferred that the Istrian rates are definitely above world average, although not as high as those in

Table 4.1. Schizophrenia rates in contrasting parts of Croatia [347, 327]

			Schizophrenia Study area	Schizophrenia Control area	Other psychoses Study area	Other psychoses Control area
Hospitalizations – One-day prevalence	1962		81	46	23	10
	1966		74	51	23	10
Hospitalizations – Discharges 1959–1960		Age 15–19	30	18	19	11
		20–39	115	68	69	29
		40+	79	32	148	58
Discharges 1965		Age 15–19	36	17	18	8
		20–39	117	77	153	27
		40+	111	54	272	78
Household surveys – Prevalence						
(a) Mixed communes		Age 20–39	644	266	196	110
		40–64	846	317	719	305
(b) Cities		Age 20–64	732	420	772	491

Rates are per 100 000 corresponding population. The „study" area comprised communes in the Istrian peninsula and neighboring littoral with approximately 500 000 population in total. The "control" communes from which hospitalization data were drawn comprise the rest of Croatia while those from which the household samples were drawn are scattered between Zagreb in the north to Split in the south.

Eire. (Allowance has to be made in such comparisons for the intensity of the case search, and household visits are presumed to be more intensive than enquiry through key informants.) Unpublished data show Istria to have higher rates than the control population for several psychosomatic diseases as well as for the psychoses, but not for other somatic disorders [302], a point which will be returned to in a later chapter.

The reasons why the Irish have a high schizophrenia rate could be essentially different from the reasons why the Istrians have one, but when one meets two examples of such a phenomenon it is normal to ask what else they have in common, and what they do not have. The two peoples have no particular genetic origins in common; they are substantially different in culture, in marriage patterns, and in diet. Among the Irish the disease most affects the communities holding most strongly to cultural traditions, while among the Croatians the people of Istria are those seen as being *least* loyal to tradition. On the other hand both the Irish and the Istrians have experienced centuries of resented domination by some neighboring power, both have experienced massive overseas emigration (plus in the Istrian case, departures of seafarers), and anthropological descriptions from each region depict much intergenerational tension which is partly linked to the question of emigration [172, 73]. Both in the west of Ireland and in southwestern Croatia the residents appear to feel envious of but also resentful toward their family members who have gone overseas, even though the remittances of these overseas members help maintain the home economy. In both locations also, there is reported to be tension and resentment directed by the rural population toward the people of the city, nominally for their abandonment of tradition but more truly for their success [47]. None of these features are true of the Croatian interior.

The fact that both groups have experienced massive emigration leads one to ask whether the high schizophrenia rates might not be due to a "sedimentation" of the less fit in the homeland while the more fit grasped the foreign opportunities. However, such a hypothesis would be contrary to Ødegaard's well-known conclusion that the schizophrenia-prone tend to migrate since they are unable to establish satisfactory roots in any community [466]; and it is also contrary to the finding of a high rate among the Irish migrants to North America. Hence that explanation does not seem acceptable. That the high schizophrenia rate in each location is related to chronic intrapsychic conflicts of whether to emigrate or not is a somewhat more plausible hypothesis. We know that although schizophrenics are often capable of carrying out arduous tasks when the instructions are sufficiently clear and straightforward, they are liable to develop symptoms when called upon to carry out apparently easier tasks which involve attention to more than one set of instructions or set of inputs at the same time [85]. Elsewhere I have argued that the same probably applies to the schizophrenia-prone person, so that the incidence of manifest schizophrenia rises when the members of a society are exposed to conflicting or unduly complex demands from their environment, i.e., to a type of "double bind" [424]. It is possible that in Ireland and Istria, a great many individuals must from childhood have been struggling with the almost impossible task of retaining the emotional advantages deriving from the mother culture and the family attachments, while striving for material advantages comparable to those obtainable overseas. Certainly it has often been described how Irishmen reproach themselves, and are reproached by others, for having taken the "wrong" decision, regardless of whether they have migrated or stayed at home, and the same seems to occur in Istria whereas it is not described in other European peoples from which there has been a massive movement overseas, people like the Dutch and Scots, the difference relating to the type of nationalism which had developed. If intrapsychic conflicts around migration can contribute directly to schizophrenia, they might also be contributing less directly, by exacerbating certain types of interpersonal conflict (e.g., between mother and son) from which other types of schizophrenia-evoking, intrapsychic stresses could arise; but such ideas must remain merely conjecture until ways are found for testing them.

2 Peoples with Low Rates: Hutterites, Tongans, and Taiwan Aborigines

Returning to more concrete facts, let us consider some characteristics of societies in which schizophrenia appears unusually infrequent. Well-researched examples of such societies are more difficult to find than examples of societies with high rates, since whereas the high rates usually cause concern and hence action, low rates do not and it is therefore only rarely that these are researched with the same vigor. Moreover, where low rates are discovered, they have often only been recorded in part of the society, and it is then possible to argue that the cases which could not be found in the studied section of the population would probably be found in another section. That last argument can be illustrated with respect to the community survey data from India which were summarized in Table 3.3. The schizophrenia prevalence rates reported for urban and semiurban populations there are lower than those usually obtained by community surveys of a similar type elsewhere in the world (the Camberwell rate given in Fig. 4.2 does not meet that qualification), but since the rates in the rural samples summarized in the same table are considerably higher, it can be argued that Indian society must encourage schizophrenics to stay in or return to the rural areas. That assumption is probably only partly true, for it is an interesting fact that in the rural surveys the schizophrenics are found mainly in the upper castes, with the rate being considerably less in the lower castes [93, 168], just the opposite of what one expects in the way of a social class gradient in a Western society. However, since there is a possibility that these urban Indian rates might have been lower than the rural ones because the urban population has more access to hospitals and since patients actually in mental hospital at time of the survey might not have been counted (something which affects the Stirling County and Midtown Manhattan survey data), it seems better to turn to other sources even though these may not provide as wide a coverage.

The best-documented example of confirmed low rates of schizophrenia relates to the *Hutterites*, a religious minority living mainly in farm communes on the North American prairies and maintaining a life style very different from that of the dominant society around them. Since the First World War or earlier, they appear to have had a reputation for good mental health among local medical personnel, but it was known that they preferred to look after their patients themselves, so that this reputation might mean little and hospitalization data would not be satisfactory. In the early 1950s, a survey of 19 Hutterite farm colonies with a total population of approximately 8 500 was undertaken by a visiting team of psychiatrists, social scientists, and assistants [161], the colonies being very cooperative in arranging for households to be screened and for persons with the possibility of a mental disorder to be examined. A total of eight cases of active schizophrenia was found in an adult (15+) population of 4 100, yielding a prevalence rate of 19 per 10 000 adults. Also, since it was reocgnized that this low rate could have arisen from the less stable members having left the communes, a special register was created of all who had been born in one of these colonies since 1874 and who had later left, and serious efforts were made to obtain news of these. However, although one of the 114 individuals who had "deserted" the movement had been in mental hospital for a few months, a second had died of epilepsy in an asylum, and a third had committed suicide, there was no evidence of any more schizophrenia. The Hutterites did prove to suffer from a special form of depression which they called *Anfechtung* (temptation by the devil) in which there were hallucinations or delusions harmonizing with their religious beliefs, but the clinical picture and recovery rate are fully in accordance with a diagnosis of depression and there is no reason to think that these cases were disguised schizophrenia. (The researchers were American, and hence were more likely to have had a tendency to overdiagnose schizophrenia than overdiagnose depression [123], as has already been noted.)

The second people in whom an apparently low rate of schizophrenia (and other psychoses) has been deliberately investigated are the Tongans of the South Pacific. (The name "Tongan" is also given to an unrelated tribe in East Africa.) The Polynesians, to whom they belong, had had a vague reputation for good mental health among anthropologists earlier in this century, as illustrated by Margaret Mead's statement that in the Manu'a Archipelago, with a population of about 2000, she came across only one case of psychosis during her 9-month stay in the 1920s, a "man of about thirty with a well-systematized delusion of grandeur" [398]. That impression was initially supported by the low mental hospitalization rates of the Maori in New Zealand, but by 1950 the Hawaiians had a schizophrenia first admission rate which was higher than that for the Caucasians in Hawaii [543], and since then the Maori hospitalization rate has also come up to that of the New Zealand Whites. Therefore, there was no reason to think that the Polynesian race had any particular resistance to the disease, but this did not exclude the possiblity of the incidence remaining low in those Polynesian societies which had retained something of the sociocultural characteristics which Margaret Mead had found.

The Tongan inquiry was more superficial than the others which have been considered in this chapter, but the most complete investigation of a low rate after the Hutterite one. It comprised three parts: an analysis of admissions of the central mental asylum over a 12-year period; an attempt to assess the incidence of mental disorder in Tongans who had migrated to the northern part of New Zealand; and a field survey of a single island with about 4500 population [445]. The asylum first admissions averaged less than 2 cases per 10 000 aged 15+ for all disorders including epilepsy, and schizophrenia comprised about 60% of those cases to which a diagnosis had been given, a third of the cases not having received any diagnosis. In the Auckland region of New Zealand, it was calculated that the Tongans would have had a first admission rate only half that of the local Whites and Maori if their population were truly what had been recorded at the census, but since it was widely believed that the census figure was an understatement, due to considerable numbers arriving as visitors and overstaying their permission, it is probable that the actual ratio was lower than that. The prevalence survey was done twice, first by an investigator who spoke no Tongan and worked only with key informants and secondly, 18 months later, by one who spoke Tongan, was known on the island, and not only interviewed key informants but examined the patients whom the latter indicated. Through this double prevalence inquiry one obvious schizophrenic and two schizoaffective cases were discovered, yielding a 12-month active prevalence rate of 14 per 10 000 adults. There was no evidence to suggest that additional cases might have been concealed or might have been able to escape public notice (assuming that social functioning was disturbed), and no reason to think that any of the other cases of psychosis, four in number, might have been schizophrenic.

The third instance of a low schizophrenia rate being found on field survey relates to the Taiwan aboriginal tribes. After Lin's well-known mental health survey of the Taiwan Chinese [512], the same approach was used among four aboriginal tribes there, employing community informants and household visiting. If one ignores the cases who were reported to have had a schizophreniform condition in the past but to be healthy at time of investigation, only four cases of schizophrenia were found in a total population of almost 11 500, yielding an active prevalence rate of 6 per 10 000 aged 14+, something still lower that in the Hutterite and Tongan samples. Whether this figure can be taken on a par with the other two is to be doubted, since (a) there were other currently inactive cases assessed to be shizophrenic who might have been active within the 12-month period; (b) there was a high frequency of alcoholic disturbances which are known to sometimes mask schizophrenia (for instance, among the Irish [30]); and (c) it is unlikely that the Chinese investigators, representing a conquering power, would have had as full a cooperation among these tribes as they received among the Taiwan Chinese. Nevertheless, if one is seeking for the lowest recorded active prevalence rate of schizophrenia, this is it. There are other instances of low rates either of hospitalizations [618] or as assessed through brief key informant surveys [436], mostly from the Pacific; but the evidence is too slight to put much weight on and will not be used any further here.

These three examples are from different races, and although genetic inbreeding might be a factor in the Hutterite case, the evidence is strongly against this in the other two. Since they also live under very different conditions, with different diets, types of intercurrent infection, etc., a shared environmental factor seems also unlikely. Regarding shared sociocultural features, the information on the Taiwan aborigins is too slight to build on and we know that although they may have little schizophrenia they are not so mentally healthy in other respects. With the other two peoples, however, one can discern a number of features which they appear to have in common and which could be interesting to contrast with the features shared by the two high-rate peoples. In the first place, they are both communalistic as opposed to individualistic, with many activities and decisions being undertaken jointly and with individual initiative being quite limited. Secondly, they are both quite hierarchically structured, with the commune patriarch or senior preacher in the one people and the aristocracy and royal family in the other being highly respected. A third common feature is a strong respect for tradition and a strong, fundamentalist type of religious belief, combined with a relatively low valuing of material possessions. A fourth feature is that they have both largely turned their back on the more technologically developed societies around them, believing their own ways of life better, and a fifth is that at the time of the psychiatric assessments they still had command of sufficient fertile land to satisfy their members' modest needs and allow for population growth without much need for competition between individuals or families.

If one compares these features with the features held in common by the two high-rate peoples, then there are immediate contrasts. The Irish and southern Croatians were short of fertile land and there was quite strong competition between individuals and families because of this. They could not, for this reason, safely turn their back on the more technologically advanced peoples around them, but had to try to earn a living from these. In both the Irish and the Croatians, tradition preached strong respect for the patriarch, but economic stresses had markedly corroded this respect so that intergenerational bitterness or strife was often sharp. In contrast to the communalism of the two low-rate peoples, the Irish put a great emphasis on privacy and secrecy, while the southern Croatians are well know in their own country for having almost completely abandoned the southern slavic *zadruga* or semicommune based on the extended family, an institution highly important in the rest of Yugoslavia.

Expressed in this fashion, the key difference between the two pairs may seem to be the economic one, with shortage of land leading to rivalry and individualism and then perhaps to the emotional breakdown of those who are schizophrenia-prone, while abundance of land makes these steps unnecessary. However, there are many peoples with an abundance of available land who have relatively high schizophrenia rates – the Cancadian Ukrainian farmers neighboring the Hutterites, for instance – while entering competitive urban life can be associated with a relatively low rate as the surveys in India (Table 3.3) indicate. An abundance of land is almost certainly an advantage as respects the risk of schizophrenia when the people are of a single mind regarding its exploitation, but there are many other matters besides the economic about which men can distress themselves. As a reminder of this fact, let us consider a couple of instances in which – although the evidence is not as good as one would like – there appears to have been a sharp rise in the incidence and prevalence of schizophrenia within a single generation.

3 Shifts from Low to High Rates: Achinese and Tallensi

In the introductory chapter of this book it was noted that Comparative Psychiatry can be concerned not just with different peoples or countries but with the same country at two or more points in time, insofar as there will often have been sociocultural changes between these periods. Over the past couple of centuries, many authorities have asked themselves whether the incidence of mental disorder – principally "lunacy" or psychosis in which one assumes schizophrenia to be playing a large part – is increasing. In the most thorough study of the question, Goldhamer and Marshall [226] concluded that between 1840 and 1930 in Massachusetts it had not been increasing in the under-50 age group but had been increasing in the over-50s. However, there were numerous factors which they were not able to fully take into consideration, notably the existence at different periods of private institutions not contributing data to the official statistics, the changing standards of what were thought to be suitable cases for admission to a mental asylum, and the effect of the foreign-born sections of the population at each period; so that the matter must remain in doubt. In other countries one could probably make similar comparisons with similarly ambiguous results. What is needed are field surveys of the same population at two or more periods, using relatively similar or easily interpreted criteria; and these can only be found for quite small populations. The instances in which this type of information is available and where there is, in my opinion, the strongest evidence of a change in prevalence of chronic psychosis (probably but not indisputably schizophrenia) derive from Southeast Asia and West Africa.

The *Achinese* (the name is spelled in many ways) are a deutero-Malay people who numbered about three-quarters of a million in 1920 and were settled on relatively abundant, fertile land in the northwest of Sumatra. Of war-like disposition they had functioned, in the nineteenth century, more as rulers and conquerors than as peasants, and this disposition led them to challenge the Dutch colonial power at a

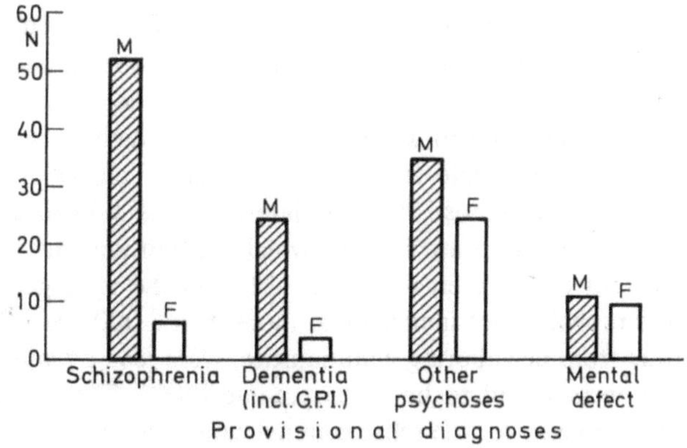

Fig. 4.3. Sex difference in the prevalence of schizophrenia among the Achinese of Sumatra at the end of their war with the colonial power 1920, as compared with sex differences in other mental disorders [629]

time when most other peoples in the Archipelago were exhibiting relatively little resistance. From this ensued a war which lasted, on and off, for 50 years, uniting the various Achinese tribes in the process but resulting in their eventual defeat. After the war, the new governor of the territory was struck by the number of insane he was encountering during this tours of the region, so that he ordered an official census of lunatics to be undertaken and followed that up by arranging for an experienced psychiatrist to investigate the situation. The census, which was known to be likely to bring news only of the most severe and communally troublesome cases (where it was not boycotted by the recently conquered people) yielded a rate of 15 cases per 10 000 *total* population [629], something which can be compared with the rates of 3.5 and 3.4 obtained by similar census methods in India in 1931 [404] and the Yunming district of China in 1942 [604]. The psychiatrist, van Loon, visited 29 villages and examined some 150 cases of psychosis, plus mental defectives and epileptics [629]. In Fig. 4.3, which analyzes his findings, one sees that there is a very marked sex difference in the cases labeled dementia praecox (i.e., schizophrenia) or unspecified dementia, but by no means as great a difference in the other psychoses (mostly of the acute reactive type) or in the mental defectives. The diagnoses of dementia praecox and unspecified dementia were only assigned if the psychosis had existed for many months and appeared chronic. Contrasting with this picture exists one given us by a physician-anthropologist who had studied the Achinese 30 years earlier and written a two-volume ethnography of them [276]. Interested in family life, psychology, and health, he informs us that mental disorder was neither common nor serious, but that it was commoner in women than in men, and he implies that many of the mentally ill were apparently being socially integrated through being given a semireligious role. Therefore, it seem highly probable that in this 30 year interval there was a significant increase in chronic psychoses in males but not in females, and that the psychosis was predominantly schizophrenia, van Loon having taken fully into account the possibility of such organic conditions as syphilitic and postencephalitic psychosis.

The second example, the *Tallensi*, are long-settled grain farmers living in the savannah zone of northern Ghana and having had a population of about 35 000 when their main ethnographer, Meyer Fortes, first visited them in the 1930s [199]. In his 2 1/2 years among them, he noted the presence of only one frank case of psychosis plus two more marginal cases, one of whom was allegedly abnormal from birth, in the population of about 5 000 within which he was making regular visits. That is roughly comparable to the Hutterite and Tongan pictures. Returning to the same communities almost 30 years later, he was able to count 13 cases within a short period, several from families which he had known well and in which such insanity had not earlier been remarked, although the total population of these communities had probably not increased to more than 6 000 over the period. These 13 cases, plus four from neighboring communities, were seen by a psychiatrist and over three-quarters were found to be schizophrenic [200]. The mean duration of illness was 4.2 (± 2.1) years for the schizophrenic cases; the sex ratio was almost balanced; the clinical pictures seem fairly typical apart from an unusually abrupt onset; but what stands out is that all but two of the cases had developed their disorder during or shortly after a visit to the south of Ghana for work, although it is estimated that only about 50 % of Tallensi in general were making that trip south, into a society speaking a language other than their own.

Using the same approach as before and asking what the Achinese and Tallensi might have in common apart from this apparent increase in schizophrenia, a first point is that they have both made a rather stressful contact with a foreign culture, and a second is that while the psychosis has apparently increased greatly in one section of the population it has not done so in another. The stressful contact with a foreign culture is unlikely to be schizophrenogenic in itself, otherwise we would have very many recorded instances of an increase in the disorder (just as we have respecting alcohol abuse under such circumstances – see Chapter 8) instead of two or three. The clustering of the patients in one half of the population might be the result of self-selection in the case of the Tallensi, but it could not have been with the Achinese. Regarding the latter, we know in general that if poorly educated persons develop a psychosis when moving to another culture in search of work, lack of preparation for the experience is of greater importance than self-selection [432], and the psychosis is an acute transitory state rather than the chronic condition which the Tallensi cases exhibited. If it is assumed that the increase in schizophrenia did actually occur in only half of each society, therefore, we must ask what it is that these halves had experienced apart from simply contact with a more dominant or affluent power, and which the other halves of the same societies had not.

The evidence on which to base any answer here is rather slight, but one possibility is that they have been confronted with the need for a change of role or life style which does not apply to or is not yet recognized by the other half of their society, and for which they also lack a satisfying model. We know that in persons such as emigrants exploring the advantages of social change, there is little evidence of real stress as long as they see themselves able to return to their previous style of life or can tell themselves that their present state is a temporary one to which no personal commitment is needed; whereas they do feel stress when a return to the former life is seen as impossible or when a permanent choice between roughly equal but competing life styles seems demanded. (European refugees after World War II exhibited little excess of mental disorder while in temporary camps, but developed a clear excess of fairly chronic schizophrenia when called upon to make a choice between equally unattractive alternatives in a country of resettlement [418]). Among the Achinese the males had for a whole generation concentrated on the role of warrior, leaving other affairs to the women, and although cultivation and trading were both quite feasible and rewarding roles for them in time of peace they had come to see these roles as undignified for true men, belonging only to women or to conquered peoples. In consequence, at the time of van Loon's investigation the women had many rewarding roles open to them while the adult men had virtually none which conformed both to traditional teachings and current realities. (Since that time, as far as I can gather, they have accepted to be traders and have become very successful ones.) Among the Tallensi the section of the society which was content to go on living as their ancestors lived had still all or most of the traditional roles open to them, since there was still ample demand for their produce, whereas, among those who went south and tasted the benefits which other life styles offered, it seems likely that there were many (of both sexes) who were no longer content simply to return to the traditional life style once they found they were not succeeding outside their own society. My conjecture is that it is this group who became most vulnerable to the schizophrenia. However, many other mechanisms could have been at work and a more systematic search for and investigation of such instances is going to be needed before we can write confidently on this matter.

4 Variations in Course and Outcome

For Kraepelin, the course of illness was an important diagnostic indicator when dementia praecox or schizophrenia was being considered, and European textbooks still imply that the disease is usually quite chronic. However, impressionistic writing from India and Africa has for long suggested that the typical case of schizophrenia there might show quite rapid recovery, more rapid than in Europe. The simplest explanation for these impressions was that clinicians were confusing acute reactive psychosis with schizophrenia, but it became apparent that if all the short-lasting cases were put into the former category, the incidence of schizophrenia in some parts of these regions would have to be very low. For instance, by following a strictly Kraepelinian line, Tewfik [612] found himself able to assign the diagnosis to only one of the 304 patients admitted to Mulago mental hospital in Uganda. Whether schizophrenia need be as chronic as Western psychiatrists are accustomed to, therefore, has become an important question.

The most thorough attempt to explore and answer this question crossculturally has been the International Pilot Study of Schizophrenia [674, 677], organized by the WHO and covering 1202 patients in nine countries. By ensuring that uniform assessment instruments were used, by including not just patients who had previously been diagnosed as schizophrenic but anyone judged to have a functional psychosis (within the limits imposed by certain exclusion criteria) and by arranging for a follow-up of these patients after 2 and 5 years, this important piece of research promised to tell us whether uniformly diagnosed schizophrenics really do suffer from a less chronic illness in Africa and India than in Europe and North America.

Table 4.2. Course of schizophrenic illness over 2 years in nine countries

Country and Center	N	1. Psychotic over 75% of the time	2. Showing severe social impairment	3. Relapsing to new episodes	4. One episode, full remission
		(%)	(%)	(%)	(%)
Nigeria (Ibadan)	63	7	5	25	58
India (agra)	89	19	18	22	51
U.S.S.R. (Moscow)	68	19	21	42	7
Colombia (Cali)	78	28	22	39	19
Taiwan (Taipei)	80	31	20	26	27
Czechoslovakia (Prague)	54	36	33	28	17
Gt. Britain (London)	58	36	38	37	23
United States (Washington)	47	47	32	16	21
Denmark (Aarhus)	48	48	33	21	6

Figures are drawn from different tables in the WHO 2-year follow-up report [677]. Not all ratings were made on all patients. Percentages refer only to patients being rated in the indicated fashion, not to total numbers.

Table 4.2 summarizes some of the key findings from this study obtained at the 2-year follow-up, the 5-year follow-up results not having been published at the time of writing but being known to have a very similar character. In the table the countries are ranked in order of increasing chronicity of the patient samples, and one can see immediately that the most technologically develloped countries yield the poorest results while the two least technologically developed yield the best. These data relate to all patients receiving a diagnosis of schizophrenia from the local teams and hence might possibly conceal international variations in diagnosis, but when only those patients adhering most closely to a "concordant" or core pattern, as assessed by computer, are chosen, essentially the same result appears. Apparently, then, the average prognosis of schizophrenia varies from country to country, with the "developed" ones having the poorest picture and the "developing" ones achieving the best, despite their poorer treatment facilities.

If this finding could be accepted at its face value and then generalized, its importance for psychiatry would be very great. Unfortunately, however, an unforeseen bias crept in at time of case selection, since the centers in the most "developed" countries happened to include patients who had (as far as can be inferred from the data) a longer average history of psychosis than those in the "developing" countries' centers did. In consequence, one can get a correlation of 0.76 ($t = 3.1$) between the national scores on an estimate of duration prior to intake and those on a measure of subsequent course [439], so that it is theoretically possible for what appears to be the result of some national influence to be only the result of the sampling method. Furthermore, since a full history of prior disorder had not been recorded at time of intake, it is possible that new calculations from the same data will still not enable us to assess whether national differences exist or not, after prior duration has been adequately allowed for, and we may need to await the results of the WHO's further study of the functional psychoses before arriving at any definite conclusion.

In the meantime, however, other more limited studies suggest strongly that, whether or not it is the level of technological development that is the key variable, there is a tendency for the lesser developed countries to have better outcomes with schizophrenia than the more developed. While we know from the Tallensi and Achinese examples cited earlier that some "traditional"societies can have quite chronic and abundant schizophrenia, it has been found in Sri Lanka that even patients with a relatively long psychotic history prior to treatment do quite well afterwards [645], and when a comparison was made of first admissions in England and in Mauritius, it was found that although the incidence rates in the two countries were very similar, the follow-up picture and course of illness was definitely better in the latter, less developed, society [444]. Moreover, in that society it was found for one of the three main subcultures that the patients showing a chronic course had actually a more acute, recent onset than the ones that recovered [506]. Hence this is definitely a subject which calls for further investigation and where international comparisons seem essential.

In the forgegoing paragraphs, the references to chronicity were such as to imply a single distinction between a continuous process and an episode but one of the additional findings from the WHO study [677] is that this is probably not true. After setting aside the patients who show a fairly continuous schizophrenic process, i.e., those referred to in columns 1 and 2 of Table 4.2, we find that countries vary considerably regarding the average course of illness for the remainder of the patients. In some instances, most notably Nigeria and India, these remaining patients have for the most part shown complete social recovery after the intake episode, with no detectable history of relapse. In other countries, most notably the U.S.S.R. and Columbia, the majority experience brief relapses. There is no apparent relationship this time to either level of technological development or duration of prior illness, but prior to the analysis of these results I had drawn attention [426] to similar differences uncovered when comparing (a) Mauritius and the United States Virgin Islands and (b) French-Canadian rural communities with different degrees of cultural uniformity. The data from the latter are summarized in Fig. 4.4.

The opinion of the WHO research team is that we may be dealing with three "schizophrenias" rather than with a single clinical entity exhibiting different courses [677], but as we will see in the next chapter an alternative solution might be to make more effort to split off schizophrenia from the more transient psychoses. My own impression is that what may differentiate societies where most schizophrenics have repeated episodes from societies in which the patients remain either chronically ill or consistently recovered is social organization and cohesion. The locations in which I have found schizophrenia to exhibit an episodic character, e.g., the "New" French Canadian communities in Fig. 4.4, are ones in which the traditional support system has broken down or where that support system is the focus of some culture conflict (as between old and new ideas). Whether such a theory could apply to the locations from which the WHO study drew its patients is a question which would require information of a much more sociological character than the reports provide; and other hypotheses are possible. However, even if the concept of three distinct schizoprenias is validated, it still remains to be explained why the international

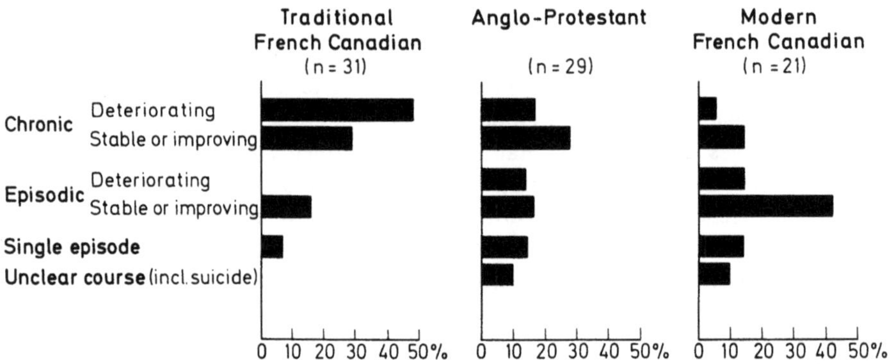

Fig. 4.4. Course of illness in the schizophrenics from two categories of French-Canadian community and from neighboring Anglo-Protestant ones. Data derive from the same study as referred to in Fig. 3.1. Relative frequency of the various types is not necessarily representative of the three subcultures, due to the small number of cases, and is shown here only as an example of a type of difference meriting further study.

distribution of one is so different from that of another, and hypotheses of the type just indicated would still be called for.

5 Types and Symptomatology

The proposal to differentiate subtypes of schizophrenia on the basis of course and outcome, although having a long history, has never been as popular as that which takes presenting symptoms as its basis and which is enshrined in the International Classification and Diseases. In the International Pilot Study of Schizophrenia, [674], the diagnosing psychiatrists were asked to assign each patient to such a subtype, and in due course the distribution of these subtypes was analyzed by country and by component symptoms. The distributions in the nine national samples proved no less varied than the course-of-illness data shown in Table 4.2, and when the countries are ranked in order of the percentage of the *paranoid* subtype in their sample, one gets almost exactly the same order, in reverse, as is shown in this table, suggesting quite strongly that chronicity is greater in this subtype than in the others and that it may be the national distribution of subtypes which has determined the national differences in mean course. Unfortunately, what seems more probable is that there are national differences in the tendency to employ these subtype labels, differences which are not soundly based on the symptomatology at all, since computer analysis of the symptom clusters detected few significant differences between the patients receiving one subtype label and those receiving another. Moreover, when the average course of illness for each subtype was calculated (something which we are not shown in detail) it is simple schizophrenia which proves to have the most chronic course, not the paranoid type. It is possible, of course, that the diagnosing clinicians were responding to more subtle clues than those which were recorded in the Present State

Table 4.3. Impressionistic associations between schizophrenic symptoms and cultural groupings [446]

Features of schizophrenia	Sociocultural correlates	Significance (*P*)
Paranoid type	MOST frequent in urban middle classes	0.05
	LEAST frequent in rural populations	0.05
Catatonic type	LEAST frequent in Euro-Americans	0.05
Hebephrenic type	MOST frequent in Japanese and Okinawans	0.05
Simple type	MOST frequent in Asians	0.01
Visual hallucinations	MOST frequent in Africa and Near East	0.05
	LEAST frequent in urban Euro-Americans	0.01
Tactile hallucinations	MOST frequent in Africa and Near East	0.10
Delusions of grandeur	MOST frequent in rural populations	0.001
Delusions of destruction	MOST frequent in Christian populations	0.01
Religious delusions	MOST frequent in Christian populations	0.01
	LEAST frequent in Buddhists, Hindus and Shintoists	0.01
Delusions of jealousy	MOST frequent in Asian populations	0.05
Depersonalization	LEAST frequent in rural populations	0.01
Flatness of affect	MOST frequent in Japanese and Okinawans	0.01
	HIGH in South American peoples	0.05
Social withdrawal	MOST frequent in Japanese and Okinawans	0.01
Negativism	MOST frequent in India and South America	0.001
Excitement	MOST frequent in Africa and South America	0.05
	LEAST frequent in Anglo-Saxon cultures	0.05
Stereotypic behavior	MOST frequent in East Indians	0.05
	LEAST frequent in Euro-Americans	0.001
Catatonic rigidity	MOST frequent in East Indians	0.01
Suicidal behavior	MOST frequent in Japanese	0.001
Temper outbursts	MOST frequent in Christian populations	0.05

Examination on which the computer analysis was based, but a re-examination of the earlier Mauritius data [506] indicates that those patients exhibiting a paranoid schizophrenia picture at first admission had no poorer a course of illness than those who did not. It is still unclear, therefore, whether prognosis will be linked to subtype around the world, once each subtype is established on the basis of internationally accepted criteria.

That there is a difference between one nation or culture and another with respect to the predominant symptomatology of schizophrenia is much more probable, since clinicians are regularly struck by this fact when they change location, and we have good descriptions of changes in symptomatology within the same society over time, even within the lifetime of a single clinician [233]. Table 4.3 summarizes the impressions of 40 psychiatrists in 27 countries in 1960, nearly all these psychiatrists having worked in more than one culture and having been asked to state how the patients in one culture compare with those in the other. The data are very "soft," but a number of the features thought to distinguish between the schizophrenics of the more and those of the less technologically developed societies surveyed are similar to ones which have been noted as distinguishing the schizophrenics in "developed" countries since 1950 from those in the same countries earlier. Thus, the differences noted respecting the paranoid and catatonic subtypes in the table parallel the fact that the paranoid subtype has increased while the catatonic has decreased throughout the Western world, even within as short a period as the 1930s to 1950s [5]. The tendency of delusions of grandeur to be found significantly less often in urban than in rural populations in 1960 parallels the fact that such delusions were reported in 17% of Heidelberg schizophrenics in 1916 as compared with only 1% in 1946 [320]. The suggestion that delusions of jealousy were less common in Euro-American populations than in Asian ones in 1960 finds an echo in the fact that they were less common at Burghölzli in 1973 than in 1912 [587].

These and other reports of crosscultural differences and historical shifts which one can derive from a comparison of records from different locations or times, or from clinicians' impressions, are undoubtedly worthwhile keeping in mind, but the possibilities of a concealed bias here are much greater than with the formal comparisons of the WHO study, and much of what is reported is rather trivial. For instance, there is an abundant literature describing the decline in religious content and increase in scientific content of delusions as people become more urbanized or westernized, but this is merely a reflection of a change in popular thought, telling us nothing about the psychopathology. Much more valuable have been the comparisons of smaller samples of schizophrenics from different subcultures within the same society, using more intensive assessments.

The pioneer work of this type was that by Opler and Singer [471] comparing young male schizophrenics of Irish-American and Italian-American origin, and it was followed by similar studies of other minorities. The advantages of this research model are that samples of patients roughly equivalent in terms of age, sex, duration of illness, location of residence, and prior treatment, can be investigated in detail, with open-ended interviews allowing the researcher to pursue clues which might be passed over with a single question if fixed-content interviews were used. Also, since the samples are small, information can be sought from relatives, the social backgrounds can be investigated in person, the symptoms can be compared with normal behavioral traits in the same subcultures [487], and the social history of the specific groups from which the patients are drawn can be obtained. (Not all these steps were undertaken in all instances.) The disadvantages of the model are that the researcher is usually left too free to impose his own interpretations on ambiguous material, that undeclared biases may have applied during the case selection, such as choosing patients who communicate easily in preference to those who are monosyllabic, and that intrasample variation may be too great to permit sound deductions regarding sample differences. It is the Irish and Italians that have been most compared here, but since the former are receiving considerable attention elsewhere in this volume, it may be more interesting now to cite some results concerning another pair of subcultures, the German-American and Polish-American. The patients were in two hospitals in upstate New York in the early 1960s, all males aged 18-44, the data coming from case records, interviews and in two-thirds of the cases from some psychological tests [494].

Table 4.4 presents the main clinical differences, probably somewhat exaggerated by the familiar research tendency to force information into simple dichotomies and

Table 4.4. Characteristics of German-American and Polish-American schizophrenics

		German-American	Polish-American	Chi^2	P
1. Subtype tendency	Paranoid	22	12	6.79	0.01
	Catatonic	8	18		
2. Somatic and hypochondriacal symptoms	Marked	10	23	11.38	0.001
	Few or absent	20	7		
3. Attitude toward authority	Passive/dependent	7	24	19.28	0.001
	Hostile/aggressive	23	6		
4. Flatness of affect	Present	17	7	6.94	0.01
	Absent or minor	13	23		
5. Tendency toward alcohol abuse	Present	5	13	5.08	0.05
	Absent	25	17		
6. Defenses	Passive/dependent	10	22	9.64	0.05
	Sadomasochistic	20	8		

Complied from various tables in Piedmont [494], with some modification of labels. Figures refer to absolute numbers, not percentages, there having been 30 patients in each sample.

pretend that a middle group does not exist. Some of the recorded differences probably derive from the German-American population having been better educated than the Polish-American one, but at a more basic level it is to be noted that the Polish immigrant group derived from a peasant society in which extended family controls were very strong, the father often feared and hated, and in which (in the United States) the mother's protection had often to be sought. The display of emotion in this society was allowed a free rein, sibling rivalry was common, and manipulative dependency on the mother important. The corresponding immigrant group from Germany is depicted as coming from a more urban background, and even when of peasant stock it was less family focused. Emotional expression was allowed less rein, independence and rationality were encouraged, and although the father was no less dominant a person in the child's life it is argued that there was more rapid internalization and more repression of oedipal feelings. Accordingly, Piedmont argues that many of the clinical differences derive from the family structure, so that the greater dependency of the Polish-American patients on the hospital personnel and on alcohol is seen as deriving from the necessarily greater dependency on the mother within their homes, while the German-American patients' greater aggressiveness and tendency toward the development of paranoid delusions is inferred to derive from greater identification with the powerful father and the greater encouragement to orientate oneself toward the wider world. The differences in the emotional content of the patients' symptoms and their use of somatization can similarly be related to family background with this type of theory.

Both the observations and the interpretations in such a study call for verification through replication, since the risk of the researcher finding the evidence that fits his theory and ignoring the evidence which does not is quite great when so open-ended an approach is used. Nevertheless, work of this type deserves to be kept in mind and related to information from other sources, for instance the suggestions in Figs. 3.1 and 4.1 that Polish Canadians have a higher incidence rate for schizophrenia

Table 4.5. Percentage frequency of symptoms of social withdrawal in young male French-Canadian and British-Canadian Schizophrenics

	Quebec		Ontario		
	Br.-Can. %	Fr.-Can. %	Br.-Can. %	Fr.-Can. %	Significance *P*
Reported of schizophrenics only					
Complains abundantly of family, friends, and associates	0	65	0	70	0.001
Feels people avoid, reject, or dislike him	12	50	10	70	0.01
Says people know of his guilt, faults, or problems	12	60	10	60	0.01
	Schizophrenia		Depression		
	Br.-Can. %	Fr.-Can. %	Br.-Can. %	Fr.-Can. %	Significance
Reported of both schizophrenics and depressives					
Feels that he has no friends	27	40	20	60	0.02

Interviews undertaken using the Mental Status Schedule [580]. Patients matched for chronicity.

than German Canadians, but perhaps not a significantly higher active prevalence rate. In the village study from which Fig. 3.1 is derived, I found that the father-son relationship did seem to be an important precipitator of schizophrenia in the Polish Canadians but that if the patient could get married and thereby escape parental dominance, the disorder terminated more completely than in other groups of patients.

With such small group comparisons, as with larger-scale studies, one can obtain greater objectivity at the possible expense of sensitivity by employing a standardized interview, and Table 4.5 shows some quite marked differences obtained in this fashion, the comparisons having been done first in Montreal and then in another part of Canada to ensure that the differences were not the accidental result of conditions at the two initial hospitals [428]. When such a standard interview schedule is used with people speaking different languages, and even sometimes if they use the same language in somewhat different fashion [580, 485], it is important to ensure that the connotations attached to a particular question or answer in the two groups are similar. For instance, this study yielded a marked cultural difference in the frequence of affirmative responses to the question whether the patient had been thinking about his own death, but whereas this was a probable indicator of psychopathology in the British Canadians, in the French Canadians it was mainly an indicator of religious orthodoxy at that time, their priests regularly urging their parishioners to do this. However, the items in Table 4.5 cannot be accounted for in such a fashion, and although they undoubtedly derive from the fact that the British Canadians are more individualistic and socially detached than the French Canadians, they would appear to tell us something about schizophrenia as well. It is often considered that social withdrawal, as an aspect of autism, carries a relatively poor prognosis. Here we see, however, that the French-Canadian patients maintained a considerable (if distorted) interest in their social environment, and yet such other evidence as we possess suggests that they are less likely to attain full social recovery than the British-Canadian schizophrenics who show greater withdrawal [428].

6 Treatment Response

When course of illness and outcome were referred to earlier in this chapter, no mention was made of the possible effect of treatment. The reason for this was twofold. In the first place it is exceedingly difficult to allow for the effect of treatment in comparative studies of the type being discussed, if the therapists are permitted to use what they think is best for each patient and if, in addition, one attempts to take into consideration not just the pharmacotherapy, as is routine, but the general therapeutic climate of each center and such social therapies as are employed. Secondly, the key findings to date indicate the best outcomes to derive not from the centers with the best treatment facilities, but from those with the most limited, so that allowing for the amount of treatment being given is not going to explain any of the findings, unless one believes that the treatment is countereffective. However, most thinking in this matter makes the elementary assumption that our key treatments are equally good regardless of country and culture, and this is not necessarily true. Research indicates that much higher doses of a given drug may be needed in one country than in another to produce not just the same therapeutic effects but the same side effects. Secondly, there is some indication that the relative susceptibility of particular symptoms to a given drug may vary from one society or culture to another, this perhaps being linked to variations in the frequency of the so-called paradoxical effects. Finally, there are almost certainly differences in response to what are called the "non-specific" aspects of treatment, the psychotherapy and sociotherapy.

The main studies indicating the required dosage of a drug used in schizophrenia to be higher in one country than in another concern comparisons between Europe and North America. Thus, New York patients required five times the dosage of butyrylperazine needed to produce a given therapeutic effect than did Erlangen (Germany) patients, and yet developed 30% fewer extrapyramidal reactions and no dystonic ones [144]. Other New York patients needed almost twice the dose needed by Liège (Belgium) patients for a given therapeutic effect, and yet had only about half the side effects [143]. Between Turkey and Germany, Turkey and the United Stated and Hungary and Canada similar differences have been found, the first-named countries' patients always needing the lower doses, and electroencephalographic (EEG) studies have shown that the differences relate not just to symptoms but to detectable influences on the brain's electrical activity [274]. It has been suspected that the patient samples were not as well matched as they should have been (in the United States/Turkey comparison true matching proved impossible) and that in the earlier studies the patients were not equally cooperative in taking their drugs, but the EEG studies with volunteers seem to dispose of these explanations. Genetic explanations have been explored [164] without much concrete support, and the favorite theory at the time of writing concerns prior exposure to other drugs, food additives, etc., which stimulate the liver's detoxifying processes, such exposure being assumed to be greater within a North American population than in a European one. Here also, however, the evidence is contradictory, since almost no significant differences were found between the responses of Javanese and German schizophrenics given injectable phenothiazines, once allowance had been made for chronicity [491], although one would have expected the former group to have had much less exposure to related chemicals than the latter. This is therefore a subject on which more research is required, research which might eventually help explain some of the differences in chronicity, although part of the Mauritius/England comparison [444] relates to patients not receiving phenothiazines.

The main evidence that symptoms do not follow the same order of response to a given drug in different peoples comes from the analysis of data from a single hospital in Djakarta [425]. There delusions and excitement disappeared significantly more rapidly in Chinese patients than in patients from an Indonesian subculture, the Minangkabau, but hostility and disorientation showed the opposite relationship under the same treatment. Differences in the nature as well as the degree of side effects, however, have been reported in other peoples, for instance between Indonesians and Germans [491]. One possible explanation is that cultures differ with respect to how much they train their members to be on guard against certain mental states. Certainly we know that they can differ with respect to how far they teach submission to the orders of a doctor or other "superior" as opposed to teaching independence, something which is relevant to the effectiveness of psychotherapy. However, they may also vary in the degree to which they encourage acceptance of specific mental experiences. Thus, the Alaska Athabaskans are reported to exhibit an undue frequency of "paradoxical" reactions during pharmacotherapy, and it has been suggested that this is due to their culture (and their life-threatening environment) teaching them to be on guard against any relaxation in alertness [260], something which the phenothiazines and anxiolytics often produce.

The third type of variance in responses to treatment, that to its "nonspecific" aspects, is very difficult to undertake crossculturally, not least because there is still so little agreement on how to assess the effects of psychotherapy. However, there are a couple of reports worth citing, both comparing United States Blacks and Whites. In the first of these, 16 carefully matched pairs of schizophrenics (plus some other pairs whom we will disregard) were given individual psychotherapy in hospital, with or without drugs, and the Black patients achieved significantly better outcome ratings than the White ones [665]. In the second, much larger, study placebos were being employed for comparison with three phenothiazines in three hospitals over a 6-week period, with standardized improvement assessments [224]. As Fig. 4.5 indicates, there were insignificant differences between the Black and White schizophrenics when the phenothiazines were used, but marked differences when the placebo was given, the Black group showing the better results in five out of the six measures on which significant differences were found. (The scales, being measures of pathology, are in the reverse order to what one expects, since the figure is designed to indicate improvements.) As one can see, the differences apply mainly between males, and the greater improvement in the Blacks is mainly in the direction of becoming more peaceful. Since this was a study of drug effects, not directly concerned either with the results of sociotherapy or with cross-cultural differences, it is extremely unlikely

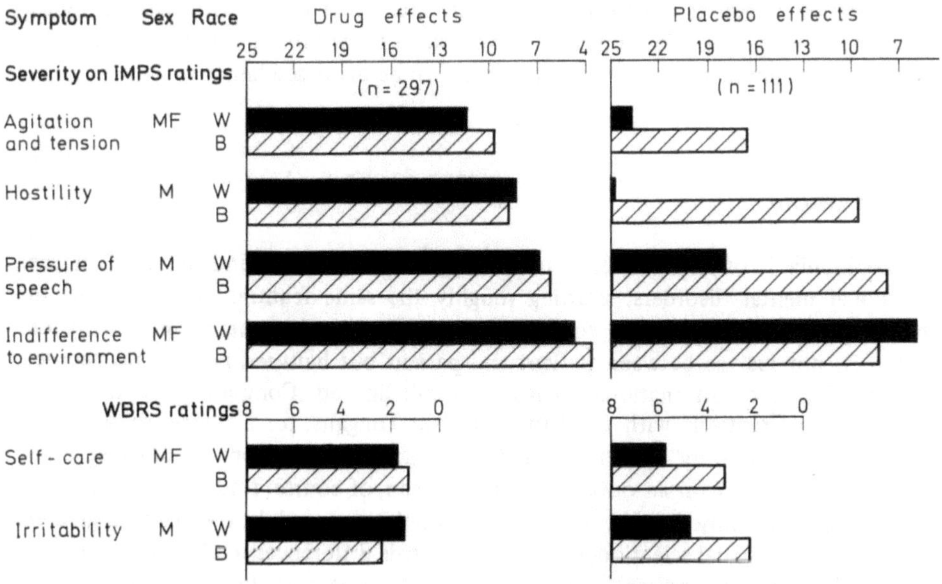

Fig. 4.5. Relative improvement of White and Black schizophrenics in United States hospitals, treated with and without phenothiazines [665]. Bars represent the decline in frequency and intensity of a given symptom over the treatment period. W, White; B, Black patient samples; following conventional United States criteria for this distinction. IMPS, Inpatient Multidimensional Psychiatric Scale; WBRS, Wittenborn Psychiatric Rating Scale. All symptom categories featured yielded significantly different results in the two racial groups when placebo was used

that the researchers' expectations would have produced such a result, but on the other hand there was no particular effort made to assess whether the two groups really were receiving the same nonspecific therapy, and the random assignment of patients to the drugs and placebo groups might have concealed initial differences between Blacks and Whites. Insofar as Blacks tend to respond more fully to nonspecific therapy of other mental disorders than United States Whites, however, we can probably take the results as meaningful, and go on to ask what meaning it is that they are conveying.

In this instance, the differences may be less a reflection of such subcultural factors as childrearing patterns and value orientations than of the relationship between the White majority and Black minority at that place and time. Blacks coming into a White-dominated United States institution have tended to be on guard against the indignities to which they were liable to be exposed by reason of their color, and if, as seems possible in those particular hospitals, they found themselves treated on a more equal footing than they expected, then it is also possible that they would exhibit a greater relaxation of tension than the equivalent White patients would do, some of the latter perhaps becoming more disturbed on finding themselves treated on an equal basis with the Blacks. In other instances, however, differences of a more fundamental, less situational nature may occur, and out of a knowledge of the cultures one can even attempt to predict, as I have done elsewhere [426], which rehabilitation measures are likely to succeed and which to fail with schizophrenics of different cultural backgrounds. However, since these attempted predictions were based only on impressions, they are too "soft" to be discussed here.

7 Conclusions

Schizophrenia is often considered to be the most distinctive and universal of the functional mental disorders, showing roughly the same features in all peoples. In this chapter I have attempted to show how much variation there can actually be within it, not just as between patient and patient but between people and people. Yet the degree of international variation is still limited. Comparing the Irish and southwestern Croations with the Hutterites and Tongans, for instance, the ratio of prevalence rates is only 4 to 1, much lower than for many somatic diseases, even those not dependent on an outside agent. One can, of course, find greater variations if one considers only limited sections of populations and hence permits greater opportunity for social selection, or if one disregards differences in diagnostic criteria. For whole societies, however, a ratio of 4/1 or 5/1 is probably as great as one is going to meet, and there is very little chance of finding a people that is schizophrenia-free, although some researchers consider this possible. Similarly, although some researchers consider this possible. Similarly, although variation in symptoms and course are substantial, they remain within certain limits (given the diagnostic criteria with which we must work today) and the common features are identifiable everywhere, although not in every patient.

These limits still provide ample scope for research and corrective action, however. If one can reduce the rate of schizophrenia in a society by half, or render its symptoms only half as distressing, or assist twice as many patients to achieve a socially complete recovery, then these are goals well worth striving for with so crippling a disease, and comparative studies seem able to provide or to corroborate indications for such action. Regardless of what may be learnt regarding vulnerability at the neurological level, the examples cited here suggest strongly that social factors affect the risk and character of the disease. These factors are not the obvious social stresses such as war, poverty and loss, or the obvious social benefits represented by prosperity, peace, and abundance of services. Often, the relation of the disease to these is in the opposite direction to what might be expected, and it has thus been argued that social stress and social protection must be irrelevant to the disease, an oversimple conclusion. To assess what constitutes a stress for the schizophrenic and the schizophrenia-prone one must study such persons themselves rather than make presumptions regarding what does and does not consitute stress; and the same is true of protective factors. Much of the needed research must be done in the laboratory, but if one compares social conditions in situations where schizophrenia is abundant or chronic with their equivalents in situations where it is rarer or milder, clues may appear which laboratory studies cannot easily yield, the reason being that the factor needs to operate over a period of years. Our knowledge of such factors is only commencing, but Table 4.6 indicates three which the material of this chapter

Table 4.6. Possible social factors affecting the risk and chronicity of schizophrenia

Precipitating or aggravating factors	Protecting or relieving factors
Strict and/or contradictory (internalized) social expectations	Liberal and/or modest social expectations
Obstacles to attainment of rewards implied in foregoing expectations	Easy attainability of rewards implied in foregoing expectations
Absence or excessive complexity of rules and guidelines for action	Simplicity and completeness of rules and guidelines for action

points to, and which might be taken as a starting point as long as it is understood that the effect of any of these factors can be neutralized by the other two.

The first factor or dimension indicated in the table, internalized social expectations and particularly expectations which conflict, has been touched on in more than one section of this chapter, but has been best demonstrated in a study not yet cited, namely Parker and Kleiner's work with urban Blacks [485]. They showed that although the migrants to Philadelphia from the southern states had lower status than the local-born Blacks on average, they had less mental disorder, including schizophrenia, than the latter, this difference being related to the fact that they had lower expectations and hence less discrepancy between what they desired and what they could reasonably achieve. The second factor in the table is also treated by these authors, and I think that they would expect the northern Blacks to have had no worse mental health than the southern ones if it had been as easy for them to attain their higher expectations. However, the expectations and facilities for gratification which are mainly compared in that study are those relating to material gains and status advancement, and it has to be realized that these may be less important than other types of need in some situations. Among the emigrant Irish and the Ukrainian Canadians, for instance, a major problem seems to be that the quite attainable upward mobility leads to a relative deprivation in other types of gratification. Studies of schizophrenic patients in hospitals and hostels suggest quite strongly that attempting to prevent a decline in social status may result in more symptoms than allowing the patient to aim at a style of life which implies quite a drop in status [448]. Finally, the value of simplicity of guidelines for the schizophrenic is well known in clinical practice, and is illustrated by the frequence with which patients who have shown good recovery within a highly organized hospital relapse when discharged to their much less well-organized, wider society. The Hutterites had very clear guidelines for all their members while the Achinese males had lost theirs; and it can be argued that the higher chronicity of the disease in modern Western societies is related to the fact that although ample rules exist, they have become very complex.

It is ideas such as these which I believe Comparative Psychiatry most usefully contributes to. The effect of genetic and other organic factors in schizophrenia is something which may very possibly affect the international distribution of the disease, and some of the differences noted in this chapter – the low rate among Taiwanese aborigines, for instance – may in future prove to be linked more to racial than to social factors. However, at the present time our knowledge of international differences in social variables is greater (although perhaps less precise) than our knowledge of differences in racial genetics, certainly the racial genetics most likely to be linked to the major mental disorder. In consequence, when an international or cross-cultural difference in schizophrenia is ascertained, it appears more promising to seek an explanation for this in terms of what we know about the relationship of the disease to social factors, than in terms of what we know about its relationship to organic ones. The theoretical design of a study which would evaluate the relative contributions which racial and sociocultural factors make to the risk of developing schizophrenia is known – see the study of coronary disease in Japanese and Japanese Americans in Chapter 9 – but its value could be small until we can identify more precisely what these genetic and sociocultural factors are.

Chapter 5 The Acute Reactive Psychoses

In discussing the course and outcome of schizophrenia in the previous chapter, attention was drawn to the fact that acute episodes of relatively brief duration and without any subsequent social disability are apparently much commoner in some countries than in others. In the WHO study these were all included with the schizophrenias, and they were not distinguishable from the more chronic cases on the basis of the symptoms recorded through the "Present State Examination" at intake [674]. However, a small number of those so classified – 52 out of the 1202 – had been diagnosed by the local psychiatrists as falling into a category other than the schizophrenias and the affective psychoses, namely within the "other psychoses" covered by the ICD (8) codes 298.1 to 298.9, and a higher percentage might have been labeled in this fashion if there had been among the centers one following the French psychiatric tradition.

Disorders which comprise less than 5% of the average service caseload (as the foregoing suggests) and which create no particular treatment problems would scarcely be expected to have a chapter to themselves in a book such as this, particularly when they carry a variety of diagnoses and receive little attention in the standard textbooks. However, the picture changes when one learns that there are societies such as Senegal [117] and Astrakhan [571] in which they are reported to be twice as frequent as schizophrenia, and other societies in which a majority of the cases which are labeled schizophrenia might equally have fitted this category. I have chosen to give these psychoses their own chapter at this point because they are close to the schizophrenias when considered only in terms of their symptomatology at any point in time, and I have entitled this chapter the Acute *Reactive* Psychoses because many of them develop subsequent to a clear, psychological or somatic stress. The international variation in the frequency and character of these disorders is probably greater than that of any other category of mental disorder apart from drug abuse, and international comparisons probably offer more here in the way of clues to etiology than they do for any other category. Moreover, the variation appears not only crossculturally at a given point in time, but historically, although one has the usual problem of interpreting just what the historical reports mean.

1 Historical Trends in Diagnosis

Temporary insanity is a condition regularly depicted throughout Western literature and in most other literatures as well, the disorder often developing as the result of an emotional shock or a god's curse. One need only to think of Ajax's brief madness after failing to be granted the armor of Achilles, or Agave's murder of her son Pentheus and her tragic recovery as depicted in Euripides' *Bacchae*. Prior to the nineteenth century it was customary for doctors to attribute most insanity either to some situational trauma such as disappointed love or financial reverse, or to an intercurrent fever or other somatic illness, in which latter case it was labeled "phrenitis" i.e. brain fever. We cannot judge today whether they were justified or unjustified in such attribution, but we do know that in the eighteenth and early nineteenth centuries, the average duration of stay of patients in mental hospitals (excluding those private ones used by families to lock away persons from whom they had taken financial power) was substantially less than it was by the end of the nineteenth century. That shift to apparently greater chronicity, which has never been adequately explained and which occurred even in as distant a location from Europe as Singapore [423], has been hypothesized to be related to the industrial revolution [124], with the suggestion that schizophrenia as we know it today only became recognizable in the 50 years before Kraepelin. Objections to this hypothesis are easy to find, although not necessarily insurmountable, but whichever view we take of the question, it does appear likely that acute transient psychoses were more common in Europe in the early nineteenth century than they were at its end.

During that century they were given a vast variety of names, many more than applied to the chronic psychoses. One authority cited by Ey [175] listed 20 such terms in 1886, not including either direct equivalents in other languages or the term which has become the most long-lived of them all since then, at least in French psychiatry, *bouffée délirante* which Magnan was only beginning to use at that time. We can infer that the greater variety of names for the short-lasting than for the longer-lasting psychoses derived in part from the fact that the latter could be observed for longer and hence had more time during which to reveal similarities which might not be apparent at first glance. However, the abundance of terms suggests that there must have been a considerable variation in the presenting clinical pictures, something which is to be borne in mind when we come to consider the current range. Most of the terms derived from French authors, and there is just possibly some significance in the fact that they attracted considerably less attention in Britain, since the industrial revolution had been longer established in the latter country and there is a theory, as noted above, that it is with industrialization that schizophrenia comes to replace the more transient psychoses.

Initially, the reactive character of these acute psychoses tended to be in the forefront, with somatic factors being stressed for "amentia" and some other categories, and with Pinel providing illustrations of the effect of emotional shock. (He cited, for instance, the case of an engineer who promptly entered a stuporous state after being told that the government had accepted his invention.) When we come to the end of the century, however, the reactive element is either less apparent or of less theoretical interest. Magnan, who has had the greatest influence on subsequent French classifications of these states, divided the acute psychoses into three broad categories: those which are predominantly affective; those which are predominantly confusional or commence with hallucinations; and those which commence with delusions ("*délires d'emblée*"). The first two of these categories were conceptually located by him within the group of the "simple psychoses" and the third in the group of "degenerative states," a division which has lost its meaning today but which on closer examination tells us something about both the psychiatry of his time and the background of the patients. "Simple" psychoses, whether inherited or not, implied no particular stigma and could happen in the best of families; "degeneracy" on the other hand was something which a family acquired through a Lamarckian process of deviant or unhealthy traits being first developed as habits and then transmitted biologically to offspring. The latter included sexual deviancy, inability to control impulses, mental deficiency, some phobias and obsessions, and an excessive susceptibility to develop delusional states in reaction to minor situational stresses (*"très grande aptitude à délirer sous l'influence des moindres causes"* [368, p 65]). These delusional states, the *bouffées délirantes*, were also seen by him as changing their character quite rapidly and as having little similarity to the forms of pathology exhibited by other members of the patient's family, a contrast to the more chronic psychoses.

From today's perspective, Magnan's division can most easily be seen as a social class one, with the *"dégénerés,"* being the chronic poor or proletariat who had received little education, were put to work as children (this was the era of Zola's *Germinal*), had little in the way of a consistent upbringing, were often accused of lawbreaking, and had good reason to feel ridden by fears of forces which they could not manage. Although this way of dividing cases may reflect a class bias, however, his descriptions (or more properly those of his student Legrain) show good clinical observation, and one might therefore have expected them to become models for the development of parallel diagnoses in other countries.

That did not happen. German psychiatry, although pursuing a few interesting psychological facets such as the relationship of some acute reactive psychoses to hysteria [55] and the existence of transient paranoid states in the absence of obvious precipitating factors [615], increasingly tended to put the short-lasting psychoses into the "amentia" category, supposedly caused by a somatic disturbance from infection, hormones or toxins, with a special place for Fürstner's "puerperal psychosis" [208]. British psychiatry, after initially showing little interest in the subject, later became obliged to do so because of the frequency with which transient psychoses were occurring in African and Indian troops, but tended to follow the German organic school in seizing on any intercurrent somatic illness as the probable cause, with the result that for a time most admissions to some Indian mental hospitals were labeled "toxic psychosis" and attributed to "toxaemia" under the influence of Overbeck-Wright [478]. (In Anglo-Saxon terminology, "amentia" was being used at this time for congenital mental retardation, a confusion which has led to the word being dropped almost entirely.) In the United States, after a brief romance with Adolf Meyer's theory that all psychotic states should be called "reactions," the major schools seized on Bleuler's claim that the "group of schizophrenias" could embrace acute, transient, as well as chronic disorders, and have applied the term schizophrenia to them ever since.

Only in Scandinavia, where there was a serious attempt to distinguish the transient, reactive "psychogenic psychoses" from the more chronic varieties, following the lead of Wimmer [661], did it seem possible that concepts would come sufficiently close to the French ones here for useful international comparisons to be possible. Unfortunately, however, important differences in theoretical approach make any such comparison very questionable. The French concept of *bouffée délirante*, as revised by Ey [175], continued to put emphasis on the presenting clinical picture and a hypothesized, constitutional predisposition rather than on the subsequent course, so that although Ey found, on follow-up, 10 out of 18 cases with this diagnosis to have developed a chronic psychosis, this did not lead him to conclude that the initial diagnosis must have been wrong [177]. The Scandinavian concept of psychogenic psychosis, although in Wimmer's time implying some vague constitutional predisposition as well as a precipitating stress, put main emphasis on the latter rather than on the clinical picture; and when cases thus diagnosed were later found to have developed a more chronic or episodic disorder, the tendency was to assume that the psychogenic psychosis diagnosis was wrong [25, 180]. (Since the work of Wimmer and Ey, further changes have taken place in the use of both *bouffée délirante* and psychogenic psychosis, but these authors remain the most representative on those concepts.)

2 International Comparisons: Europe, Africa, and the Caribban

Today the range of labels used for the acute reactive psychoses is narrower than it used to be, thanks in part to the development of therapeutic tools which can be used on most types of schizophrenia-like symptoms, and in part to the increasing dominance of North American psychiatry. The concept of hysterical psychosis has been rediscovered [266] and the Second World War with its consequent movement of refugees brought us "alien's paranoid psychosis" [309]; while a few other terms have had a limited existence; but it cannot yet be said that the terminology here is sufficiently uniform for satisfactory international comparisons. One may speculate regarding whether the differences between the national schools with respect to their approaches to the acute reactive psychoses are due purely to their different theoretical positions or have arisen in part from a difference in the clinical syndromes which they have come in contact with, but for an answer to that we must look to the future, not the past.

At present, about all that one can say at the international level is that there are certain similarities in the percentages of patients receiving diagnoses belonging to this group which may not be mere coincidence, and certain differences which invite attention. Thus, the proportion of Wimmer's Danish patients given the diagnosis of psychogenic psychosis [180] was almost the same as the percentage diagnosed as *bouffée délirante* by Ey [176], namely 5%, and in each location roughly half the patients were later found to have a more chronic condition. In contrast, 29% of the patients seen by Field at healing shrines in Ghana were placed by her into the categories of "fear psychosis" or "anxiety psychosis" [187], and this is almost identical with the percentage of patients assigned the diagnosis *bouffée délirante* in Senegal, a country which shares some of the same peoples as Ghana. In the French Antilles, it is only 15% who are reported to receive the latter diagnosis [121], a figure approximately the same as in Cuba [605]; and in North Africa both Tunisia [17] and Algeria [50] come closer to the European proportion, with 4% and 9% respectively.

These statistics and others of a similar nature, if taken with enough latitude, can be read as indicating that the acute transient psychoses occupy an increasingly important part of the psychiatric field as one moves from the more to the less technologically developed societies. However, to put them together in this fashion demands that we ignore some apparent exceptions and make doubtfully justifiable assumptions regarding the equivalence of diagnostic criteria, availability of services, and follow-up information. In Indochina, where the medical staff were French trained, the diagnosis of *bouffée délirante* was applied to only 5% of patients between the two World Wars [234], and in Ruanda-Urundi it was given to only 7% [635], although these locations would seem to have been no more developed than Senegal was in the 1960s. A preference for more organic diagnoses might account for these figures, but the tendency for the more dramatic psychoses to steal the limelight from the more insidious and chronic forms is also a factor which one needs to allow for when one moves from societies which are rich in psychiatric services to those which are poor. Accordingly, there seems little point in attempting to build on so uncertain a base. If we are to use comparative studies to understand these acute reactive psychoses better, we need either to examine specific instances where the clinical picture is fully described and analyzed, or to look to multicultural societies in which the access to services, diagnostic criteria, and record-keeping are roughly the same for each culture.

3 Comparison in Multicultural Societies: Singapore and Austria

To derive useful conclusions from multicultural settings such as those just described, it is necessary that the diagnostic classification in force enables us to make a rough division between the acute and the more chronic psychoses, and it is preferable that we can calculate incidence rates as well as the relative frequencies of the different categories of mental disorder within each subculture's patients. In Table 2.2 (p.30) was provided one such set of data from Russia, with the proportions of acute reactive psychoses ranging from 8.8% to 34.8% and with actual incidence being calculable if desired. As was pointed out there, however, the hospital was obviously serving some sections of the population much better than it was serving others, and this makes interpretation of the data very difficult. In preference I have chosen to use data from Singapore in the 1950s and Austria during the First World War, each set having particular advantages and particular disadvantages.

In Singapore, the main diagnoses covering the acute psychoses at that time were "toxic psychosis" and "puerperal psychosis." Figure 5.1 depicts their relative incidence in the main cultures. In the 1950s, Singapore's mean rate of first admissions to mental hospital was very similar to that in England and Wales, its population being relatively small and its services relatively abundant. The "toxic psychosis" diagnosis was supposed to be applied only to conditions in which there was strong reason to suspect a somatic (infectious, hormonal, or drug) origin. However, a review of case records revealed that it was principally being given to cases that showed confusion, abrupt onset, and fluctuations in symptomatology, and for whom no other diagnosis seemed more suitable. Also, the prevalence of somatic illness in this group was scarcely any higher than its prevalence in the rest of the patients. "Puerperal psychosis" was applied to conditions developing during pregnancy or the puerperium in patients who had no history of psychosis or borderline state except at a previous pregnancy.

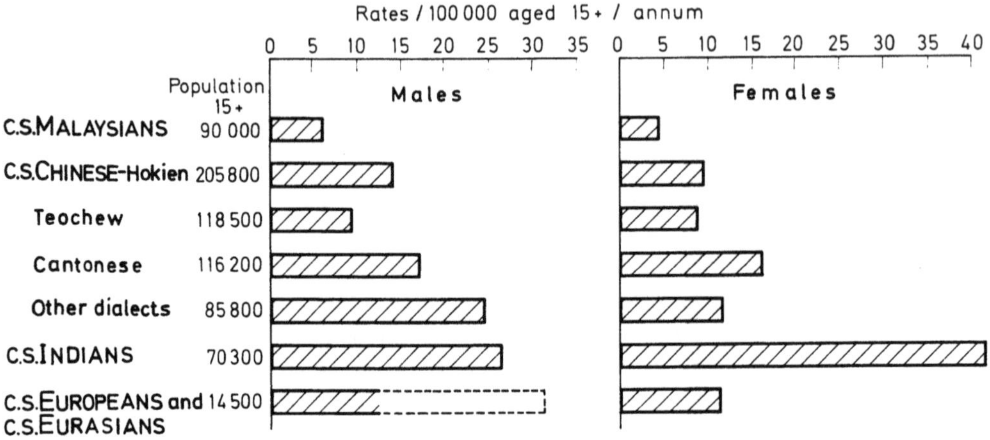

Fig. 5.1. Singapore first admission rates for "toxic" and "puerperal" psychoses, by cultural group and sex, 1950–1954. The European male rate is distorted by the large number of sailors being admitted from passing ships, acute psychosis being the type of condition which appears to require immediate hospitalization at the nearest port of call. (Own data.)

The clinical pictures overlapped those labeled schizophrenic, but abrupt onset was more common than in the latter and 45% of cases (excluding those dying soon after arrival) were discharged within 3 months as compared with 20% of schizophrenics.

There are three points at which statistically significant differences arise in this figure, namely between the Indians and the Chinese, between the Chinese and the Malays, and within the overall Chinese group between the two largest dialectal groups and the collection of small ones – "other dialects." (The difference between the Indian and Malay rates is statistically significant as well, of course.) Regarding two of these differences, namely that between the Indians and Chinese and that within the Chinese dialectal groups, there appears to be no cause for doubt; the hospitalization rates probably reflect the incidence within the community fairly uniformly. Whether there is a genuine difference between the Chinese and Malay rates, however, is uncertain, since the latter people were more inclined than the former to use their own healers (*bomohs*) as a first resort for many types of mental disease, and were slower to go to a modern hospital.

Considering first among possible etiological factors behind these differences the relative vulnerability of the cultural groups to somatic infection or other illness, it can be said that the most vulnerable were the Malays, due to their more traditional life style and relatively lower protection against infection. Indian males were more prone to misuse alcohol and hence to develop an alcoholic psychosis (included in the "toxic" group) than Chinese males, and they also had a greater vulnerability to some of the chronic psychosomatic disorders, but they did not have any greater exposure to infection and on the female side there should have been no difference in exposure either to drugs or to infection. The Europeans and Eurasians should have had the best protection against infection, but they abused alcohol more and the male rate is distorted by seamen being hospitalized from oceangoing ships. There was no reason to think that the Chinese dialectal minorities were more exposed to any relevant somatic factor than the dialectal majority were.

Turning to psychosocial factors, the situation of the Indian women would appear to have a direct bearing on their high rate, a clue to this lying in the fact that almost half of their cases were "puerperal" whereas less than a fifth of the Chinese female ones were. Among the Indians, it was customary for women to return to their parental homes for their first and sometimes subsequent confinements, but the majority of young married Indian women in Singapore at this time had their parents in India, their husbands having gone back there to seek a bride, and their husbands might not be able or willing to pay for their return to their parents in accordance with custom. Given the fact that most of these women would not really have known their husbands before their marriage and had then immediately to move to a place where not merely the husband but the neighbors and the whole style of life was different, there is no doubt that such women would be under severe stress and that this would become much greater if the expected return to the parental home for confinement was not feasible. The possibility of these attacks being allowed to develop for the purpose of persuading the husband to send the wife to her home is real here and hence some of the cases might better have been given the diagnosis of hysterical psychosis, but although the Indians were more prone to hysterical and dissociation states than the other Singaporean peoples [421], I see no reason to call these pseudopsychoses. Also probably pertinent (and echoing Magnan) is the fact that the Indian households were the least cohesive, resulting in them having by far the highest rate of juvenile delinquency [422], as was shown in Fig. 2.3. The other stressor which seems relevant to Fig. 5.1 is minority status. I have demonstrated elsewhere [420] that there is a significant, inverse correlation between relative group strength in the population and the incidence of suicide and of certain other mental disorders when the seven main Singapore Chinese dialectal groups are compared. Two aspects of minority status appear to be at work: the emotional support of neighbors sharing one's background, something which was important mainly for the women, and the competitive advantage of having people of one's own background at each location where one sought either work, customers, or collaboration, something which was important mainly for the men. As we see in the figure, the relationship of the toxic psychoses to dialectal group size affects only the male rate ($r = -0.74$ when seven dialectal groups are considered) and therefore it seems likely that it is the stress of economic competition which is relevant here rather than emotional stress. This last inference is strengthened by the fact that on the female side it is the Cantonese who have the highest rate, since at that time most Singapore Chinese women worked only within their own homes, whereas those of the Cantonese subgroup went out to work, even as road laborers.

These Singaporean comparisons seem reasonably valid if one is considering cases that last more than a few days, since except among the Malays it was the custom to seek help for a patient from all types of source, traditional and modern, almost simultaneously, and since the ratio of hospital beds to population was adequate by European standards. However, as was noted earlier, the Malay rates are suspect due to the greater availability and repute of their *bomohs*, and in all groups there were almost certainly cases of short-lasting psychosis which never came to medical attention. If one wants to cover even the shortest-lasting psychoses in one's comparisons – although, as will be discussed below, there is a problem deciding just how long a state of confusion or excitement should last before it merits the label psychosis – the best source of information is one in which all members of the population are constantly under official supervision, i.e., something like a prison or an army unit. Army data are the more representative, particularly when there is national conscription, and the intake screening and limited age span can impose a helpful uniformity. However, a common problem with such military statistics is that one cannot obtain satisfactory figures regarding the population-at-risk. I have been unable to find any data relevant to this chapter from a military or similarly controlled population which yield both a denominator and breakdown by subcultures, but the figures which Pilcz [496] reported regarding Austrian Army psychiatric casualties during the First World War are interesting and seem worthwhile republishing. Table 5.1 summarizes them, with the cultural groups being placed in order of the percentage of patients receiving the diagnosis of "amentia". (Other military data are given in Chap. 10.)

Taking the order in which the cultural groups are placed, the first thing which is likely to strike the reader with a little knowledge of this region is that the most urbanized and educated groups are at the right and the most rural and little-educated on the left. In other words, the risk of getting amentia relative to the risk of getting some other mental disorder is inversely associated with education, urbanization, and sanitation. In the Austro-Hungarian Empire at that time, sanitary conditions in Vienna and the other main cities were reasonably good and certainly much better than in the Empire's outer marches, so that it is reasonable to suspect that the rates of amentia are causally linked to sanitary conditions at home, i.e., to the likelihood of the soldiers bringing some infectious or dietary disorder with them. However, if that were the case one would expect the percentages for amentia to be inversely related to those for *each* other category of mental disorders, whereas that is not so. As one can see in the second row, the groups with the highest rates of amentia are also those with the highest rates of schizophrenia and paranoia. Moreover, when soldiers from different regions are all mixed together in the same barracks, it is often those from the more sanitary backgrounds that are the more vulnerable to infectious disease, not those from the more insanitary. Hence the variance in percentages diagnosed as amentia does not seem to be adequately accounted for in terms of exposure to infection, and some relationship to education seems the more likely.

Formal education enlarges one's knowledge of the world, makes one readier for what one may meet when one is moved to another location, and also provides greater confidence in the face of unfamiliar problems. When we compare groups of immigrants, it is a general rule that the mental health of those with a good, formal preparation for what they will meet – i.e., with a good education – is superior to that of those who have only a little knowledge of what they will meet, and the term "alien's paranoid psychosis" has been given to a particular type of disorder with relatively good outcome which is met in the latter [309]. However, if the situation were merely that the least educated had the greatest chance of breaking down under the stress of unfamiliar conditions, one would expect, as before, to find each other cate-

Table 5.1. Percentage distribution of psychiatric diagnoses in seven subcultural groups: Austrian Army Garrison Hospital, 1914–1917, Vienna [496]

	Croatians Serbians Slovenians	Poles Ruthenians	Hungarians	Germans	Czechs	Jews	Austrians (Viennese)
"Amentia"	13.9	9.8	7.8	7.8	4.1	3.6	3.0
Schizophrenia and paranoia	25.5	23.7	22.1	20.1	21.9	23.0	14.2
Manic and cyclical psychoses	4.4	2.9	2.6	3.6	2.2	4.6	2.6
Depressive psychoses	11.9	18.8	9.7	7.9	7.8	3.0	3.8
Alcoholic psychoses and drug abuse	6.1	3.9	3.9	11.6	12.0	1.6	21.0
Chronic organic psychoses (incl. G.P.I.)	11.9	8.9	16.6	16.4	11.3	13.2	15.1
Mental deficiency	9.0	12.2	12.3	13.0	10.4	7.0	8.5
Neuroses	6.4	12.5	17.3	9.5	17.1	19.0	11.9
Other diagnoses (incl. "simulation")	10.9	7.3	7.7	10.1	13.2	25.0	19.9
Total	100.0	100.0	100.0	100.0	100.0	100.0	100.0
Number of cases	341	590	308	1453	1071	498	916

Cultural groupings are as used in the original and Pilcz does not state how they were arrived at. It is therefore unclear whether "Viennese" refers to birthplace or some other characteristic, and whether the "Germans" are Austrian citizens or citizens of Germany. I have assumed the "Viennese" refers to citizens of today's Niederösterreich and "Germans" to those of Oberösterreich, but the point is not important gory of mental disorder to increase proportionately as the percentage given the diagnosis of amentia declined; and that is not the case. What one finds instead is that it is neurosis and the personality disorders (the latter constituting the main part of "other diagnoses") which increase their percentages as those for amentia decline. Accordingly, there is a suggestion in this table that as education increases, what had been a risk of developing an acute reactive psychosis turns into a risk of developing a nonpsychotic disorder. Obviously, this is only a suggestion since we do not know the actual rates. Nevertheless it is a point worth bearing in mind.

The group with the highest relative proportion of cases diagnosed as amentia is the Southern Slavic one. In the Singapore material the high-rate group was the Indian one. In the previous chapter it proved helpful to ask what, if anything, the different high-rate groups had in common, and although we do not know for sure that the Southern Slavs had the highest actual incidence rate for amentia it could still be interesting to ask what else, if anything, these two people have in common vis-à-vis the groups with which we have been comparing them. At first examination there is almost no similarity. The Indians were not, on average, less educated than other Singaporeans, and the Southern Slavs did not have less cohesive families than the other Austro-Hungarian peoples. On the contrary, they had probably the strongest family structure, certainly the most patriarchal. The Southern Slavs, like many Singapore Indians, were far from their parental homes; but that was true of several other subcultures within the Austrian Army as well. The Indians misused alcohol more than other Singaporean groups except possibly the European, but in the Austrian Army there were cultural groups which did this much more than the Southern Slavic one did. The only real points at which there does appear to be a possible similarity relates to a hysterical predisposition and to somatization.

It was mentioned earlier that the Indians suffered a greater risk of hysteria and of psychosomatic disorders than other Singaporean peoples. Information on these conditions among subgroups of the Austrian Army during the First World War is thin, but during the Second World War reports of such predispositions did come out of Yugoslavia whereas they did not come from other parts of the region. Toward the end of this war there was an extensive epidemic of what was called the "partizan sickness" affecting at least 3 000 individuals [482]. This was a pseudo-epilepsy somewhat similar to the "Puerto Rican Syndrome," and it affected both sexes. Moreover, it has been recorded that in Yugoslavia and Italy during and after World War II, "Men from Yugoslav Dinaric areas showed a striking instability of mental equilibrium... Previously brave fighters were scared by trifling organic sensations and seemed entirely lost in their organic nervous symptoms." The same source states that doctors from these regions "maintained that the soldiers from strict patriarchal settings had no resistance to illness when separated from 'their own,' meaning kin, clan brothers, tribe members or at least men from their own community" [172 pp 386–387]. The most vulnerable in these respects were not the Southern Croats whose high rate of schizophrenia was discussed in Chap. 4, but men whose culture showed an Albanian influence. "Their psychological resistance to illness was nil and the percentage of fatal cases, especially of pneumonia, was relatively high" [172 p 386].

These quotations are instructive in three ways. They point to a possible similarity between the Southern Slavs and the Singapore Indians as respects a tendency to develop hysterical or depressive features in the face of somatic illness or other stresses, features which might become psychotic in extreme cases. They give us some reason to think that the Southern Slavs may have had a genuinely high rate of amentia during the First World War as well as a high percentage of psychiatric patients receiving that diagnosis. And they give us a slight clue to etiology. The fact that vulnerability was particularly high among men from "strict patriarchal settings" brings to mind the fact that the Singapore Indians had come predominantly from villages in which a strict hierarchy – although of caste rather than of generation – also existed. These two peoples can therefore be recognized as having one more thing in common, namely that they had moved out of a setting where many personal problems were expected to be brought to community elders for decision, into a situation where these problems had to be handled largely alone. We will see below that there are other settings in which the acute reactive psychoses appear to be related to problems of balance between communal and individual decision-taking.

These inferences are about as much as one can draw from the Singapore and Austrian data just presented, and there may be readers who would hold that I have gone too far in even attempting them, based as they are on so many assumptions. It can be argued that one should first be sure that the disorders which one is discussing fit a uniform set of criteria (whether or not they receive the same diagnosis) before going on to make assumptions about relative incidence. My own view is that it is useful to draw inferences from even quite weak data, so long as one does not put much weight on them, but it is certainly also useful to look at the clinical pictures in more detail than has just been done, and to assess whether one is truly dealing with specific clinical entities. This can be undertaken, within the Comparative Psychiatry context, both with respect to conditions which are said to be culture bound, i.e., found with extreme rarity if at all outside a given culture, and with respect to conditions which are considered universal but are assumed to occur with different frequencies in different peoples. We will move on to these further steps now, commencing with the question of whether the diagnosis of *bouffée délirante* is being employed in the same fashion in settings where it is reportedly common as in settings where it is reportedly rare.

4 *Bouffée Délirante:* France, Senegal, and Guadeloupe

The metropolitan French literature on *bouffée délirante* is extensive and varied, but there is broad agreement [121, 176] that the criteria for this diagnosis should be:

a) Acuteness of onset;
b) Intensity of the delusional and hallucinatory experience;
c) Kaleidoscopic shifting from one mental state to another, both at the ideational and at the emotional level, without consistency of delusional content;
d) Fascination of the patient by his delusional experiences;
e) Termination of the episode and return to prior state within a short period (e.g., 3 months), but not necessarily without later relapse.

The disorder is to be distinguished from the affective psychoses by (b) and (c), from schizophrenia by (c) and (d), from simple confusional states by (b), and from the simple hallucinosis by (a). Some authors think the disorder particularly likely to occur in mental defectives and persons with psychopathic or sociopathic, impulsive tendencies, and although emotional shocks may precipitate it, as with Wimmer's psychogenic psychosis, these (and other precipitants such as infections or drugs) are usually considered of much less importance than the constitutional "ground" or "reactive threshold" assumed to underlie the process. The disorder is usually thought to affect mainly the young, with women more vulnerable than men. Ey's theory regarding it is that it represents a crumbling (*déstructuration*) of consciousness or of the ego [175], and although it may have a positive side through allowing expression of powerful but repressed feelings [198] it is usually regarded as pathological, with the longer-term prognosis uncertain even though temporary recovery occurs.

As noted earlier, such psychotic states occur in only about 5% of mental hospital admissions in France but are claimed to constitute 30% in Senegal, despite the fact that the latter's hospital is unlikely to see the more short-lasting cases since those would recover before the help of modern medicine was sought. It is therefore of particular interest to know what sorts of conditions are included under this diagnosis in Senegal, information which is provided in a long paper by Collomb with 32 case illustrations [118], and in additional papers by some of his associates. On first impression, the Senegal cases fit the criteria listed above very well. Thus, 77% have acute onset, there is in all cases a rapid fluctuation of mood, of insight and of hallucinatory or delusional experiences, all patients are deeply immersed in these experiences, and recovery occurs within 3 months [118]. The fact that onset is quite often with hallucinations rather than delusions does not seem an important difference even though Magnan had made a distinction here, and neither does it seem so important that the patients cover a considerably wider age range than is usual in France. An occasional case from among the 32 might seem better to merit the diagnosis of affective psychosis than of *bouffée délirante*, but the same holds true of cases reported from France itself. Judging only by the clinical presentation, therefore, there seems no reason to think that these patients are suffering from anything different from what would be called *bouffée délirante* in France.

Where a difference does appear is when one looks beyond the patient to his milieu and examines his delusions from that angle. In France the delusional content appears to have no uniting theme; in Senegal the same is true to the outsider, but it often does have a unifying theme in the eyes of the local culture [475]. To take an illustration, Collomb's fifth case [118] is that of a young married woman who successively expressed the belief that (a) sorcerers had buried objects where she walked; (b) her mother was not her mother; (c) it was dangerous to go into the house; and (d) her clothing was being stolen. These elements become much more coherent when one realizes that the first and last stemmed from a socially endorsed fear that one of her co-wives was trying to bewitch her, while the other two elements are expressions of her belief that her mother, with whom she was living, was not doing enough to protect her against such bewitchment. A second point of difference is that whereas in France each patient is wholly alone in his delusional beliefs, in Senegal there are always likely to be some persons around the patient who think that these beliefs might be true, and it is possible for the patient's whole milieu to agree with this. That is not to say that the patient is merely expressing a shared illusion and has been falsely labeled psychotic, something which can happen when the medical staff are insufficiently informed of the background; for these patients were often dangerous to themselves or to others in ways which their society did not condone. But while the milieu will view these acts as both forbidden and irrational, it will not view as irrational the fears and some of the beliefs which led to the patient abandoning self-control and embracing his private delusions. This is a point which appears to be crucial for the course of the illness.

West African societies have been alleged by more than one authority to have a paranoid or persecution complex, and in illustration of the claim Field has recorded 134 inscriptions from trucks travelling the Ghanian highways, inscriptions whose commonest themes she interprets as paranoid apprehension and paranoid boasting [187]. Insofar as this is not a misunderstanding of these societies, we might say that the climate of mistrust must be producing the apparent excess of psychoses, but we could also say that it is the relative abundance of psychotics which is producing the mistrust, or we could look for a third factor underlying both. Let us look at another part of the world where *bouffée délirante* is reported to be relatively common, and see if that helps us to understand the West African picture.

In the French Caribbean, as noted earlier, the proportion of mental hospital admissions receiving the diagnosis of *bouffée délirante* has been about the same as that receiving the diagnosis of acute reactive psychosis in Cuba, namely 15%, and one could add that it is probably about the same as that which has been diagnosed as acute paranoid schizophrenia in Haiti [381]. In all three territories, moreover, it appears likely that many of the other patients admitted with a diagnosis of alcoholic psychosis are exhibiting essentially the same syndrome. The most complete study of these acute psychoses in this region is that by Constant [121], who covered 112 cases in Guadéloupe. In conformity with the standard criteria for *bouffée délirante*, all his cases exhibited sudden onset, a brief stay in hospital (average 4 weeks), a clinical picture dominated by gross delusions, and recovery without relapse in 80%. Ninety percent had delusions of persecution, 80% had hallucinations, and in 70% the delusional content made some reference to magic or witchcraft. Narcoanalysis of cases with hallucinations demonstrated the latter to be genuine and not hysterical confabulations. The delusions proved on investigation to cohere around a single theme, as in Senegal, and as with most *bouffée délirante* cases anywhere the patients seemed fascinated by their own productions; but there were significant differences from both the European and the African cases with respect to affectivity, the precipitating events, and the involvement of the patients' milieux.

The first difference lay in the fact that the patients related their hallucinations and delusions with relatively little affect, something which proved on closer examination to be not an indifference but a passivity. In other words, these Caribbean patients appeared to be feeling that they had handed over their problems to someone else and therefore need not worry much about them any more, even though they might have been so panic-stricken by them initially. This could have been due to the treatment which all the cases had received prior to the research interview, but seems likely to have a more basic cause. The second difference was that although the great majority were clearly "reactive," in the sense that there was a link between the symptomatology and a recent stress, that stress was as often internal as external, for instance some sexual conflict relating as much to the patient's Catholic upbringing as to a fear of spells and of "bad luck." Finally, although the patient's milieu was certainly involved in attempting to find a medical, religious, or magical cure, this involvement seems to have been more on behalf of the patient as individual than on behalf of a family or wider social unit as would often be the case in Senegal. The public seemed to feel that anybody could be driven into such a mental state by "bad luck" or some largely unexplainable attack, and that therefore one ought to provide help in case one might need similar help oneself, this attitude being distinct from what one would usually meet in Europe, where the average person would not think himself liable to such an affliction, or in West Africa, where the individual's illness would be more often seen as the symptom of a communal disorder. A final, lesser, difference between the Guadeloupean cases and others is that before hospitalization the patients had often refused food, although their delusions never contained a fear of poisoning, and had created a confrontation with their families by this means quite as much as by the obvious psychosis.

Comparing both the West African and the Caribbean cases of *bouffée délirante* with the cases described in France, a point which probably comes out more clearly in the case histories than in the present summary is the degree to which the behavior of the former appears directed to mobilizing either the immediate milieu or the social powers to take action. In a certain sense these psychoses are attention-getters in the same way as hysterical behavior is attention getting. However, in neither location is there the self-centeredness which one finds in the hysterical patient, and the enjoyment in playing the role; rather there is in both sets of patients a striving to be reintegrated into a social group. In West Africa that reintegration is symbolized by the rites which take place at the healing shrines in Ghana [187] and the Ivory Coast [493]; and the patient is an active participant. In the Caribbean the patients are much more passive but their desire to be taken care of by society is clear. Their passivity as they recount their hallucinations and delusions, linked to the refusal to eat, clearly suggests regression to a passive oral stage, and it is significant that in Cuba the patients with these acute reactive psychoses were quite disproportionately still living with their own parents, when compared with neighbors of their own age groups [88]. In West Africa, Collomb has pointed out [118] that most such patients come from the recently developed urban conglomerations and not from the traditional villages although it is in the latter that the communal beliefs which have been called paranoid are strongest; and in Cuba J.A. Bustamante has for long been insisting that these acute psychoses arise not from underdevelopment but from rapid social change [87]. That is a comment which brings us back to European experience, although not with *bouffée délirante* as such, since it is the acuteness of the social change and the separation from comrades which is supposed to be behind the "alien's paranoid psychosis."

However, there is a second point which seems to differentiate the African and Caribbean cases of acute reactive psychosis from European cases, and this is the nature of the underlying conflicts which can be uncovered when enough care is taken by the investigator. Although many of Constant's cases seem to be reacting simply to some minor event of frightening supernatural significance, still more appear to have become psychotic at a moment of crisis in some internal conflict, a conflict which in Europeans would be expected to give rise to a neurosis rather than a psychosis. In West Africa the same can be said of some of the delusional cases described in the book *Oedipe Africain* [476], and we have an admirably clear picture of the transition from what we would call psychotic to neurotic mechanisms of defense in an Ivory Coast patient described by Zempléni [684]. One can interpret these facts in many ways, but one possible link is to the relative emphasis given to individualization. The more a person is taught to be independent of others, the more he must develop psychological mechanisms which will permit him to remain functioning independently in the face of difficulties. The more a person is brought up as a member of a mutually supportive group, on the other hand, the more effective his defenses are likely to be if they depend on the strengths of that group rather than on himself. Regardless of theory, however, this is a field in which international comparisons seem worthwhile.

5 The Psychoses of the Puerperium: West and North Africa

The foregoing comments on *bouffée délirante* have suggested that in societies where this disorder is relatively common, it may be a substitute for neurosis and may also represent an attempt (not conscious) to summon group help and solidarity in the face of a threat which is often perceived as supernatural. In societies where *bouffée délirante* is much less common the syndrome may not carry the same significance, and there are other acute psychotic syndromes which can be relatively common in some societies and in which this symbolic meaning appears absent. Such is the case not only when the psychosis is an incoherent confusion, but when the psychological basis of the disturbance is more individual. We will now briefly explore cross-cultural differences in two such forms, namely amok and some of the psychoses of puerperium.

"Puerperal psychosis" was initially conceived by Fürstner [208] and by Aschaffenburg as a brain disorder arising from the normal but more particularly from the pathological (puerperal fever, eclampsia, etc.) stresses of childbearing. However, as maternal morbidity and mortality declined during the present century while the rate of puerperal psychoses remained the same in most countries [246] or even mounted slightly [291], the original hypothesis was difficult to maintain and it then came to be recognized that the psychoses developing during the puerperium were really no different from various psychoses developing at other times, so that the original term has been dropped from most official terminologies. It remains agreed that there is a reactive component in the psychoses of the puerperium, since the risk of onset is considerably higher during this period than at other times, and it is also agreed that the onset is usually acute, but other distinguishing features are lacking and in most medically advanced countries it is not found that these psychoses are any more transient than average; in fact, Hemphill reported from Britain that puerperal schizophrenia tended to be above average in chronicity [254].

In Europe and North America the psychoses of the puerperium constitute between 2% and 8% of female mental hospital admissions, a range which appears to be accounted for as much by differences in definition as by differences in actual risk.

However, in West Africa up to a third of female psychiatric admissions are reported to take place during the puerperium [63] and in North Africa between 10% and 15% occur thus. Moreover, on that continent the disorder appears to be relatively brief so that, for instance, over half of a Nigerian sample were able to be discharged within 3 weeks [162], and it thus seems justifiable to regard the majority of such conditions in these countries as belonging to the acute reactive psychoses.

At first glance, the above-cited differences in proportions between Europe and Africa might seem explainable on the basis of the latter continent's higher birth rate, since the average African woman must spend considerably more of her life in the puerperium than the average European, but such an explanation assumes that every pregnancy during a woman's lifetime carries the same risk of psychosis, and although this may be true in some societies it is not at all true in others. In the United States, Black women have been shown to have twice the rate of psychoses of the puerperium that White women have, and they also have a considerably higher birth rate. However, when psychotic samples from the two racial groups were compared with each other and with control groups of other pregnant women of the same age and race, it was found that 56% of the Black psychotics were in their first pregnancy as compared with only 17% of Black controls ($P \leqslant 0.001$) [479], whereas no significant difference of this type appeared between the White psychotics and controls. Furthermore, as Fig. 5.2 indicates, this difference applied regardless of age. (For details of this complex study the reader is referred to the original articles.) Given the weaker social organization of Black as compared with White society in the United States, one could interpret this difference along the same lines as was done for *bouffée délirante*, namely by arguing that the Black primiparae were likely to be in the greatest need of social support and had learnt no more effective way of summoning it. However, when one turns to developing countries one can find similar differences respecting the proportions of patients becoming psychotic during their first pregnancy, and the same argument does not hold. Table 5.2 presents data from four such countries

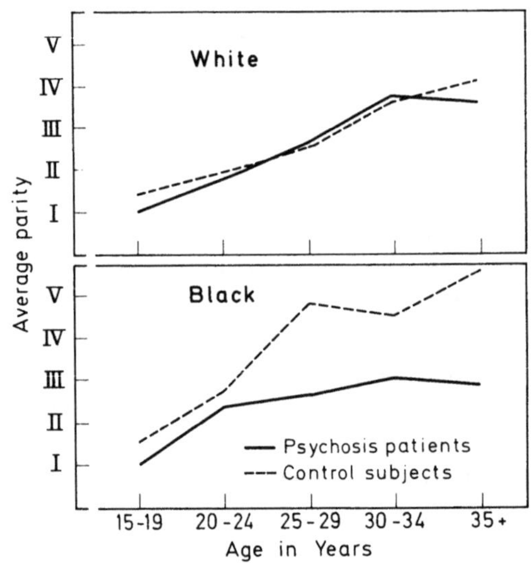

Fig. 5.2. Black and White patients with a psychosis of the puerperium, Ohio, 1940–1958, as compared with control groups in terms of parity and age [479]

Table 5.2. Psychosis of the puerperium related to parity in four countries

		India [558]	Senegal [159]	Morocco [106]	Algeria [377]
Number of cases		76	213	100	37
Parity	1st	47%	43%	29%	14%
	2nd	18%	17%	24%	19%
	3rd	6%	14%	19%	27%
	4th and over	29%	26%	28%	40%

$Chi^2 = 18.12$; d.f. = 3; $P < 0.001$; comparing first pregnancy with remainder

and one sees that in North Africa the proportion of primiparae among the puerperal psychotics is significantly lower than the corresponding proportions in India and Senegal, although national birth rates suggest that they should all be about the same. Nearly all the women in the table were delivered in Western style hospitals, so that marked differences in physical exhaustion should have been avoided, and in each of the indicated societies a woman's first pregnancy receives much attention from her milieu, more so than occurs at later pregnancies. Accordingly, these primiparae should not have felt any need for more social support and intergration. We know in Western society, however, that in the psychoses of the puerperium a relatively common symptom is fear of harming the newborn baby, something which is regognized to be a disguised expression of rejection or hostility towards what the infant symbolizes, and in East Africa there is a popular belief that recently delivered mothers can be inflicted with a strong desire to eat or otherwise kill the infant [131]. Rather than interpreting the puerperal psychotic reactions reflected in the table as a means of seeking greater social integration and support, therefore, we might think of them as an expression of rejection, and we can ask what it is in these societies that the primarae, in particular, might wish to reject.

The answer to this question is twofold. Giving birth to a first child means on the one hand the abandonment of the role of dependent child, a role which can persist after early marriage when the latter has been undertaken between families rather than between individuals. It can also mean assuming the specific roles of wife and mother in a way which might only partly have been accepted till then. We have seen that in the Caribbean, the acute reactive psychoses seem most likely to occur in individuals showing signs of overdependency or a desire to regress to an oral-dependent phase. It could be that in North Africa societies, the childrearing practices (particularly those directed at girls) are less prone to produce fixation at an oral-dependent level than the equivalent practices in India and West Africa. It is my impression from anthropological reading that this is the case, but the evidence is too debatable to build on. It could also be that the particular role of wife-mother is less attractive in Indian and West African society than in North African ones, and this likewise seems quite possible. In North Africa, although there is so much male dominance, the women have formed an almost closed and highly interacting society, with little of the isolation which has been so often described as afflicting the young Indian wife, and without the interference in the mother-child relationship which Collomb reports to be so significant in Sengalese family life [119]. In West Africa there also appear to be traditional beliefs leading the pregnant woman (but not just the primipara) to think of the forthcoming child as a danger to herself not just physically but spiritually, and these have also been alleged to play a role in producing the abundance of puerperal psychosis [159]. Whether all this is true is very difficult to assess, and still more difficult is to assess the presence of similar but apparently inoperative factors in other societies, but the evidence does suggest that where the psychoses of the puerperium are frequent, this may be because they symbolize a rejection of what adult female roles are offering in the given society.

6 Amok: Malaysia, Indonesia, and Laos

Rejection of a particular role and of the society which attempts to impose it is not an idea that lies too far from normal thinking. Neither is the idea of ending one's life and thus being freed from obligations, or of taking revenge against particular persons who have injured one. Seeking one's own death while attempting to kill *random* members of that society at the same time, however, is definitely far from the thinking of the vast majority of people in most societies. Hence, when we find such a desire being acted out during a brief psychotic episode, and when such episodes occur much more in some societies than in others, it is a puzzling and potentially instructive aspect of psychopathology.

In its strict sense, the term amok refers to a sudden, homicidal attack which is directed against people whom the amoker (person running amok) has no particular enmity towards or affection for, and which then continues against additional persons until the amoker is restrained or killed. The typical attack occurs in the absence of any prior or subsequent signs of psychosis, it endangers the amoker's own life either directly or by retaliation, and there is usually amnesia both for the event and for prior feelings of hostility, although a desire for death may be admitted. In a much looser sense the word amok has also been applied to psychotic attacks against individuals who are conceived by the patient to have personally injured him, who are hallucinated to be devils or persecutors, or whom the patient seeks to free from real or imagined suffering in the present world (the Jonestown massacre in Guyana, for instance). However, the latter type of behavior can arise in association with many states, psychotic or otherwise, and it is only with amok in the strict sense of the term that I am concerned here.

In every large society, if one searches the records thoroughly enough, one can find one or two instances of persons running amok in the sense being used here, but these instances are extremely rare, occurring only once in many million man-years, and it is often uncertain whether the term should really apply. During the 1960s, however, attacks of amok were occurring in Vientiane and surrounding Laotian towns at a rate of between 6 and 12 per year [649], and in parts of the Malay peninsula and archipelago in the early nineteenth century they were occurring, as far as I have been able to estimate, at a rate of at least one case per 1000 adult males per annum over 1 or 2 decades [427]. (For purposes of comparison, let it be realized that the latter rate, which does not include other forms of homicide, is about 10 times the average suicide rate in males today, or five times the rates of suicide and homicide combined.) In Laos, where the hand grenade was the main weapon, there was an average of over 12 persons injured in each episode, the social impact being so grave that the government had to forbid the holding of certain traditional festivals since it was at these that the attacks particularly occurred. Roughly half the Laotian amokers lost their own lifes in the event, and among the nineteenth century Malays the proportion was probably higher.

Amok is about as exclusively a male disorder as puerperal psychosis is a female one, and when we ask what else distinguishes the amoker form others of his own society the relatively few features which one finds mentioned with fair consistency from the nineteenth century to the present are surprisingly similar to features which have already been noted as characterizing persons vulnerable to other acute reactive psychoses. Amokers tend disproportionately to be persons from rural communities who have been conscripted into the army or have moved to town in search of work, and seem to have been overwhelmed by what they met. Sometimes they are stated to have complained of homesickness. Although some have functioned quite competently as soldiers, they are rarely described as having an aggressive tendency. Rather, the neighbors and relatives of the Laotian sample (who were relatively young) described many as being "emotionally labile, irresponsible, childish or excessively reliant on others" [650], and nineteenth century papers referring to older amokers sometimes describe them as having been relatively quiet and timid. In nearly all cases there were recognizable precipitators, but these were usually not such as one would have expected to produce such a violent outburst – for instance, losses at gambling, quarrel with a girlfriend or a painful ulcer on the leg – and there was often a prodromal period of withdrawal or brooding lasting hours or days before the attack broke out. Beliefs in magic or the supernatural appear to play virtually no role either in predisposing to the attack or in the attack itself, something which distinguishes amok both from the main forms of *bouffée délirante* which we have been considering, and from the sometimes homicidal but more chronic Windigo psychosis of the Algonquians [608]. There is virtually never any claim that a spirit ordered the amoker to kill, or statement by onlookers that he seemed to have been hallucinating, or subsequent evidence of panic-linked delusions of being bewitched.

Whether the amoker is apprehended or escapes, his psychosis is usually of quite brief duration, measured in hours or days rather than weeks or months, and cases with typical behavior but with signs of a more chronic psychosis have been few. In fact, some of the episodes are so brief that if the social consequences had not been so grave they might have been labeled hysterical or dissociative. However, hysterical episodes, and even hysterical psychoses, are typically attempts to manipulate society, and simple dissociations, including such pseudo-amok states as the Wild-Man syndrome in New Guinea [110], typically conform to socially established limits. With amok there is very rarely any evidence of an attempt to manipulate society, and although those who survived used to be regarded as heroes, the typical case is clearly seeking his own death rather that that title. As we have just seen, the Malay and Laotian male who was liable to run amok was the sort of person who would be liable to develop another type of acute reactive psychosis, but there is nothing in his situation or in the precipitating factors which would seem to conduce to this type of psychosis rather than something like *bouffée délirante* (which seems relatively infrequent in village Malays), apart from the fact that he belongs to one of these cultures. With reference to amok-like cases in New Guinea, Burton-Bradley has stated that the thinking behind the act probably runs as follows:

> I am not an important or 'big man', I possess only my sense of personal dignity. My life has been reduced to nothing by an intolerable insult. Therefore, I have nothing to lose except my life, which is nothing, so I trade my life for yours as your life is favoured. The exchange is in my favour, so I shall not only kill you, but I will kill many of you, and at the same time rehabilitate myself in the eyes of the group of which I am a member, even though I might be killed in the process [82].

That line of thinking, derived from interviews with persons who have committed homicide of this type, probably reflects something of what goes on at a less conscious level in the mind of the true amoker, even though the latter does not direct his attack against one set of people rather than another and has not suffered from what he consciously labels as an "intolerable insult." It is a line of thinking which we can easily classify as narcissistic, but we still have to explain why the result among the Malays and Laotians is amok rather than a more innocuous psychosis or drunken pseudo-amok which would give the subject a better chance of social rehabilitation.

Part of the probable explanation is historical. From the fifteenth to at least the eighteenth century European travellers describe amok as being an extreme but deliberate and socially useful way of reacting to unacceptable injury or insult, or to a lesser extent a way of seeking an "honorable death" in place of slow death by disease [427]. At that time the amoker avoided attacking persons he liked, he was not thought of as insane, and if he survived the event he was likely to be treated as a hero both in life and in legend. When European powers imposed relative peace and a new concept of justice in the region in the later eighteenth century, the social usefulness of the tradition (which had lain in making petty rulers afraid to be too arbitrary in their use of power, and in providing suicidal shock troops during battle) waned and what had previously been a conscious act became a dissociated or psychotic one, with claimed amnesia both for the event and for any desire to be aggressive; but the heroic legend remained and offered a model frequently acted on. In the 1840s that model received a severe blow from a British judge in the Straits Settlements (Malaya) who, in a widely publicized judgment, held up the amok tradition as evidence that the Malays were savages and not worthy to associate with civilized people; and from then on the rate in European-influenced territories dropped sharply while the cases that came to medical attention there increasingly exhibited signs of a more chronic psychosis. In Laos such a history is lacking, but elders report that cases did exist in the past and the people did have the more recent image of the heroic, self-sacrificing Montagnard guerilla fighting against the French during the present century.

A socially communicated model similar to those which teach "drunken comportment" [364] (see p 193) is therefore part of the explanation, and there can be an epidemic spread of amok just as of simple suicide. However, many societies have legends of self-sacrificing warriors without such a model being able to overcome man's general abhorrence of casual homicide, and the aggressive feelings referred to in the quotation from Burton-Bradley above are usually displaced intrapsychically or defused socially. Ajax hallucinated cattle to be the Greek princes and slaughtered the former in place of the latter. In parts of the Solomon Islands today one of the familiar ways in which a psychosis erupts is by a patient rushing around slashing down the fruit- and nut-bearing trees of all and sundry. In New Guinea itself, although the thinking described by Burton-Bradly results in homicide in some tribes, there are in other tribes various institutionalized forms of "Wild Man " behavior in which amok-like attacks of fury occur but where the public is amply warned and no real harm is done [110]. Why should such displacements not be employed by the Malays and Laotians?

On the Laotians we possess too little information to draw conclusions from, but the rich literature on Malay and Indonesian community life offers a variety of clues. In many subcultures within that culture realm, the individual is taught, from infancy, to divorce his behavior from his underlying feelings and to make the former conform to what is "proper" in the give social setting [210]. Moreover, there can be a very rigid separation of sex roles and a rigid code of conduct for males [102], something which in the sexual sphere can give rise to the neurosis called *koro* (see p 273). In some of these subcultures escape valves exist, for instance participation in the Balinese temple plays, but in others the only escape for repressed resentment in a male appears to have been going to raid en enemy, something which happened often enough at one time. Accordingly, chronic irritation tended to be bottled up until it either weakened or exploded. Moreover, when one considers the ways in which infants were trained to separate their behavior from their underlying feelings, one finds something relatively similar to what psychoanalytic theory would say is likely to lead to excessive narcissism [316]. The infant has been described as getting little feedback from adults to his attempts at self-expression; he is used as a puppet so that differentiation of self and other is impeded [36]; and the tantrums which this treatment regularly produces are then ignored, with no help being given the infant to handle his own rage. (The provoking of tantrums in children also occurs among the subcultures from which the Singapore Indians largely derive, and seems likely to contribute to their later psychopathology, but among them there is not the same insistence on separating feelings from behavior.)

If a clear relationship could be established between the tendency to use these interacting childrearing methods and the risk of amok, psychoanalytic theory with respect to the nature and origins of narcissistic rage would be given substantial backing, and we would also have a plausible explanation why this particular type of acute reactive psychosis arises mainly in these peoples. When ego and alter are insufficiently differentiated in infancy, any suicidal tendency in later life, particularly one arising from narcissistic rage, would seem likely to distinguish insufficiently between the killing of oneself and the killing of others. However, by the time that childrearing practices in different Malay subcultures came to be studied, amok had become rare among them, and we cannot say today whether the subcultures in which amok was commonest during the nineteenth century were ones in which the above-mentioned childrearing methods were common, or whether they had in fact a much more empathic parent-child relationship, such as that reported in the Singapore Malays [152]. Amok behavior does appear to fit, in more exaggerated form, the model which we have of narcissistic rage, and what has been stated regarding Malay training in propriety gives some indications why that rage should assume psychotic form, but the links in the etiological chain are still weak.

7 Conclusions

The material brought together in this chapter makes it clear that the acute reactive psychoses vary markedly from one society to another, and that this is not due simply to the wide variation in terminology. In fact, the material suggests that if a more uniform way of identifying and classifying these psychoses were arrived at, the international and crosscultural variation would be much more evident than it is at present, although some of the apparent crosscultural variations in schizophrenia (not the variations mainly stressed in the previous chapter) might thereby be reduced. We can regard the various acute psychotic syndromes – and there are many of these, as the historical review indicated – as essentially different diseases, some of which might be "culture bound," or we can regard most of them as essentially the same disease with a strong pathoplastic element. The choice depends partly on what we choose to regard as a "disease" in psychiatry, but if it depends also on the presence of common features then the present review, limited though it has been, suggests that we might be thinking of a single disease in various guises.

The common features are social, but in a certain way they can be considered as constituting a "ground" in the same sense as Magnan and his successors in the French school thought of there being a constitutional or inherited "ground" out of which various acute psychoses could spring. The first of the features is a tendency to dependency on others, and a second is separation from the community on which the dependency has focused, perhaps as simple a separation as marrying into a previously unknown family. The acute reactive psychoses are almost certainly rare in societies (including many Eskimo) which put a high emphasis on independence and individualism, but they are also probably rare in societies which promote dependency and interdependency, whether these have low rates of schizophrenia, like the Tongans and Hutterites discussed in the previous chapter, or whether they have high rates of that disorder as was the case with the traditional French-Canadian villages (see p 60), always assuming that members are not obliged to leave the communal shelter. The third common point relates to education. Broadly speaking, the more education an individual receives, the more he is likely to have some forewarning of what he will meet when he leaves his own community, and how he should cope with it. The groups in which relatively high rates of acute reactive psychosis seem to occur are all ones with very limited formal education, and if, as seem likely, there was a decline in the incidence of these psychoses in Europe and North America between the 1880s and 1930s, the rising standards of education could be one factor in this.

In contrast to these socially predisposing factors, the nature of the precipitating stress, the family history, and somatic influences all acquire less importance when one employs the Comparative Psychiatry approach. A person with congenital mental deficiency or under the influence of a drug such as cannabis will probably be more liable to develop an acute psychotic reaction when confronted with a disturbing experience than someone who has normal, unimpeded intelligence, but if that experience is met in the company of familiar others, the risk of such a reaction will be comparatively low, regardless of whether the intelligence is impeded or not. Coming from a Singapore Chinese family in which there is a history of psychosis increases the risk of developing a psychotic reaction during one's first puerperium, but is of less prognostic importance than being a recently arrived Indian who finds Singapore life still bewildering and whose parents are a thousand miles away. Finding signs that someone is attempting to bewitch one is more likely to result in a psychotic reaction than finding a thief in the house, but the former is also very unlikly to have any such result if one has been educated to be a true nonbeliever in witchcraft or if one's family is believed to possess strong countermagic.

When the Austrian Army data were examined, it was noted that education probably correlated inversely with the proportion of amentia cases seen, but directly with the proportion of neurotic ones, and it was later suggested that some of the acute reactive psychoses might arise from factors which in a more educated (or perhaps more individualistic) population would give rise to a neurosis or personality disorder. Moreover, it has been suggested that in Senegal and Guadeloupe, the attacks of *bouffée délirante* were sometimes an abandonment of ego control for the purpose of getting the milieu to take over control on behalf of the patient. It can be asked, therefore, whether these acute reactions deserve the title of psychosis, or whether they are not semi-conscious forms of ego defense against pressures from the id and the exterior. This question cannot be satisfactorily answered, since there are no sufficiently international and detailed criteria whereby to differentiate the psychoses from other abnormal mental states. More detailed investigations of these acute reactive psychoses in different societies would probably help us to arrive at a more satisfactory conceptualization of the meaning of the term psychosis than we have today, but a few remarks may not be out of place here.

When we come to consider suicide we will meet a type of case in which the simple division between true suicide and parasuicide breaks down, i.e., where the act would undoubtedly lead to death if other persons did not intervene, where a chance has been given for others to intervene, but where there remains a serious risk that they will not do so in time. The simplest way to interpret these cases is to assume that the act is the product of two forces or desires, one for death and the other for greater social integration, with the patient's final thinking being "if they are not concerned sufficiently about me to protect me from death, I do not wish to live." A similar compromise between different forces may apply with some of the acute reactive psychoses – "reality is too painful to face and I am withdrawing from it, but I will return to it if people make it less painful or if my self-esteem is sufficiently solaced." In the Indian Army, men unable to return home for certain important events would enter catatonic states with rocking and head-banging, states leading to chronic psychosis or to serious head injury if untreated but relieved very rapidly if ECT were given or if news were brought from the family that the return was not necessary [140]. Because chronic psychotic states can result, it would seem quite wrong to view such behavior as merely hysterical, but that does not mean that it cannot be manipulative. It is largely the jurists who have imposed on psychiatry the myth that each person can be regarded as being of a single mind which either is functioning, in which case that person is responsible for his acts, or nonfunctioning, in which case he is not held responsible but is (usually) labeled insane. We need to give more attention to the fact that a person can abdicate reponsibility for his own acts and own safety, and that societies can differ greatly both with respect to the internal obstacles to, and the external advantages of, such abdication. Becoming temporarily psychotic may, in terms of survival, be a reality-oriented act, and in some societies there are many more gradiations in the process than in others.

Chapter 6 The Affective Disorders

In the previous chapter, a major problem in attempting international comparisons was the large number of apparently discrete categories of acute psychosis which had received separate diagnostic labels in the past, categories which were often recognized only by particular national schools. In the present chapter an overabundance of psychiatric terms is no problem, since the terms melancholia, depression, and mania have a long and relatively stable history; but the opposite problem arises since the first two of these have been overinclusive and psychiatry is still not agreed on how to subdivide them in a logical fashion, while the differential diagnosis of mania depends greatly on precision of observation.

Depression (and its predecessor melancholia) can refer to a disorder, a symptom, or a mental state falling within the limits of the normal variation. As a disorder, moreover, it extends all the way from a psychotic state in which social functioning is completely abandoned to a reaction to loss which is only slightly greater than what is considered normal in the given society; and there are no agreed ways of subdividing that continuity. We have had divisions into two, three, four, or more categories of depressive disorder [299], but the way in which these have been applied have rarely been sufficiently consistent for it to be clear that the same criteria have been applied at two or more centers, or even at the same center, at different times. Also, since even quite severe depression may not give rise to much social disturbance, it is difficult to know what basis was operating in a given society at a given point in time to separate depressed patients given hospitalization (or outpatient treatment) from those that were not given it. It is even difficult to get a clear picture of what had constituted a "case" of depression in a community survey and thence to assess whether two such surveys are comparable in this regard.

For these reasons the present chapter will make little attempt to measure the incidence of any given degree of disorder, and will focus more on impressions, symptomatology, and ratios.

Viewed from one angle this can be taken as meaning that less is going to be claimed respecting differences in the frequency of the basic affective disorders and more attention paid to the pathoplastic elements of that disorder. Viewed from another angle it means exploring whether what is called depression in different societies is likely to have the same underlying psychopathology throughout, or whether different pathological processes might be involved. There appears no need to go into the history of the main terms which have been used to describe the affective states, since their meanings have been unusually stable and there are numerous papers on the ways in which these terms have been employed across the centuries. However, the very fact that the terms have so long a history means that it is possible to pick up variations which have lasted for decades, thus disposing of the possibility that they are temporary accidents. There are a couple of such examples worth nothing.

1 Historical Symptom Changes in Europe: The "English Malady"

In 1733, an Edinburgh-trained physician, George Cheyne, commenced a book entitled *The English Malady; or a Treatise of Nervous Diseases of all Kinds* with the statement that "The title I have chosen for this treatise is a reproach universally thrown on this island by foreigners, ... by whom nervous distempers, spleen, vapours and lowness of spirits are in derision called the English Malady. And I wish there were not so good grounds for this reflection ...[since] these nervous disorders being computed ... [affect] ... almost one third of the people of condition [i.e., the upper and middle classes] in England" [104]. As the title indicates, he is including "nervous diseases of all kinds" in these remarks; but it is clear from his later pages and case illustrations that after "what ought only to be called Vapours (if that name be proper at all) ...," the more serious and next most common category of mental disorder that he is referring to comprises a combination of psychosomatic complaints and "a deep and fixed melancholy, wandering and delusory images of the brain ..., loss of memory, despondency, horror and despair." In this second most common class of mental disorders, he noted also that there are "sometimes unaccountable fits of laughing, apparent joy, leaping and dancing; at other times crying, grief and anguish" [p 199]. It is fairly clear that it was mainly affective disorders that he was referring to, either depressive or circular, and there is corroborative evidence that people in continental Europe were calling this the *maladie anglaise* and thinking the English to be particularly prone to it.

Since melancholia was a condition well known to continental European physicians at this time and earlier, the only reasons why it should have been given the title of "English Malady" would seem to be either that it had genuinely become much more common among the English than among other European peoples, or that the form which it was taking among the English was somewhat different from that observed elsewhere. There is reason to think that both may have been true. On the one hand Hunter and Macalpine [271] state that melancholia had been particularly associated with the English since Elizabethan times; a physician called Blackmore wrote in the early eighteenth century that what he called the English "spleen" was seldom found in other lands [56]; and a statistical study has shown both suicide and lunacy to have increased in frequency in London at the beginning of the eighteenth century [582]. On the other hand there is rather striking evidence that it was during the seventeenth century, and in England, that there began the change which converted the predominantly somatic picture of medieval melancholia into the predominantly psychic picture of the disorder described by Kraepelin and his immediate successors.

That change is documented in two once very widely read texts: Burton's *The Anatomy of Melancholy* [81], which was first published in 1621 and which has remained a classic of English literature until the present day; and Baxter's *A Christian Directory* [37], which was published in 1673 and remained widely read until the beginning of the twentieth century, although now largely forgotten. Both authors were members of the clergy who had medical training or experience but who did not see medicine as claiming their prime allegiance. Both may have themselves been mildly affected by depression (as Cheyne was, more seriously) but a reading of their texts makes it clear that this had very little influence on the picture which they described. Burton drew on all the relevant medical texts of his time and earlier, so that from a medical angle he was a compiler or summarizer rather than an original observer, although his text was highly original. Baxter drew almost completely on his own experience, first as the only person with some medical knowledge in a rural district where he was a nonconformist minister for 10 years, and then as a church leader who had acquired a reputation for being able to help depressed persons and who in consequence received patients from all over the country. Both authors used very systematic ways of describing the syndromes which they were writing about, the first in a table and the second in a list of signs and symptoms ranked in order of frequency.

Tables 6.1 and 6.2 summarize these descriptions, and there are two main points which stand out when they are compared. The first is that whereas the earlier description shows melancholia to have had more somatic than psychological symptoms, the later suggests it to have almost exclusively psychological ones. The second point is that whereas the psychological symptoms described by Burton are of a very mixed

Table 6.1. Symptoms of melancholy according to Burton (1621), by subtype [81]

By type of disorder	*Symptoms in the body*		*Symptoms in the mind*	
Common to all types	Ill digestion Wind Hard belly Much walking Leaping (twitches) in many places	Crudity (undigested food) Dry brains Thick blood Heaviness of heart Palpitations	Fear without cause Suspicion Discontent Irksomeness Restless thoughts	Sorrow without cause Jealousy Solitariness Continual cogitations Vain imaginings
General melancholy	Black (swarthy) Broad veins Most part lean	Their hemrods commonly stopped (constipation with hemorrhoids)	Averse from company	Hates light
Hypochondriacal or windy melancholy	Rumbling in the guts Heat in the bowels Shortness of wind Sour belchings Cold sweat	Bellyache Suffocation Much spittle Singing in the ears	Troublesome Lascivious by reason of wind	Suspicious Anxiety Affected by fits
Head melancholy, (incl. love and religious melancholy)	Headache Heaviness Lightness High colour	Binding Vertigo Singing in the ears	Solicitude Anxiety Perpetual cogitation of such toys they are possessed of	Superfluous cares Thoughts like dreams

Table 6.2. Symptoms of melancholy according to Baxter (1673) [37]

Symptoms	
Common	Occasional
Exaggeration of fears and dangers (1, 2)	Ruminations (16)
Gloomy mood and frequent weeping (3)	Circularity and confusion of thought (18, 19)
Self-reproach regarding cheerfulness (3, 4)	Inaction; tendency to keep to bed (17)
Self-accusations (5)	Obsessive scruples, rituals, prohibitions (20, 21)
Despair regarding future salvation (6, 7, 8)	Accusatory hallucinations (25)
Identification with others' miseries (9)	Coprolalic and blasphemous urges (26)
Belief in the uniqueness of own case (10)	Intense guilt over blasphemies (27)
Rejection of comforting attention (11)	Delusions of demonic possesseion (28)
Conscience is punitive (12)	Hallucinations, visual (29)
Loss of religious beliefs and habits (13, 24)	Suicidal tendencies (30)
Peevishness and resentment (14)	Paranoid ideation (31)
Avoidance of company (15)	Mutism (32)
Inability to control own thoughts (22, 23)	Loss of insight (35)
	Relapses or intransigeance (33, 34)

The numbers in parentheses indicate the order in which Baxter placed the symptoms

and unfamiliar character, while lacking any real reference to self-accusations and exaggerated guilt feelings, those described by Baxter involve several aspects of self-accusation and are almost immediately familiar to the twentieth century clinician, even though he may think that they fit patients seen earlier in this century better than patients seen today. Elsewhere I have discussed in some detail how far these two authors can be taken as representing their respective times [434], and have concluded that the somatic emphasis and virtual absence of reference to exaggerated guilt feelings by Burton truly reflect the clinical descriptions of the previous 50 years, while the emergence of self-accusations and exaggerated guilt feelings which Baxter describes was also representative of his time, although his omission of somatic symptoms is probably due to the context in which he was writing and although the self-accusations were probably more common among members of his own moderately Protestant church than in members of either the anglo-catholic or the puritan wings of the religious spectrum. Clinicians such as Sydenham were still in Baxter's time reporting a form of melancholia closer to what Burton had described, but the picture was changing and in the eighteenth century the features on which the psychoanalytic school has put such emphasis during the twentieth century were coming to the fore in Britain. Cheyne, although retaining a quite medieval theory of the causation of melancholia – he saw it as due to "a glewiness, sizyness, viscidity and grossness in the fluids" [104, p 6] – states that during his own depressive illness, "I went about like a malefactor condemned, or one who expected every moment to be crushed by a ponderous instrument of death, hanging over his head" [p 327].

In the early eighteenth century, melancholia was increasingly being regarded by English physicians and laymen alike as a disorder of the mind with the somatic complaints being secondary. This can be seen in the passages quoted by Hunter and Macalpine [271], and was most probably due to symptoms having become predominanty psychological rather than somatic. In continental Europe at the same period, however, the symptomatology seems to have remained predominantly somatic. The anonymous author of the article on melancholia in Diderot's Encyclopedia stated that its origin is in the abdomen with the brain being only secondarily affected [586]; and although authors like the French Lorry [360] and the German Medicus [402] show some departure from the old humoral theories in the 1760s, it is toward the somatic nervous system that they turn rather than to more psychological concepts. It is not really until one gets to Pinel at the beginning of the nineteenth century that continental European physicians appear to have espoused a psychological view of the disorder, and by that time the term "English Malady" was virtually forgotten, presumably because the condition was no longer affecting the English more than other peoples.

Why should there have been an association between English society and depression at this time and why, also, should there have been the change in symptomatology which is illustrated in the lists from Burton and Baxter and which was later to spread through most of Europe? If one assumes that the period during which the English had an excess of this disorder extended from Elizabethean times until about 1750, then one finds oneself in precisely the location and period which historians and sociologists have identified as the most important for the rise of Capitalism and the birth of the Industrial Revolution. Moreover, the author who gives us the first real picture of the symptom change, Baxter, is also one whom Max Weber regularly cites as an authority and a leader in the matter of the changed attitudes of Christianity towards the accumulation of capital and the striving for success within this world [646]. It would seem a reasonable working hypothesis, therefore, to suspect that there could be a connection between the forces in English society which contributed to the rise of capitalism, and those which contributed to the changed character and frequency of melancholia. Taking current theories regarding the etiology of affective disorders into account, there are three such forces or movements which come to mind. The first is Protestantism, bringing not just the new attitude towards personal striving which Weber highlights, but a new, more awesome and potentially guilt-ridden relationship between man and God. The second is the change in childrearing patterns which Philippe Ariès described [22], leading not just to a greater emphasis on the molding of the future adult but to a more consistent parent-child relationship. The third is the marked increase in geographic mobility and elective economic individualism, resulting in a reduction of close social ties and hence of sources of emotional support, something which can be akin to bereavement.

Each of these changes or forces seems unlikely, by itself, to have produced both the increase in melancholia and the shift in symptomatology with which we are concerned, but in combination they might have had such an effect. Both an increased fear of an all-seeing God and a shift to a more consistent parent-child relationship (with its greater potential for superego formation) appear capable of producing symptoms of guilt, but the timing and location do not harmonize well with the clinical change, seventeenth century England being less affected than sixteenth century Geneva and Edinburgh by preoccupations regarding man's relation to God, and no more affected than France by the new moral ideas regarding children's education. Geographic mobility was recognized shortly after that time to be associated with a pathological form of nostalgic mourning for their native communities on the part of Swiss soldiers who hired themselves out to foreign powers [23]; and we have had ample further evidence that people from rural communities moving to the city tend to develop depressions, for instance the case of Peruvian Indians moving to Lima [206]. But in most instances such depression is not accompanied by delusions of guilt. A fourth factor which could have affected the symptomatology at that time but was unconnected with capitalism is the spread of Cartesian ideas regarding body-mind dualism, since this made it increasingly difficult to attribute spiritual or mental anguish to bodily causes and led people to look within their minds rather than within their bodies for the causes of their melancholy.

There are therefore a number of interesting pointers to possible connections between affective disturbance and sociocultural forces in that history, but no one cause to which the changes in frequency and symptomatology of depression can be attributed.

2 High Incidence Rates: European Jewry, 1895–1930

For the second historical example we must pass to the beginning of the present century. By the end of the eighteenth century the English had lost their reputation for being particularly prone to melancholia, and in the nineteenth century, when the Danes acquired a reputation of this [46], it seems to have been only temporary and the result of a political reverse. By the end of the century, however, manic-depressive insanity was being associated, along with some lesser mental disorders, with the Jewish culture and political situation. Already by 1858 it had been noted that around what was then Königsberg in eastern Germany, the Jews had four times as many patients in mental asylum as Catholics or Protestants had [135], in proportion to the population; but it was also recognized that the Jews tended to live predominantly in towns, and that the urban/rural difference in rates was still greater than the religious difference, so that these figures did not necessarily mean that Jews had a higher vulnerability. However, by 1901, Fishberg in New York [194], Pilcz in Vienna [495], and others had been collecting statistics from a number of sources suggesting that Jews must have an excessive vulnerability to mental disorders in general, despite their virtual immunity to those associated with alcohol, and Pilcz stated that his attention had first been drawn to the fact when he was studying periodic (manic-depressive) psychoses. Over the next 30 years there then appeared – according to Becker who compiled a most helpful bibliography on the subject [42] – over 150 articles on various aspects of Jewish mental health, most of them indicating this people to have an excess of mental disorder when compared with the populations around them. A part of this excess was certainly due to their being more urban, and probably a further part to their being a minority, since in New York at that time the Jewish mental hospitalization rate, although higher than that of native Americans, was lower than those of other immigrant groups with smaller populations [581]. But when one looks at specific diagnoses within the European reports, it is principally manic-depressive psychosis which shows the greatest excess of Jewish rates.

Table 6.3 summarizes findings from the three most detailed studies of the subject in the first part of this century, each representing a different country and a different relationship of psychiatric services to population. The Frankfurt data concern an ur-

Table 6.3. Manic-depressive psychosis in Jews and Non-Jews: Vienna, Frankfurt, and Poland

	Populations		Rates				Ratio	
	Jews	Non-Jews	Jews		Non-Jews		Jews/Non-Jews	
Diagnostic Category			MDP	Other	MDP	Other	MDP	Other
Source	('000s)							
A. University Psychiatric Clinic, Vienna, 1898–1901 [495]	146	1502	1.3	7.8	0.56	8.1	2.3	0.96
B. Frankfurt City Asylum, 1897–1907, (annual mean) [567]	22.4	278	37	144	10.6	180	3.5	0.8
C. Poland (47 Hospitals and Mental Asylums), 1929 [41]	2968	27 440	7.2	75.5	1.6	27.6	4.5	2.7

Admission rates per 100 000 total population. In Vienna the University Clinic only provided a relatively small part of the total psychiatric care, which accounts for the low rates for all categories there, and the figures given for manic-depressive psychosis (MDP) comprise the combined rates for depression, mania, and periodic psychosis in the original table. The Frankfurt Asylum took some cases from the surrounding region, so that the populations are an underestimate. In Poland the population figures refer to the whole country, but it is clear that some parts, notably in the east, hospitalized almost no mental patients.

ban population which was relatively well served, the Polish data draw from both urban and rural sectors and represent a lower ratio of services to population, while the Vienna University clinic drew disproportionately from the middle classes. In the last two columns of the table one sees that the ratio of Jewish to non-Jewish rates of manic-depressive psychosis is consistently above the theoretically expected unity, while the same is not true respecting other admissions. A similar excess of affective disorders can be inferred to have been occurring among Amsterdam Jews between the two World Wars, if one combines information on incidence from one source [321] with information on diagnostic distribution from another [232].

These ratios do not by themselves necessarily indicate that Jews had a greater vulnerability to manic-depressive psychoses than the surrounding peoples at that time; they may merely indicate that the Jews were readier to arrange for persons with the milder varieties of such conditions to be hospitalized, and although that seems unlikely in view of their unexceptional admission rates for other mental disorders, one must remember that the rarity of alcoholic psychoses in Jews distorts the latter picture. Fortunately, there are two papers providing clinical details on the manic-depressive psychoses in Jews, one based on a survey of case records from 1855 to 1940 [267] and the other on direct observation [333], both from Germany.In these we learn that the Jewish disorders tended to commence earlier in life, to be more profound, and to last longer than their equivalents in non-Jewish patients, almost half requiring over 12 months stay in hospital. Agitated depression and the circular type were commoner than simple depression, while the "benumbed" (erstärrte) melancholia was uncommon but there was also considerably more somatic or hypochondriac symptomatology. Presumably, therefore, the hospitalized Jewish cases were at least as severe as the non-Jewish ones, and the higher incidence in the Jews can be taken as geniune.

Why should this be? A genetic factor is made unlikely by the fact that in New York, Jews of the same stock did not have higher rates of hospitalization for manic-depressive psychosis than other immigrants in the 1920s [372] and 1950s [375], although they did have an excess of cases during the years 1939-1941, an extremely stressful period for them [374]. A cultural factor extending far into the Hebrew tradition itself is made unlikely by the same token, and because Grewel has claimed that when the Ashkenazim in Amsterdam were showing an excess of affective disorders, the Sephardim were not [232].

Turning to the social situation of this people at that time, the most obvious hypothesis is that the excess of affective disorders represented severe grief reactions in persons who had lost relatives in the Russian pogroms or similar antisemitic uprisings. However, one would have expected the case illustrations provided by the psychiatrists at that time to have mentioned this fact, which is not the case in the papers I have read, and one would also have expected a decline in the frequency of melancholia among the Jews over the nineteenth century, accompanying the decline in attacks on Jews, whereas the literature tells of an increase which one writer [472] classifies as marked. Although antisemitism almost certainly contributed to the development of affective disorders in European Jews during the period under discussion, therefore, it seems likely that other factors were also involved. When one looks for such other factors, that which comes most readily to view has striking similarities to one which we were considering in relation to the "English Malady." This is geographic mobility and the severance of earlier communal ties.

Prior to Napoleon, most European Jews lived in urban or rural enclaves where they had their own elders through whom the Christian rulers operated; and they had no civil rights in the wider Christian society. Napoleon made them common citizens of the lands he conquered, and although his laws were overturned after his retreat, the European Jew was invited to become a second-class citizen of the society in which he lived rather than a foreign body, and there was a massive migration of Jews from the ghetto and the shtetl into the wider urban community. For instance, Jews increased from 18% to 35% of the Warsaw population between 1830 and 1880; they came to comprise over half of the population of a number of other large Polish centers over the same period; and they became involved in national politics as never before. After 1870 this elicited a gradually increasing reaction from German and Polish nationalists, but before and during that reaction we can infer that in the process of mixing with the Christians and freethinkers the Jews were losing the communal warmth and supportiveness to which they had become accustomed within their enclaves. It has been argued that European Jewish culture, in the centuries of ghetto and shtetl life, became overprotective as a compensation for the long history of persecution, and that its members became overdependent [541]. Whether that is true or not, it seems almost certain that the individual Jew who left the ghetto or shtetl for wider citizenship at that time was reducing his sources of emotional support, and that he could therefore be expected to be more vulnerable to the rejection and ostracism from his Christian neighbors which the new nationalisms promoted, than were people who had not known the protection of ghetto life or had never left it.

3 Recent Hospitalization Rates: Subcultures in England and Mauritius

The two examples employed so far in this chapter have the advantage of relating to a whole generation or more, so that – as with some of the data on high schizophrenia rates – one can be reasonably confident that one is dealing with more than just an incidental or minor phenomenon. However, it can be objected that the condition which the seventeenth century English and the pre-1935 Jews suffered from is not necessarily the same as that which we call depression today, so that these examples are of doubtful relevance to present needs. More recent pictures, which are easy to find but not so easy to interpret, thus need to be examined. We will for the present stick to hospitalization data, since these presumably still reflect a certain uniformity of admission criteria, but at the end of the chapter we will examine some results from community surveys.

Figure 6.1 represents a range of rates from England and Wales which have the disadvantage of referring mainly to immigrants who may not be representative of their societies of origin, but they provide the challenge of apparently conflicting with what was said earlier here regarding the link between affective disorder and migration. It was stated above that migrants tend to be more vulnerable to such disorder than nonmigrants, owing to having recently suffered separation from sources of support, and it would seem to follow that recent migrants should suffer more in this

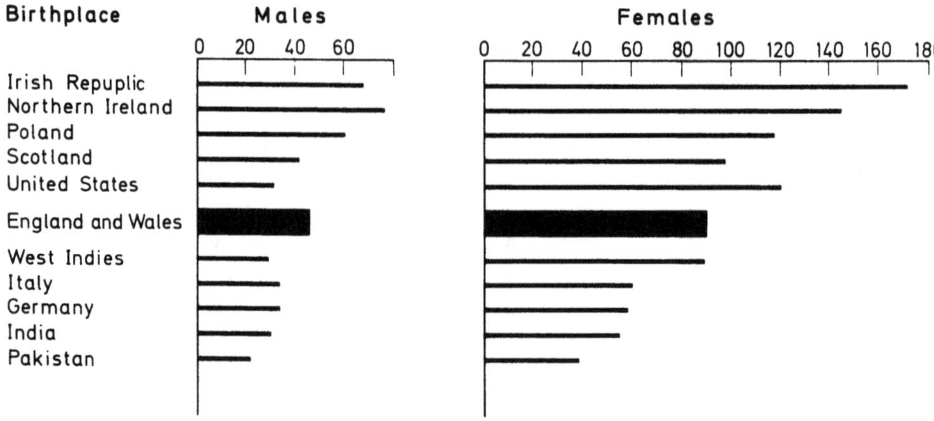

Fig. 6.1. Rates of admission for manic-depressive psychosis and involutional melancholia to mental hospitals in England and Wales in 1971, by country of birth and by sex. Rates are per 100 000 aged 15+ [112]

fashion than persons long established in the society, and foreigners more than those linked to it. However, the groups with the highest rates in this figure either are closely allied to the English in terms of culture or, in the case of the Poles, had been in the country for many years, whereas the groups with the lowest rates had relatively few of their members more than 10 years in the country, and their cultural backgrounds were usually very different from that of the English.

The figure relates to patients given a diagnosis of manic-depressive or involutional psychosis, but not to those diagnosed as depressive neurosis or as simple depression, which in any case would be likely to be treated on an outpatient basis rather than in hospital in the 1970s. A partial explanation for the more recent immigrant groups having the lower rates in this figure, therefore, could be that the strains and isolation of migration conduce to a reactive, nonpsychotic, depression and that the true manic-depressive psychoses are unaffected by the migrational experience. That, with its implication that these psychoses are unaffected by environmental factors generally, would be a valuable finding if it were proven true, but unfortunately the broader picture suggests a different explanation. Fully aware that the Asian immigrants might avoid mental hospitalization, Cochrane and his colleagues explored their mental health by a community survey and other methods [113, 114], and discovered that the group as a whole had not just a low rate of psychoses but a low rate of minor mental disturbance, with fewer depressive symptoms than their British neighbors. The low rate of manic-depressive psychosis thus proves to go hand-in-hand with a low rate of minor depressive symptomatology rather than being independent of the latter as was hypothesized above, and another reason for the Asian immigrants' few hospitalizations must therefore be found.

Let us set aside for the moment the possible reasons for this apparent immunity on the part of the Asian immigrants, and look at the manic-depressive psychoses in other groups in the figure. Do the Irish and Poles with significantly higher-than-average rates and the Italians and Germans with significantly lower-than-average ones in

Britain have above- and below-average rates elsewhere? In Canada, the Italian- and the German-origin sections of the population do have significantly below-average rates for the manic-depressive psychoses [435, 440], while the Polish origin have above-average ones (own data). However, the Irish-Canadians have manic-depressive rates which are slightly below average, which is out of harmony with Fig. 6.1; and since these psychoses only comprised 2.3% of mental hospital admissions in Poland itself during the 1960s [273], it seems likely that the true incidence rate among nonmigrating Poles must be relatively low. In Northern Ireland and the Republic of Ireland, admissions classified within the broad manic-depressive psychoses category run at a much higher rate then Fig 6.1 indicates, and one may guess that they are truly higher, but since a diagnosis of simple depression leads to classification with the psychoses in the Republic but with "other disorders" in England a direct comparison is impossible.

It does not seem to be justifiable to argue for a particular cultural factor with respect to the German, Italian, and Polish groups included in Fig. 6.1, since selective factors had been at work. The German and Italian migrants to Britain are mostly people interested in seeing more of the world, and they can easily return to their homelands on feeling depressed, so that they are only likely to stay if they are comfortable. The Polish immigrants, on the other hand, were largely people who did not feel themselves able to return to Poland, and who often thought of themselves as exiles. With the Irish the matter is somewhat different, since the homeland rates are probably at least as high as those among their emigrants, and since if they were beginning to suffer from a pathological nostalgia it would have been extremely easy for them to return to their native communities.

Although Irish susceptibility to affective disorders has been recognized, it has not received the attention which has been given their susceptibilities to schizophrenia and alcoholism. Explanations for the former are therefore largely lacking. If one reads descriptions of Irish life such as those by the anthropologists Brody [73], Messenger [407], and Scheper-Hughes [538], one gets the impression that the rural Irish child (other than the favorite son) receives a relatively cold upbringing, such as would – according to psychoanalytic theory – predispose to regression; and on the other hand he is not taught self-sufficiency; so that this might be one factor. Another potential factor is the guilt-laden character of Irish Catholicism [231]. The distribution of affective disorders in the Republic of Ireland is not the same as that of schizophrenia, being less in the west where schizophrenia is most frequent, and more in the southeast where this brand of Roman Catholicism has tended to be strongest. The fact that in Canada the rate of manic-depressive admissions is relatively low could be accounted for, within the same argument, by the greater emphasis which all subcultures there need to place on self-sufficiency. However, the character of depression among the Irish needs more study before one can develop justifiable theories to explain it.

Returning to the low rates of affective psychoses and symptomatology among the Asian immigrants to Britain, the three most obvious reasons for this occurring are that (a) they come from races and cultures resistant to affective disorder; (b) they could have undergone positive selection during the process of deciding to emigrate; and (c) they could still be in the state of temporary euphoria which is known to affect most recent immigrants. None of these reasons appears plausible on closer examination. The first is unlikely in view of the high rates of affective mental disorders among the Singapore Indians, both Hindu and Moslem (see p 139); the third unlikely in view of the fact that migrant euphoria rarely lasts more than a few months [624]; and although the possibility of positive selection must be kept in mind it is diminished by the fact that from some villages in Pakistan almost every able-bodied man seems to have taken part in the move [305], with the families following. A fourth possibility is that under harsh homeland conditions these people have been trained to withstand emotional deprivation and loss, and have found conditions in Britain not more depriving but more supportive, due to the financial gains and to settlement in groups. While it is generally true that emotionally supportive ties are stronger in small rural communities, even in poor countries, than in urban conglomerates, one must not romanticize village life or forget that where basic necessities are lacking, villagers may be forced to compete fiercely against neighbors and even against members of their own families. This has recently been described from India [262]; it has already been implied as having existed in Ireland; and we will see that it applies in Mexico. Moreover, even when there has been a loss of emotional support for the Asian immigrant, he may still receive relatively more of this than the average British native and European immigrant do, because of the latters' much greater tendency to strive for individualism and independence, and hence to abandon social ties.

The last remarks are mere conjecture and the paradox of the low rates of affective disorder in the Asian immigrants to Britain is not likely to be resolved until the mental health of the families and neighbors whom they left behind has also been assessed. However, to bring a little more light on the subject and particularly on the apparent contradiction between these low rates and the high rates which Indian immigrants exhibited in comparison with other Asian peoples in Singapore, it may be helpful to look at another situation in which peoples of Indian origin can be compared with others, this time in a generation which is not immigrant.

Figure 6.2 gives the rates of first admission for affective disorders to the sole mental hospital serving Mauritius, an island whose population derives in the most part from India several generations ago, but which has also a large, predominantly urban, Christian minority of mainly African origin. The rates in this figure are not comparable with those in the last, in the first place because they concern first admissions rather than total, and in the second place because the strict distinction between manic-depressive psychosis and unspecified depression was not employed in Mauritius. However, some comparison is possible with the Republic of Ireland and Northern Ireland, where this distinction was not as strict, and the adult first admission rates for affective disorders in these three territories in 1971–1972 prove to be as follows:

	Males	Females	Total
Mauritius (all ethnic groups)	75	73	74
Republic of Ireland	62	96	79
Northern Ireland	48	80	64

Although one always has problems in attempting to compare admission rates from different countries, and although this comparison is not really just since Mauritius

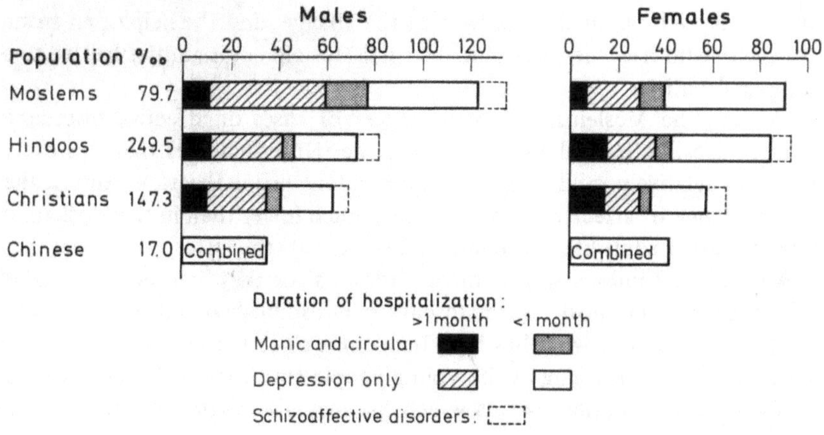

Fig. 6.2. Affective hospitalizations in Mauritius. Incidence of first admissions for affective disorders in four cultural groups, 1972; for two categories of disorder and two lengths of hospitalization (own data, unpublished). Rates are per 100 000 aged 15+, with extensions indicating how far they would increase if schizoaffective psychoses were included. Duration of hospitalization includes all periods of readmission during the 5 years subsequent to first entry. Significance levels of differences between rates for total first admissions with affective disorders, both sexes combined, are: Moslem-Hindoo, 0.05; Moslem-Christian, 0.01; Hindoo-Christian, 0.05; and Moslem-Chinese, 0.01. When only patients requiring more than 30 days in hospital are considered, the differences are all within chance range

had fewer outpatient services than Ireland did, these data at least dispose of the idea that Indians might have an unusual resistance to affective disorders, for either genetic or cultural reasons. Following up one argument offered earlier to explain the low Indian and Pakistani rates in Britain, it should be pointed out that Mauritius in 1972 was poor, with much unemployment and with a per capita GNP of only $300 compared to $1580 for the Republic of Ireland and $2600 for Great Britain, so that its inhabitants might also have found Britain relatively comfortable and supportive if they had gone there. However, Fig. 6.2 is offered less for the purpose of comparison with Britain than for the internal comparisons which it offers. There are three main points of interest in this figure, namely that the male rates are as high as the female, that the Hindoos (local spelling) and Moslems who are mainly rural have rates exceeding those of the Christians who are mainly urban, and that the Moslem males have an overall rate considerably higher than that of the Hindoos. The first of these points will be discussed in the next section but the other two can appropriately be discussed now.

In a previous analysis of Mauritian mental hospitalizations for the year 1956 [506], the Christians had rates significantly higher than the Hindoos and Moslems, while the two latter where insignificantly different in this respect. This was no surprise to us, since the Christians had a less cohesive family structure and their members were more liable to belong to broken families. The marked increase in Moslem as compared to Hindoo rates by 1972 was a surprise, however, and the deterioration of the latter as compared to the Christian rates was puzzling. Analysis of the data by age and by district has shed some light in the change, and the help of an anthropologist colleague who had been studying the rural Moslem communities has led to some possible explanations.

Among the Moslems, the main excess of cases of affective disorder occurs in young males, both rural and urban, and the figure indicates that this excess is comprised of relatively mild cases not requiring long hospitalization. Among the Hindoos the incidence of affective disorder is still much lower than in the Moslems and Christians in earlier adult life, but considerably exceeds the latter's rate from the age of 45 onwards. The Hindoos are the most traditional of the three peoples, and in the past have accorded the most respect to culturally established status, including the status attached to age; but what has been happening since the 1950s is that this respect for status has been declining as the young people find that their elders cannot provide them with the material rewards which the media advertize. It thus seems not unreasonable to link the relative increase in affective disorder among the older Hindoos since 1956 to the fact that the young are not according them the respect and support they had looked forward to. The Moslems probably confronted this problem earlier, by reason of being a minority, and after some physical confrontations during which their minority status was made very clear to them they seem to have turned to a more constructive form of competition with the other subcultures and among themselves. In the rural areas there is rivalry among them to see who can build the best house, reap the best crops, and place a son in the best urban employment, whereas this is still largely absent among the Hindoos. The impression is that this rivalry is reducing the camaraderie to which they had been accustomed, and forcing the young men to abandon previous friendships, but that recovery from any resultant depression is rapid and new alliances are formed. If this impression is true and if it has any bearing on the frequency of affective psychoses, this could be a situation analogous to that which was discussed respecting the seventeenth century English.

4 Sex Ratios: Mauritians, West Indians, and French-Canadians

The third main feature of Fig. 6.2 is the slight excess of male over female rates, something which is almost never met among Western societies where the male rate for affective disorders may be only half as great as the female one. Does this mean that the sex ratio for such disorders depends wholly on sociocultural factors rather than on something more fundamental?

Probably not. Among patients coming into care in India, both in hospital and private practice, a similar excess of male over female cases has been reported [553], but the picture is reversed when community surveys are undertaken. The most likely explanation in both locations is that in this cultural tradition, medical care for a male is sought more rapidly than medical care for a female since the family's survival is thought – rightly or wrongly – to depend on the man's labor so that impairment of his health is seen as more of a threat to that survival than impairment of the woman's health. (In Western societies where medical attention is sought for lesser health problems, the reverse tends to be the case, with women going more quickly to the doctor than men do, even when both have employment outside the home [259].)

Among the Mauritian Christians the attitude towards medical care for each sex is less clear cut, and it is possible the the incidence of affective disorder in men and women is relatively similar, but in view of data from other societies I am not prepared to claim that there is a true excess of male cases in that population,

When surveys have been done in representative community or general medical populations, women always seem to report more depressive symptoms than men do, even in societies which do not use alcohol. (Where alcohol is consumed, males tend more than females to use it as a mask or defense when depressed.) The male rate can come close to the female one, as among the Serer of Senegal [45] or among social welfare recipients in some Western societies, but it never seems to significantly exceed the latter and hence one has here, in my opinion, an example of a predominantly biological effect. For Western societies it has been argued that such an effect could also arise from the different types of relationship which boys and girls have with their opposite-sex parents [352], but if this were the primary influence I would have expected to find somewhere a society in which childrearing patterns were sufficiently different for the sex ratio of affective disorders to be reversed, and that I have not found. Accordingly, when international and crosscultural differences in the affective disorders are being considered, a probable biological factor influencing the sex ratio must always be kept in mind, and it is something which seems to relate to the minor symptoms of depression as much as or more than to the manic-depressive psychoses.

The fact that there is probably a biological basis for the sex differential in this group of disorders does not mean, however, that that ratio cannot vary in association with sociocultural factors. One can see an example of such variation in Fig. 6.1, where the female rates in the West Indians and the United-States-born are over three times the male ones, while among the Germans, Italians, Indians, and Pakistani the female rates are less than twice the male. These are not just chance differences. There is adequate evidence that the stresses on West Indian women and the types of affective disorders which they produce in Britain are considerably different from those affecting the Pakistani women there [357, 113]. Moreover, this difference is equally clearly linked to their culturally based life patterns, since the West Indian woman is much more likely than the Indian or Pakistani one, whether in Britain or in the homeland, to be self supporting and either living alone or supporting children whose fathers have disappeared, these children sometimes being left with a grandmother while the mother seeks employment elsewhere, something almost unknown among East Indians.

Another example, but more interesting for the way in which a male rate almost reaches the level of the female one, can be found in Canada. There the M/F ratio for manic-depressive psychoses (setting aside the depressive neuroses) first admitted to hospital in 1961 was 2/3, but in the Prairie Provinces the rates for French Canadians were 28 and 29 per 100 000 adult males and females respectively, a significant difference from the average ratio. The most probable reason for this is that a substantial minority of the French Canadian male population in these provinces consisted of men who had moved west in search of work while leaving their family and friends in Quebec. The French-Canadian female population in the same provinces contained few women who moved independently in this fashion, but a substantial minority who married men from another subculture or who joined their husbands after the latter found work. The French-Canadian male migrating in search of work is no more isolated than his counterparts from other Canadian subcultures, but his attachment to his home community and his vulnerability to isolation appear considerable greater, for cultural reasons, and this is the most likely explanation for the unusual M/F ratio.

5 Ratio of Depression to Mania: South Africa, New Zealand, and Fiji

Another ratio of considerable theoretical interest with respect to the affective disorders, but one which has received surprisingly little attention, is the ratio of depressive to manic or mixed states. Psychiatric theory has at times viewed mania as something quite distinct from depression, as a state which alternates with depression by reason of certain neurobiochemical processes, and as a psychological defense against depressive feelings without any biochemical change being involved. Accordingly, one might have expected more writing on the question of how frequently mania replaces depression or appears in its absense, than is actually to be found. The main reason for the neglect of this ratio is presumably a distrust of diagnostic consistency in these disorders, a distrust which applies not just to depression, as was discussed earlier, but to mania as well, as the US/UK Diagnostic Project [123] has proven justified. (The staff psychiatrists at two United States hospitals had assigned the diagnosis of "manic-depressive psychosis, manic type" to only 2 of the 28 patients so diagnosed by the – largely British trained – research team.) International differences in the ratio of depressive to manic or mixed affective psychosis (D/M ratio) are easy to find, for instance among the nonschizophrenic cases recorded in the WHO's IPSS project [674]. In that, Moscow reported only one case of manic depressive psychosis, manic type (296.1) as compared with ten of the depressed type (296.2), whereas Agra (India) reported 20 cases of the former to five of the latter. But the diagnostic uncertainties require us here, as with previous questions, to ignore such wide international variations and look for comparative data stemming from single psychiatric services in which there is likely to have been reasonable uniformity of diagnostic approach. We have just been considering one such set of data, since the D/M ratio in Mauritian Moslem female patients was over 7/1 whereas in Christian female patients it was only about 2/1. However, on the male side the range of D/M ratios is considerably narrower and more extreme examples affecting both sexes are preferable. Instances where the rate of depression very greatly exceeds that of the manic and mixed states are difficult to find, since under these conditions statistical reports usually combine all under a single heading, so that only informal information is available. Where the D/M ratio is close to or below unity, however, quantitative differentiation is commoner.

One quite striking example of a difference in D/M ratios comes from South Africa and a lesser one can be found in Fiji, each example overlapping culturally the Mauritian comparisons just discussed, since there is a certain similarity of background between the Mauritian Christians and the "Cape Coloured" of South Africa, and since in Fiji a majority of the population, as in Mauritius, derives from India, their ancestors having been brought there at about the same time as the migration to Mauritius and for the same purpose, to work in the cane fields.

In South Africa, although psychiatric services to the Bantu population are very different from those provided the Whites, so that a comparison between the two which depends on cases coming into care makes little sense, the "Cape Coloured" theoretically have the same access to mental hospital as the Whites do, and have very similar (nonprivate) mental hospitalization rates after the rural-urban distribution and age structure are taken into consideration [331]. The "Cape Coloured" are people of mixed European and African origin, of lower social status than the Whites and lacking some of the latters' legal privileges, but they possesses considerably more privileges than the Bantu and this cuts them off from the traditional healers which the latter have continued to make much use of. Table 6.4 indicates the numbers of cases of affective disorder admitted to one psychiatric hospital during 1944–1946, with a more detailed diagnostic breakdown of the 88% of such patients remaining in hospital more than 8 months. (It is clear that only the most severe mental disorders were sent to mental hospital at this time, as was true in a number of other countries, and the author presumably felt that those who stayed in hospital more briefly were under observation too short a time to justify stating whether their condition was what we would today call unipolar or bipolar.) Diagnoses were made retrospectively, with the later course of illness taken into account.

What is striking about this table is that no "Cape Coloured" patient admitted under the age of about 45 (i.e., the involutional period) and kept under hospital observation for at least 8 months had either a simple depressive psychosis or a manic state which shifted into the depressive phase later, whereas there were 22 "Cape Coloured" patients who entered hospital with a manic psychosis and remained manic for 8 months or longer without showing a shift into depression, and 32 White patients who developed a depressive or mixed psychosis in the same hospital over the same period. In the involutional stage, the "Cape Coloured" did produce cases of melancholia, as the table indicates, but even here the author tells us that these disorders were always of the agitated variety, and never showed the psychomotor retardation which was relatively common in the White involutional melancholias at the same hospital.

Table 6.4. Cases of manic, depressive, and mixed affective psychosis in White and "Cape Coloured" patients, South Africa [331, 332]

		White		"Cape Coloured"	
Estimated population aged 20+ at risk	Urban	84 000		99 000	
	Rural	250 000		217 000	
Cases of affective disorder admitted 1944–1946		72		36	
Studied cases with more than 8 months in hospital		68		27	
Involutional melancholia		18	(26%)	5	(19%)
Depression only		12	(18%)	0	
Mixed manic-depressive		20	(29%)	0	
Manic only		18	(26%)	22	(81%)
Males			(29%)		(19%)
Females			(71%)		(81%)

The low D/M ratio in the "Cape Coloured" echoes in much more emphatic fashion the relatively low ratio in the Mauritian Christians, but it could in part have arisen from the former having a tradition of keeping even severely depressed persons at home. It is fortunate, therefore, that we also possess the results of a community mental health survey carried out among the "Cape Coloured" [220]. No case of manic-depressive psychosis appears to have been uncovered among the 500 adults surveyed but the interview, based on that employed in the Stirling County survey, did elicit at least one depressive symptom from 12% of the sample, and this can be compared with the 7% reporting such symptoms in Stirling County itself and the 29% in the corresponding Nigerian survey (see Table 3.5). This indicates that the "Cape Coloured" are prepared to recognize and report depressive symptoms in themselves, something which might not have been the case. However, since this population was very aware of their disadvantaged status in comparison with persons of equivalent education in other African countries and among the South African Whites, by the time of that survey, it appears to me that 12% is a low figure and that this people must be quite resistant to depression. The interview was not such as enabled the researchers to assess the frequency of hypomanic symptoms, and hence we cannot judge on the basis of that survey whether this people have a tendency to employ a manic or hypomanic defense against feeling depressed; but it does seem likely that they have a genuinely low D/M ratio, at least until the involutional period.

The last qualification was prompted by the fact that the "Cape Coloured" did hospitalize 5 cases of involutional melancholia, something which raises the question whether in discussing the D/M ratio we should confine ourselves to disorders commencing at an earlier age and treat the involutional melancholias as a separate diagnostic entity. Mania developing first after the age of 45 is regarded as rare [607], and it would seem of some theoretical significance to know whether in peoples prone to manic states in early life, depression increases and mania declines in the involutional age.

There are data from New Zealand which seem to answer that question. The New Zealand Maori in the 1960s had mental hospitalization rates relatively similar to those of the rest of the population, being higher for schizophrenia but lower for the psychoneuroses and disorders of old age [463]. When the ratio of depressive to manic and circular psychoses is calculated in three age groups for each people, the results are:

Age groups	10–29	30–49	50+
Maori	1.13	1.10	1.09
Other New Zealanders	3.55	4.65	7.71

While the D/M ratio varies markedly for the rest of the population, therefore, it does not shift significantly within the Maori, and age can thus not be assumed to alter the relation of mania to depression.

The final point which I wish to make regarding the D/M ratio concerns education. It is a common observation that that ratio increases with increasing education (perhaps as a result of greater self-criticism) so that, for instance, manic outbursts are more commonly expected from lower-class than from middle-class patients in most

Western societies. In the illustrations just cited, the groups with a higher D/M ratio in New Zealand and South Africa had also the higher mean level of education, and although that is not true with respect to the Moslem and Christian women in Mauritius, we might doubt whether the latter observation should be given weight since on the male side the D/M ratios in Mauritius do not significantly differ. Therefore, the question arises whether crosscultural differences in D/M ratios are anything more than a reflection of educational level, and this question is of some theoretical significance since if education were a major factor, this would argue strongly for a psychological or interactional explanation of the D/M ratio as opposed to a purely biochemical one. Can we find a marked difference in D/M ratios which is not linked to education?

An example is available from Fiji. There, where approximately half the population is of East Indian origin and most of the remainder derive from Melanesian or Polynesian stock, there is only a negligible difference between the mean educational levels of these two moieties and they have almost identical hospital admission rates for total psychiatric disorder. However, while the East Indians sent slightly more cases of depression than mania to the sole mental hospital in the country during the years 1972–1975, the remainder of the population hospitalized only one case of depression for every four showing a manic or mixed state [442]. (There was also a psychiatric outpatient service for the never-hospitalized to which the milder depressions could be referred, something which probably explains the overall difference in D/M ratios between Fiji and Mauritius hospital admissions.) Moreover, this D/M difference between the Indians and the rest of the Fiji population is echoed in the suicide and crime statistics, for the Indians have a suicide rate which is many times higher than that for the rest of the population [290], but they are less involved in attacks on other people. It seems, therefore, that it cannot only be the self-criticism induced by higher formal education which determines whether an affective psychosis will tend to assume a manic or a depressive form; and neither does it seem likely to be the informal education which is operative, since a Fijian is at least as restrained and as selfcritical as a Fiji Indian with the same level of schooling. The door is therefore reopened to the possibility of a neurobiological (in this instance perhaps racial) explanation for differences in the D/M ratio, although it is not necessarily closed to other explanations of a social character. For instance, the following differences between the main Fijian peoples as respects internalization and response to unhappiness might be considered pertinent.

The average Fijian (Melanesian) child has a warm upbringing which continues until puberty; the average Fijian woman can expect to spend her whole life among relatives who are mutually supportive; and the average Fijian man has been taught that the way in which his ancestors acquired or regained prestige and communal support was through contributing to the prestige of their community, perhaps by attacking an enemy [522]. One can say, therefore, that the Fijian is unlikely to have a punitive superego and that when feeling unhappy he is likely to act in such a way as he believes will make his community think well of him. The average Fiji Indian child is more likely to have an erratic childhood, as is the case in India itself; the Fiji Indian woman is liable (although less than in India itself) to feel isolated and exploited by her husband's family; and on the male side the Fiji Indians have been taught to suppress irritation and aggression, since it was only by being docile laborers that their ancestors were able to obtain the chance to settle and thrive in Fiji [219]. Accordingly, the Fiji Indian is more likely to have a punitive superego and is less likely to believe that whatever loss or unhappiness he feels will be corrected by the members of his milieu if he acts positively towards them, although he may still feel that if he can forget his unhappiness for a time, circumstances will change and it will disappear. If one wished to sponsor a "social learning" theory to account for variations in the D/M ratio, therefore, one could argue that the Fiji Indian is more trained to internalize frustrations and to be self punishing, while the Fijian is more trained to act in a positive or seemingly cheerful fashion when feeling depressed, in the expectation that his milieu will give him the support which will then banish that depressive feeling.

6 Abnormal Guilt and Self-Depreciation: Eastern and Western Religions

The etiological model just proposed has at least one major flaw. The theory which links depression to the internalization of aggression and to a punitive superego was based on the observation in the earlier part of this century that serious cases of melancholia usually suffered from delusions of guilt and self-depreciation. However, the depression exhibited by the Fiji Indians does not usually have exaggerated guilt feelings as a presenting symptom, and neither did European depression before the seventeenth century, as we saw at the beginning of this chapter. The hypothesized punitive superego, therefore, would seem to be irrelevant not just ot the Fiji picture but to depression generally, and excessive guilt feelings would seem to be quite secondary symptoms. Yet the psychoanalytic work relating depression to evidence suggestive of a punitive superego cannot be ignored, and neither can the fact that when delusions of guilt are present the prognosis for a depression is considerably poorer than when they are absent. This has been recorded by many nonpsychoanalytic writers, including Kraepelin himself, who saw "ideas of sin as playing the largest part" [319, p 18] in "melancholia gravis" but much less part in lighter depressions. A North American study has shown that patients subject to depression can have stricter consciences (and hence presumably stricter superegos) than the average person without this being expressed in excessive feelings of guilt [14], and the matter is obviously quite complex. An examination of the international distribution of guilt feelings and related symptoms in depression would therefore seem called for here, and the result might assist us in explaining the Fiji data.

Table 6.5 provides a suitable starting-point for such an examination. In the early 1960s, an international survey of psychiatrists' impressions regarding the symptomatology of endogenous depression was undertaken, with the latter being defined as a condition characterized by dejection, early morning waking, diurnal mood change, and neglect of the social environment [447]. Respondents were provided with a list of other symptoms and asked to indicate whether each of the latter was usually, occasionally or only rarely present when that basic picture of endogenous depression was found in their society or in particular subcultures within it. They were also asked certain questions regarding the society or subculture from which their patients stemmed, and when the answers relating to the symptoms of guilt and self-deprecia-

Table 6.5. Frequency with which guilt and self-depreciation are judged to be "usual" in cases of depression, as related to society's religious affiliation and orientation [447]

Religious Orientation	Affiliation		Numbers of societies reported on	Percentages of societies in which depressed patients "usually" show: Abnormal guilt feelings	Abnormal self-depreciation
Active or devout	Christian	RC	12	67%	67%
		Other	7	57%	86%
	Hindu and Moslem		7	0	0
	Buddhist, etc.		3	0	0
Less devout	Christian	RC	20	20%	15%
		Other	17	29%	29%
	Hindu and Moslem		9	11%	33%
	Buddhist, etc.		15	13%	53%

tion were analyzed in relation to the information on the different societies, they proved to covary much more strongly with religion than with anything else. It is this covariance which Table 6.5 shows, with a distinction between religious affiliation and what the respondent judged to be the intensity of the society's involvement with the dominant religion. One can see that exaggerated guilt feelings are much more often regarded as "usual" in depressed patients of devoutly Christian societies than in those of other societies, and that they are never regarded as "usual" in the depressed patients of societies assessed to be active in their involvement with a non-Christian religion. Self-depreciation follows the same pattern in the religiously active societies, but gives quite a different picture in the less active ones.

These findings concerned only impressions, not carefully measured data, and Table 6.5 presents only the most easily identified of the variables with which these symptoms could be linked. Since that time, more precise research in numerous countries has indicated that the depicted, double association with religion is broadly true but that there are sufficient exceptions to suggest that religion of itself is probably not a primary factor. For instance, one can find active Roman Catholic societies in which delusions of guilt rarely accompany depression [27], and non-Christian societies such as India in which marked regional differences in this symptom appear [609]. Although still not as comprehensive as required, recent studies give some indication of what the more basic factors determining the distribution of this symptom may be.

The most superficial but easily identified factor is probably the degree to which the voicing of self-criticisms and criticisms of others is encouraged by the local culture. It was remarked in the previous chapter (p 103) that some West African societies have what has been called a paranoid complex. There, people are encouraged to attribute all sorts of misfortunes and unhappiness to witchcraft, and in consequence both depressed and most other types of patient will exhibit what appear to be paranoid symptoms, not blaming themselves. In other parts of West Africa, healing shrines have been springing up at which clients are called upon to confess their sins, and at these shrines the people with depression, like the other clients, may accuse themselves of sin in a stereotyped manner without the self-accusations having anything to do with their psychopathology [187, 493], and without the shrines necessarily reflecting a Christian influence. In traditionally Christian societies the same can occur, depending on how far religious leaders are urging their parishioners to identify and confess their sins; and such influence need not be confined to this symptom. In Montreal in the early 1960s, most of our French-Canadian patients, regardless of diagnosis, admitted to "thinking about their own death" when asked about this by the clinician; but that was because their priests had been urging them to do this as a sound religious practice. In most Western societies since the 1940s, parents, priests, and teachers have been talking much less confidently about sin and guilt, and this is almost certainly relevant to the marked decline in the frequency of delusions of guilt in the 1970s, i.e., in the new generations.

A second, related factor affecting the reported distribution of delusions of guilt is the tendency for Western-trained psychiatrists to assume that when accusations against others are voiced, delusions of guilt are likely to be absent, since if hostility can be expressed against others then according to some psychoanalytic theories that hostility is not turned against the self. That assumption is untrue and deceiving. It took an Egyptian psychiatrist to point out that at his clinic, two-thirds of the depressed patients who were complaining about others turned to criticizing themselves when allowed to talk longer [165], and since then we have been reminded that in societies which believe in witchcraft, depressed persons quite often accuse themselves of this at the same time as they are accusing others [493]. Such accusations, although often called paranoid, prove in the African depressive to be considerably different from the accusations of schizophrenics and paranoiacs. With the latter they tend to be against distant powers – police, Jewish capitalists, foreign witches, etc. – whereas with the depressives they tend to be against intimates, suggesting that the symptom is not so much a projection-denial of hostile feelings as a complaint against the "we", analogous to the European patient's complaint against the "I". Such an idea is much more plausible for African societies than for most others, since a very different concept of the self reigns there (see the collection of papers in *La Notion de Personne en Afrique Noire* [101]) from what is common in Europe and North America; and it can be harmonized with psychoanalytic theory, if desired, through the use of the constructs "group ego" and "group superego" or "clan conscience" [439, 483]. However, it is not only in Africa that such a concern for the "we" rather than for the "I" appears in depressive symptomatology. Kimura [307] has shown that in Japan, what are commonly labeled as guilt feelings are different from those in Europe, being more concerned with family and social roles and less with personal needs.

In the types of society just referred to one can say, as El Islam [165] has done, that depression usually involves self-accusations and that it is only the clinician's lack of time or insensitivity which prevents the accusations against the "we" from being recognized as such. Moreover, in such societies one can sometimes see a shift from the "we" to the "I" as individuation increases. For instance, at the Ghanaian shrines mentioned earlier, the older depressives tended to express only stereotyped confessions whereas those under the age of 40 expressed much more personal and idiosyncratic self-accusations [187], the change apparently being linked to a shift from communal subsistence farming to private cash-crop farming in the previous generation. But in many societies the average depressive patient does not seem to accuse either himself or his milieu. As with the medieval melancholic, his symptoms are mainly somatic, in part what we might call the basic manic-depressive complaints of insomnia, loss of appetite, and psychomotor retardation but also hypochondriac or less dramatic attributions of disorder to the heart, liver, spine, kidneys, etc. This picture can predominate in Christian societies (particularly Mediterranean) in which the confessional is an old tradition, and there must therefore be a further factor influencing the distribution of self-accusations (against "we" or "I") in depression, apart from those which have been mentioned.

One conceptually parsimonious way of interpreting the variability here is to interpret hypochondriacal complaints in depression as complaints against the body as a part of the self, just as accusations against intimates can be interpreted as against the group as part of the self. If we divide societies into those in which the body is more and is less likely to be accepted as part of the self, then the data regarding bodily preoccupation obtained from the international survey on which Table 6.5 was based [447] fit such a theory. Cartesian dualism, which virtually denied the body any part in the self, penetrated popular thinking in southern, Catholic Europe much less thoroughly than it did that of northern, Protestant Europe, and it was around the Mediterranean that the respondents to our questionnaire survey reported somatic preoccupation to be the most "usual," while it was from northern, Protestant Europe that the groups showing the least somatic preoccupation were reported. Also potentially supportive of such a theory is the fact that somatic symptoms appear to have been increasing in northern European and North American depressives during the 1960s and 1970s, in parallel with the reacceptance of bodily needs and bodily enjoyments in these societies during these decades. However, reports on depressive illness in some less developed societies suggest that it may occur in the absence of what can be interpreted as complaints against the corporeal, psychic, or social self, and in more developed societies the question must be raised whether the conventional psychiatric method of trying to elicit symptoms from patients may not result in them being reported as present when this is not really true.

7 Responses to Treatment: Anglo-Canadians and French-Canadians

The question whether accusations against the self are a basic feature of depression is not merely academic. Researchers continue to note that when delusions of guilt are present, the depression is more severe than when they are absent, just as in Kraepelin's time, and the same is sometimes found with respect to somatic preoccupation, i.e., another possible form of complaint against the self. We need to know whether, in societies in which depression occurs relatively frequently without one or other form of self-accusation, affective disorders recover more rapidly with standard treatment than in other societies, as some reports suggest. However, this question of response to treatment is particularly difficult to assess with the affective disorders, due to the fact that spontaneous remission occurs and is more likely to supervene in patients whose disorder has been running for many weeks than in those who come for treatment early; and in international comparisons it is rare that one can be sure that there is not a marked difference in the mean duration of illness in the two samples before the treatment starts. Hence although there is an impression that recovery can be unusually rapid – for instance, after two or three sessions of ECT – in patients from societies in which accusations against some aspects of the self rarely accompany depression, this is a point on which the evidence is still inadequate. The best evidence which I have been able to find regarding a cultural difference in response of affective disorders to treatment relates to relatively mild cases, and the presence of self-accusations is not necessarily relevant.

The evidence derives from a drug trial involving Anglo-Canadian and French-Canadian patients in Montreal [425]. The former exhibited more frequent feelings of guilt at the beginning of the study, and they also responded less well to each of the two drugs being compared than the French-Canadian patients did, after allowance was made for sex, age, dosage, and duration of symptoms, as would be expected from what has just been stated. However, it was not only in their overall improvement that they did less well than the other patients. When only the symptom of excessive guilt feelings was considered and when allowance was made for the level of this symptom at the start of the therapy, there was still significantly less improvement than among the French-Canadians. In other words, French-Canadian patients exhibiting excessive guilt feelings did better than Anglo-Canadian patients exhibitng such feelings. Because the two sets of patients were not all rated by the same clinician, and because there could in theory have been differences between them with respect to absorption of their medications and even to taking the latter as prescribed, these differences should not be taken as proven. Nevertheless, these findings, which had not at all been expected, suggest that a possible relationship between culture and the chronicity of depression should be looked for, regardless of whether there are differences in the symptomatology.

8 Depressive Symptoms in Community Surveys: Sarawak and Mexico

Virtually all the foregoing comparisons of the affective disorders have employed data regarding patients coming for treatment, but it was pointed out at the beginning of this chapter that persons with feelings of depression can vary greatly in the degree to which they will seek aid for this, and that doctors also vary greatly, even within a single culture, in their tendency to regard such feelings of depression as pathological or as needing specialist care. If one encounters an unusually high rate of hospitalization for depression, and if the mental hospitals are accustomed to admit only persons unable to look after themselves, as was the case in Europe at the beginning of this century and in Fiji in the 1970s, then this high rate can reasonably be taken as indicative of a high morbidity level even if one has no idea of the prevalence of less severe cases in the population. However, when one encounters an unusually low rate of hospitalizations for affective disorder, then this does not necessarily indicate a low level of affective morbidity, since cultural traditions or the social situation may result in quite severe cases of depression never being brought for treatment. Up to a point, the probability of a low hospitalization rate signifying a low morbidity can be assessed by considering the suicide rate for the group in question, if that is available, since although depression and suicide do not run fully parallel, there can be a correlation. But a better way to check on the possibility that a people with a low rate of hospitalizations may have a genuinely low morbidity is to enquire directly about symptoms from a sufficiently large sample of the population, since if the symptoms are rarely reported, the syndrome is probably (but not necessarily) also rare. We have looked at one instance of such a check being made on a people with a low hospitalization rate, namely that on the East Asian immigrants to Britain, and there the hospital findings were corroborated; but since that immigrant population might have been self-selected for tough-mindedness we cannot draw conclusions from it regarding the degree to which a normal population can be free of depressive symptoms. Hence it is desirable that we look for a different example of hospitalization and survey data combining to indicate a low frequency of affective disorder, before we attempt to infer how unsusually low frequencies of such disorders occur.

Figure 6.3 provides such an example, combining in rather complicated fashion data from mental hospitalizations, suicide statistics, and a community survey and then contrasting these with comparable data on neighboring peoples and on one with a very different response style. Part I derives from what has probably been the largest community mental health survey ever carried out, but one which few psychiatrists know about since its results are unfortunately still unpublished at the time of writing, more than 10 years after the field work was completed. In this survey, organized by Dr. K.E. Schmidt at the Kuching mental hospital, a range of Sarawak communities representative of three of the four main peoples in the territory was selected, and three sets of lay interviewers, one from each people, were trained to administer a three-part questionnaire, the first part being addressed to the individual members of the household, the second to the head of the household regarding its members, and the third to the interviewer himself regarding the impression made by each respondent. All adults in all households in each community were contacted, with a very low refusal rate thanks to prior arrangements for obtaining the support of each community's leaders; and if the interviewer thought on the basis of the answers or of a subject's behavior that someone seemed in any way mentally disturbed, it was arranged for that person to be interviewed by the research psychiatrist, who then recorded whether he considered him to constitute a "case" of mental disorder or not. Approximately 2.3% of the over 20 000 subjects were judged to be "cases" in this fashion, and these are kept separate in the figure. Among the 30 questions about symptoms addressed to each respondent were six which are often associated with depression. These six are listed in the Figure legend.

On all six symptoms, the 97% of Sarawak Malays who were classified as "normal" gave only about a tenth of the positive responses to each of the depressive symptoms which their "normal" Chinese and Iban neighbors did, and the few who were classified as "cases" also scored lower on these symptoms than the corresponding Chinese and Iban, as can be gathered from the figure. By itself, the first of these differences might mean nothing more than that Malays tend to say "No" to all questions when interviewed in this fashion, just as the Mexicans shown in Part III probably have a tendency to say "Yes." (The Mexican part of the figure – which uses the same scale – has been included mainly to indicate how wide a range of responses can be obtained

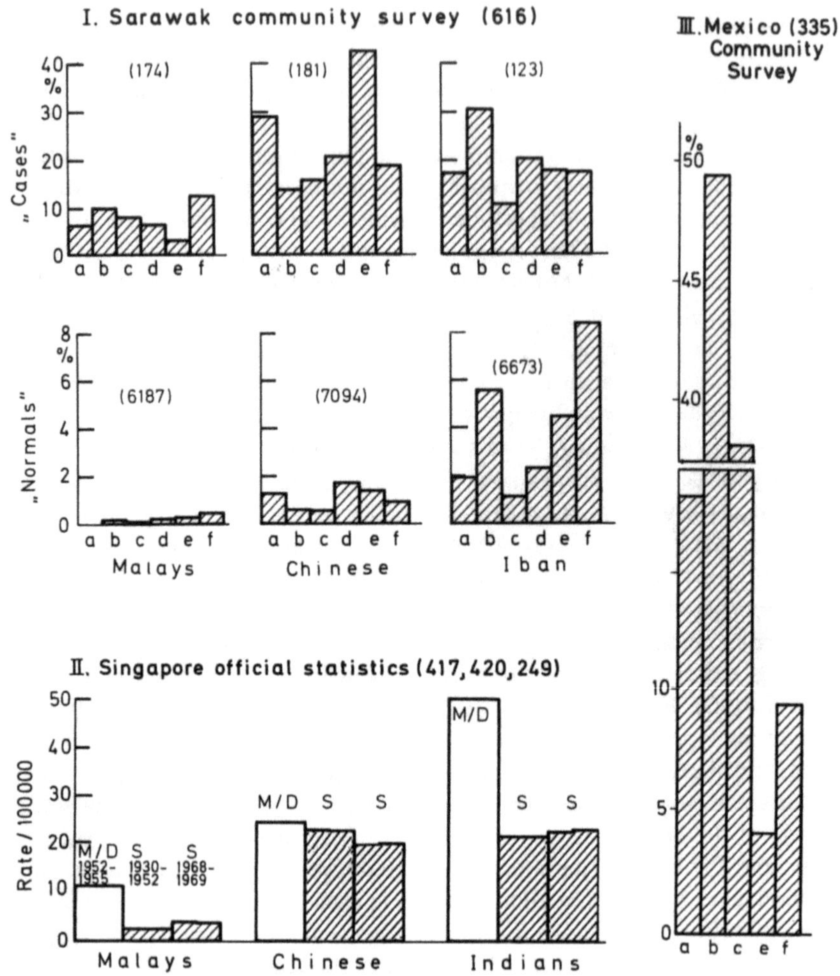

Fig. 6.3 Parts I, II, III. Depressive symptom levels, manic-depressive psychosis, and suicide in Malays and Chinese, with comparative symptom levels from Mexico. **I** Sarawak community survey. These data represent rates per 100 persons aged 15 to 59, divided into those whom the research psychiatrist judged to have a definite mental disorder (all diagnostic categories) and those judged not to have such disorder. The number of persons surveyed are shown in brackets above each set of columns. The letters *a* to *f* below the columns refer to the following questions: (a) "Are your spirits low or are you depressed?" (b) "Do you feel it is difficult to get going?" (c) "Do you feel as if nothing turns out properly?" (d) "Do you fell life is not worthwhile living?" (e) "How is your appetite?" (poor) and (f) "How is your sleep?" (poor). **II** Singapore official statistics. These data represent rates per 100 000 aged 15+ per annum. Mental hospitalization rates refer to first admissions diagnosed as having a manic-depressive or involutional psychosis in the years 1950–1954; the first set of suicide rates refers to three periods of approximately 3 years each between 1930 and 1952 regardless of ascribed cause; the second set of suicide rates refers to equivalent data for 1968–1969. **III** Mexico community survey. These data represent combined rates per 100 persons aged 20 to 59 in Tehuantepec and three social strata in Mexico City, the questions posed having been almost identical with those cited for Sarawak

to a community mental health survey, when peoples of different backgrounds are involved, as was noted also regarding Puerto Ricans on p 52) However, the responses of the Malay "cases" indicate that any tendency to say "No" to such questions cannot be too strong, and the fact that the overall "caseness" among the Sarawak Malays was as high as that among the Chinese shows that the former must have been giving sufficient positive answers regarding other categories of symptom or disturbance. Moreover, although neither mental hospitalizations nor suicides can be satisfactorily compared in Sarawak itself, since medical and police services are very limited in comparison with the size of the population, Part II indicates that in Singapore, where the Malays and the Chinese have similar characteristics to their fellows in Sarawak and where official data are satisfactory, the Malays have very much lower rates of suicide than the Chinese (and Indians), and also significantly lower rates of mental hospital admission for affective psychosis. These different sets of data, in combination, suggest strongly that certain Malay peoples have unusually low rates of affective disturbance, whether of a severe or of a mild character.

The finding is not one which can easily be attributed to a general racial resistance. My own experience with Indonesian students going to foreign universities is that they are unusually susceptible to depression of the nostalgic type, and Professor Kusumanto Setyonegoro, head of the University of Indonesia's department of psychiatry, has told me that he needs to take particular care in screening persons for overseas training, for this reason. Earlier, there had been recorded 11 cases of suicide or of (mainly affective) psychosis within a 20-year period among the first 250 graduates from the new medical school at Batavia (Djakarta), which is a relatively high rate, and Pfeiffer has more recently [490] described a form of depression in persons who have not been able to maintain "face," which is relatively common in the west-coast Indonesian island of Nias. Suicide which is discreetly private appears to be relatively infrequent throughout the culture region, but it was noted in the previous chapter that amok, which belongs predominantly to the same region, was historically viewed as an approved form of suicide in designated circumstances, and the history of the archipelago also contains a number of dramatic and admired episodes of mass suicide. Insofar as the Sarawak and Singapore Malays have genuinely lower rates of affective disturbances than most peoples, therefore, this has to be attributed to local subcultural or social factors rather than to the influences of race or of the cultural traditions over the whole region. It may therefore be profitable to look briefly at the ways in which the Singapore and Sarawak Malays differ from other peoples in the region.

Anthropological information on the Sarawak Malays is slight, but the Singapore Malays have been quite extensively studied, and a number of ways in which this people differs from the Javanese, Makassarese, Batak, and some sections of the majority population of Western Malaysia can be identified. The most obvious is that they put proportionately less emphasis on propriety and the need to maintain status in competition with others of the same or a different culture. While sensitive to insult, the men of this group react less strongly than is true of many other Malaysian peoples, and they tend to withdraw from situations which might later expose them to conflict and insult rather than defend what they could rightfully claim as their own. (This, which can be inferred to have been learnt during European colonial rule, was shown by the way in which an important economic activity, that of taxi-driving, was largely ceded to Chinese drivers when it appeared that the occupation could only be retained either by fighting or by accepting insults [641].) In some other cultures of the region, as Pfeiffer has pointed out [490], the feeling of having lost "face" is liable to result in depression, whereas this is a considerably less important element in the peoples under discussion. More important, however, are probably the very close and warm relationships which the subculture encourages between parents and off-spring, something which results in small children being bought sweets and toys when there is not even enough money to buy adequate food [559], and in wives demanding and receiving divorce when they are called upon to move to a place from which they cannot easily visit their parents [151]. Children who are orphaned are made a great fuss of by the other villagers and given many presents, while adults who have grand-parents alive are considered to be particularly fortunate, since this adds a further generation with which gratifying emotional interaction can take place [150]. The little which we know about the Sarawak Malays suggests a similar picture, and it is my impression that it is the individual's care to keep himself surrounded by persons with whom he can have warm relationships which results in the lower rate of affective disorder here. (It also results at times in poverty and malnutrition, since time which needs to be spent in earning one's bread is spent in emotional gratifications; but that is another matter.)

Returning briefly now to the Mexican data in Fig. 6.3 Part III, it needs to be added that the very high frequency with which depressive symptoms were reported by a supposedly representative sample of Mexicans may not be entirely due to a tendency to answer "Yes" to any such enquiries. These subjects answered "Yes" to an unusual extent to the other items of the questionnaire as well, but another study using the same Midtown Manhattan scale showed that the depressive symptoms were acknowledged much more than the rest [179], and the work of Diaz-Guerrero [148], Maccoby [365], and Fromm [207] has shown that this people do possess an unusual tendency towards depression and various forms of passive dependency. They were not cited earlier in this chapter as an example of a people in which affective disorders are particularly high, because we do not possess good data with which to compare the frequency of manic-depressive psychosis in them with that in other peoples. However, a comparison of Mexican-American with Anglo-American patients at the Arizona State Mental Hospital showed that the former, particularly on the female side, had a considerably heavier depressive symptomatology than the latter [399]. When one compares Mexican social life, whether village or urban, with that of the Sarawak and Singapore Malays, one finds that although the average infant is warmly cared for, there is a marked change after weaning and in adult life there is much competitiveness and distrust of others. Fromm and Maccoby [207] felt it necessary to introduce a social experiment to assess whether the villagers with whom they worked were capable of cooperation, so doubtful did this seem at first sight, and it is interesting that others have found it necessary to undertake the same type of experiment in the west of Ireland [73], where a high level of depression is also found. From a comparison of the family and social life of the Mexicans and Malays, one gets the impression that the former would like to be as warmly trusting and interacting as the latter, but that scarcity of fertile land forces them to cut the ties which they have with others, whereas the Malays (but not their kin, the Javanese) have still ample land from which to earn a living.

9 Conclusions

The main point at which the majority of the studies cited in this chapter converge, and which has perhaps not come forward as much in other epidemiological studies of the affective disorders, concerns individual striving. With the seventeenth century English, the Jews at the beginning of this century, and the Mauritian Moslems more recently, we have evidence that these disorders became more manifest after there had been a shift from a social setting in which there was much mutual supportiveness or acceptance of ascribed statuses, towards a way of life in which there was more competition between individuals. Conversely, among the Sarawak and Singapore Malays an unusually low level of affective disorder and symptomatology appears linked to an avoidance of competitiveness, and the same seems to have been broadly true among the Mauritian Hindoos under the age of about 60, although a different factor increases depression above that age. The association with competitiveness overlaps the more familiar association with urbanization but does not derive from it, since the higher Moslem rates in Mauritius arise as much in rural as in urban districts.

This link with competitiveness and thence inversely with the number of people to whom one has close supportive ties, however, cannot be absolute. The Asian immigrant to Britain is in many ways more competitive and striving than the average Briton or the average Irish migrant, and although the seventeenth century English were followed by increasingly individualistic generations, the latter are reported to have lost the excess tendency towards melancholia, most probably because they had learnt to be more self-sufficient [23]. Accordingly, a second variable seems implied here, namely the level of individual need or expectation respecting emotional support. Brown and Harris [74] borrow the term "assumptive world" to describe one factor in the vulnerability of London women to depression, and it is in part this which is being referred to now, with the women's assumptions being considerably determined by the culture. However, the high vulnerability to the Irish to depression, and probably of the Mexicans as well, despite many generations of obligatory competition among neighbors and family members, would seem to mean that it is not just what life teaches them to expect which is important here. There must also be a more basic vulnerablitity or need for social support which can vary from one people to another, and although this could very well be genetic in origin, as the sex difference presumably is, a social explanation is also possible. The descriptions which we possess of Irish and Mexican village life, and more particularly of the childrearing practices there, are such as to lead one to expect regressive tendencies in the psychoanalytic sense; and these might be pertinent.

The increased rate of affective disorders which had developed in the Mauritian Moslems in association with greater individual striving comprised mainly short-lasting states, and the Moslem rate of more chronic states was not significantly higher than those of the other Mauritian groups. From this one might be tempted to deduce that it is the milder, reactive form of depression which is mainly affected by the greater individualism, and that manic-depressive psychosis remains relatively independent of that sociopsychological change. However, the Moslems have an excess of manic and circular disorders, even though brief ones, as well as depressive disorders, and we can infer that the excess of disorders in the Jews related more to the manic and circular psychoses than to the simple depressions usually found in their German Christian neighbors. Hence it is the more complex forms of affective disorder which are particularly associated with this variable, not the less. The present material does not support the idea that affective disorder can be divided into endogenous and reactive categories either on the basis of relative chronicity or on the basis of a distinction between simple depression and the mixed or manic states. In Singapore, the relatively few Malay cases of hospitalized affective disorder contained essentially the same proportions of long-stay (over 2 years) and short-stay (less than 6 months) categories as the Indians who had so much higher a hospitalization rate [419]. Among both the Mauritian Moslems and the European Jews there were proportionately more cases exhibiting mania than in the groups with which they are each compared, but whereas this higher frequency of mania was associated in the Jews with a greater-than-average chronicity (as is true of most European peoples), in the Moslems it was associated with a lower-than-average chronicity, as far as can be judged.

The latter point brings us to the question of the relationship between symptomatology and chronicity. In Africa and India it is the general impression that when indigenous but Westernized patients exhibit European-style delusions of guilt, their disorder is more persistent than that of patients without this symptom, just as in Europe and the United States. However, the symptoms which stood out in the more chronic Jewish patients were not delusions of guilt but hypochondrical complaints about various bodily systems, plus complaints against the persons whom the patients believed could cure them. (The involvement of the body in the self, in European Jewish society, was brought home to me in the refugee camps after World War II. Jewish concentration camp survivors stood out from other ethnic groups not through their frank grief or their expressions of guilt, but through their demands for unnecessary surgery, i.e., for a socially approved way of punishing or mutilating thir bodies [418]). Similarly, when one turns to clinical descriptions of non-Westernized African patients, one gets the impression that those expressing direct accusations against themselves have a better chance of early recovery than those directing accusations against a family or community which has rejected them (see "Justine ou la confession interminable" by Andras Zempléni in the reports on the Ivory Coast healing shrine [493].) Taken together with psychoanalytic commentaries on depressed patients, these observations suggest that a major factor affecting the chronicity and resistance to cure of an affective disorder, whether the latter has or has not an obvious social precipitant, is the presence of a conflict between one part of the self and another part of the self, regardless of whether these parts are purely intrapsychic, involve the body, or involve a social group with which the patient so closely identifies himself that he thinks of "we" rather than of "I."

This chapter is entitled "the affective disorders," but it has nowhere been stated just what I think these disorders are. In the foregoing conclusions it has been indicated that a division into endogenous and reactive, unipolar and bipolar, or some other dichotomy does not appear useful when comparisons of the type undertaken

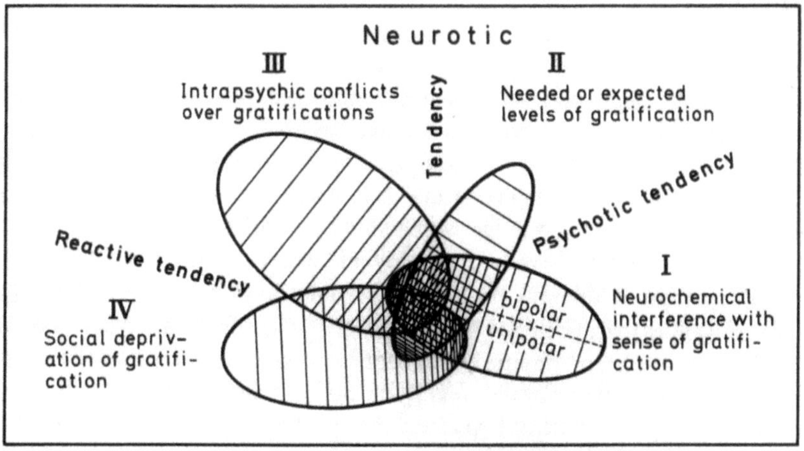

Fig. 6.4. Hypothetical model of factors influencing the risk and severity of affective disorders. Each factor is assumed to vary from mild (widely spaced bars) to intense (closely spaced bars). Risk is assumed to increase with intensity of overlapping factors, and severity of disorder is indicated by density of shading. No particular significance is attached to the size, shape, or placing of the areas assigned to each factor, and they are all conceived as being orthogonal to each other, as if in four dimensions

here are attempted; and I know of no other method of classification which can link observed clinical features to hypothesized etiological influences in any more satisfactory yet simple way. What appears to fit the international and cross-cultural comparisons best is not any division into discrete entities or distribution along a single axis, but rather some multiaxial model of the type suggested in Fig. 6.4, with a different factor operating by small increments along each axis. At their strongest, some of these factors, or perhaps all of them, may be able to produce a manifest affective disorder even when the others are relatively weak, as is intended to be indicated by the variations in shading, but the great majority of such disorders are going to be the result of adverse forces of varied strength along several axes. The main etiological factors are likely to be:

I) An *organic* one, concerned with the neurobiological (neurochemical processes whereby experiences are labeled by the brain as gratifying, so that a genetic or other defect affecting these processes will reduce the sense of gratification obtained from normally satisfying intakes;

II) An *intrapsychic* one, concerned with the level of gratification which is needed to maintain psychic functioning and/or is expected on the basis of past experience, so that a high level of need or of expectation will result in a sense of distress when the level of perceived emotional gratification drops only moderately;

III) A second *intrapsychic* one, concerned with the reactions which a loss of gratifications is likely to elicit, such as denial, hostility towards others, or hostility towards parts of the self;

IV) An *environmental* factor, concerned with the access which individuals have to emotionally gratifying experiences in their social environments.

As far as international and cross-cultural comparisons are concerned, the neurological influence of race or gene pool should be assessable by comparing the percentages of manic depressive patients in different races whose relatives, of a given level of consanguinity, also have had a manic-depressive disorder; but I have been unable to find suitable reports for this. In Bulgaria, family linkages is reported for 60% of cases [410], but the treated incidence rate is low and the criteria for diagnosis and linkage are too vague for one to judge which study of a different race or genetic pool would be truly comparable. Levels of intrapsychic expectation are fairly easy to assess, and would seem to be relevant to the age distribution of cases among the Mauritian Hindoos as well as the difference between French-Canadian and other male migrants to the Prairies. (A systematic study of expectations was carried out by the Dutch Government among persons prior to emigration [509]; but there was unfortunately no sufficient follow-up to enable one to assess the association between these and later mental health.) Levels of intrapsychic need, as distinct from expectation, can only be hypothesized on the basis of debatable theory, but the apparently high rates in the Irish and the Mexicans might be best explained on such a basis if a generally accepted theory were developed.

The influence of one type of reaction to loss can be inferred from the ratio of mania to depression, if one remembers that mania can be a direct response to loss [606], something which is sometimes forgotten in northern Europe; and some sociocultural factors underlying that choice of response were considered with respect to Fiji and New Zealand. The influence of another type of response, namely that of directing hostility towards the part of the self believed responsible for the loss of gratifications, has traditionally been discussed only with respect to guilt feelings, but our comparative material suggests strongly that cultural background can guide that hostility toward the body or toward persons with whom the subject identifies so completely that it is as if they were part of a group self. Finally, variations in the access which people have to emotional gratification and support from their environment are easy to relate to the incidence and prevalence of affective disorders and symptoms, and comparisons yield the expected differences.

However, the understanding of any given difference is likely to be much better if one considers the various axes or dimensions together, rather than separately as has just been done.

Chapter 7 Suicide and Parasuicide

In contrast to what has been repeatedly noted regarding the psychoses, satisfactorily comparable data on suicide are abundant, in fact so abundant that I had thought to omit the subject from the present book since covering it requires a book in itself. However, although the literature is so extensive and in places so rich, the way in which psychiatry uses it has remained confused, in part because of an insufficient distinction between consummated suicide and parasuicide (suicidal attempts which have failed by reason of something more than mere accident) and in part because suicide resulting from clear thinking is insufficiently distinguished from that resulting from disturbed thinking. Psychiatry is concerned with the latter but not usually with the former. Also, purely sociological theories of suicide, such as those of Durkheim, are sometimes applied to mental disorder and it is desirable to assess how well these theories are based. The purpose of this chapter is to make clearer, with the aid of international and historical comparisons, the different forces motivating suicide and parasuicide and the lessons which psychiatry should be able to draw from the theories to which the study of suicide has given birth.

1 Eighteenth and Nineteenth Century Trends

The collecting of national data on suicide started in Sweden (which then included Finland) in 1749; the first text to give some statistics on the subject [79] appeared in 1761; and the first text discussing international differences in rates was probably that by Falret [181] in 1822. As additional countries started publishing similar data, it could be seen that these international differences were marked and that the higher rates tended to belong to the richer societies, something which was quite disturbing to that century's idea of progress. Moreover, as the century drew on, it became apparent that the rate was rising in most countries, but particularly in those which were making the fastest progress in terms of wealth and eventually industrialization.

This is illustrated in Fig. 7.1, which summarizes the longest series of national statistics on suicide which we possess, those from Sweden and Finland as given by Verkko [634], and compares them with those of their Scandinavian neighbors, Denmark and Norway. The rates in any such comparison should not, as was discussed in Chap. 2, be regarded as precise, but the relative positions of national groups on such a chart can be taken as valid, since we know that when their members move from Europe to Australia (see Fig. 1.1) or to the United States [533], the rank order of suicide rates remains about the same.

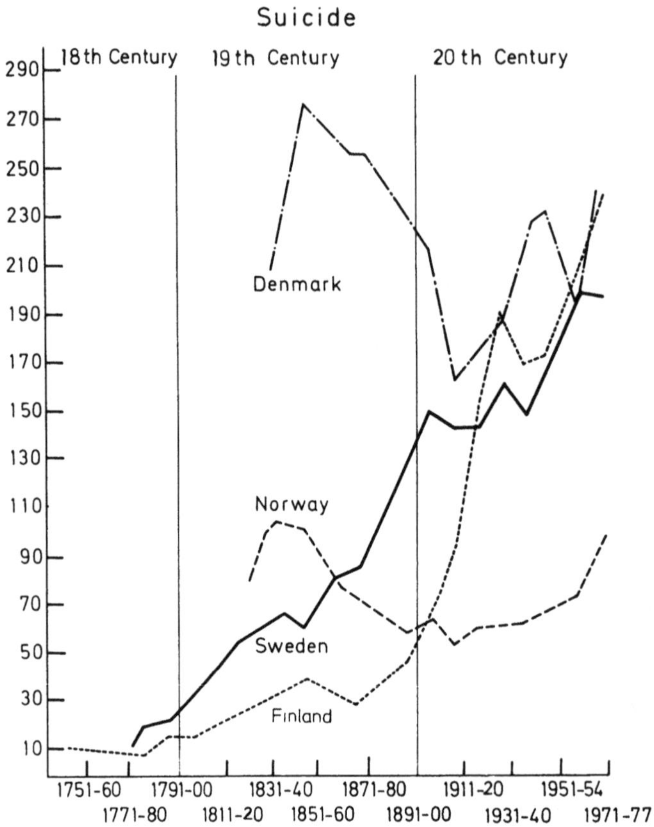

Fig. 7.1. Historical changes in the suicide rate, 1750–1977, in four Scandinavian countries, per 1 000 000 inhabitants. From Verkko [634], supplemented by more recent data from *Health Statistics Annuals*

The most striking points in this figure are the wide difference between the Danish and Swedish rates in the earlier part of the nineteenth century, and the sharp rise of the latter as the century progressed; but other data from Denmark suggest that suicide had also shown a sharp rise there prior to 1850 [540]. These increases paralleled increases in prosperity. At the end of the eighteenth century Denmark had a very primitive economy, due to the "bonding" of farmers to their landlords and the lack of interest by the latter in agriculture; but the freeing of the bondsmen at that time and the loss of Norway in 1814 brought about a dramatic change which turned Denmark from one of the poorest to one of the richest countries in Europe by the middle of the century. Sweden made the change later, since in the 1820s it had almost no middle class, trade, or manufacturing industry, if one excludes the massive distillation of alcohol from potatoes. In subsequent decades, however, the revival of agriculture and then the exploitation of rich mineral resources with the aid of the new Bessemer process sent this country likewise on the road to economic prosperity so that, for instance, bank deposits increased by 500% between 1860 and 1875 alone [414], although it continued for long to remain poorer than Denmark.

Outside Scandinavia, similar associations between recent economic prosperity and a raised suicide rate were also to be found. For instance, in Germany around 1880 the following association was to be found:

	Saxony	*Prussia*	*Würtemburg*	*Bavaria*
Bank deposits per capita [414]				
(in British shillings)	83	39	30	10
Suicide per 100 000 population [383]	39.1	17.4	13.5	12.7

However, there were exceptions to the picture, notably the low rates in England and in Belgium, the richest countries (with Holland) in the continent for most of the century, but countries which had made the shift to a capitalist economy earlier. (England probably suffered higher suicide rates between 1720 and 1750 [664, p 266].)

Whether these increases in suicide signified a rise in mental disturbance or whether they were a purely social phenomenon occasioned much debate. Prior to the nineteenth century, suicide had been thought of as mainly a 'moral' disorder, not a mental one, and hence the increase in rates was not initially seen as a problem for psychiatrists. However, in 1845 Bourdin published his book, *Du Suicide considèrè comme Maladie* [62], and other psychiatrists came increasingly to claim that although it did not seem correct to regard suicide as a single psychiatric entity (as Bourdin implied), it did seem appropriate to regard most suicidal acts as resulting from one or other of a variety of mental disorders. In making this claim, they were undoubtedly thinking more about their patients who had survived a suicide attempt and the injustice that was caused by suicide being treated as a criminal act in many countries, than about incidence rates. However, some authorities, notably the sociologist and Czech national leader Thomas Masaryk [383] did link suicide rates to mental disorder and deduced that the increase in suicide was merely one aspect of an increase in mental disorders which was affecting the whole civilized world, and was the result to too much freedom and excitement. Masaryk wrote: "We find these incubators of mental derangement among people who throw off the yoke of authority, among people who form associations, seek to make their own laws, and have a literary calling; in nations where an incessant impulse drives men to flee the sphere circumscribed by their birth" [383, p 110]. "Civilized man finds himself in the pathological state of a general nervousness ... which leads on the one hand to psychosis, on the other to suicide" [383, p 113].

Although the evidence favoring this theory was slight – it rested particularly on Esquirol's comments [173] on cases he had seen in 1830 – it was quickly espoused by people who saw a need to return to stronger government and less revolutionary strife, and it correspondingly became an anathema to those who desired to move on to a freer, more egalitarian social structure. Among the latter were many of the relatively recently enfranchized Jews, including Emil Durkheim. He tore this theory to pieces in his book on suicide, brought together a variety of somewhat better data to show that there is "no relation between variations of the two phenomena [suicide and psychosis] with sex, age, faith, country, degree of civilization" [160, p 400], and poured scorn on psychiatrists for claiming suicide to be mainly within their sphere.

In actual fact, there was no great difference between the views of Masaryk and Durkheim regarding the nature of most suicides in their late-nineteenth century European society, if one sets aside their opinions regarding the relationship of suicide to mental disorder and regarding what needs to be done. Masaryk held that miseducation was developing new needs in people before they had sufficiently learnt the forms of self-control and social control which are required to guide these needs. Durkheim saw contemporary suicide as increasing either when society was encouraging new goals without setting sufficient limits to them (anomic suicide) or when the bonds between the person and his society – his social integration – became too weak and his individualism became too great (egoistic suicide). However, neither of these sociologists explained the mental processes which led from the hypothesized social situation to the act of self-destruction, and neither Masaryk's view of the process as essentially psychiatric nor Durkheim's view that it as essentially non-psychiatric fitted the facts available to them.

If Masaryk's theory had been correct, the majority of persons committing suicide should have been recognized to have been mentally ill (in a nineteenth century sense) prior to the act, regardless of whether the suicide rate was high or low. If Durkheim's theory of most variations in suicide being independent of mental disorder were true, then one would expect the rates of suicide associated with mental illness to vary independently of the rates of suicide not associated with such illness. Neither was the case. When one examines the proportions of suicides recognized at that time as having been mentally ill, one finds, as is shown in Table 7.1, that they constitute only a minority and that the percentage remains roughly the same whether the society has a high suicide rate (Saxony) or a low one (Belgium). What is striking about the data in this table, and is the reason for it being presented, is that despite the marked differences in rates between Saxony, France, and Belgium, the proportions of cases assigned to the different categories of 'main cause" are very similar. Insofar as anomic and egoistic tendencies in societies affect the risk of suicide, therefore, they seem to do so regardless of what are seen by police or other officials as the main underlying causes in individual cases.

2 Durkheim's Fatalistic and Anomic Types in the Twentieth Century

Durkheim's theory and typology of suicide remain the most widely credited of all the many that have been formulated, and in the present century his concept of anomie has been taken up by a host of social scientists working both on suicide and on other subjects. However, it is something of a paradox that whereas he arrived at these ideas mainly through comparing the relatively crude suicide rates in different societies during the nineteenth century, his followers have done very little in the way of international comparisons using the more detailed and probably more accurate twentieth century international data. The latter have been used by his followers to extend his argument regarding the tendency of suicide rates of decline during wars and other national crises, a tendency which is easily linked to the greater social integration which usually occurs within nations at such times and which has been much more striking during the two World Wars than previously, as the Japanese rates in

Table 7.1. Causes attributed to suicide in Saxony, France, and Belgium in the 1840s–1850s, by sex and with incidence rates for related years

	Both sexes			Males		Females	
	Saxony	France	Belgium	Saxony	France	Saxony	France
Suicide rate per 100 000	25.1	11.0	5.5				
Total cases reviewed	5497	24 462	2428	4317	18 713	1180	5749
Main attributed cause	%	%	%	%	%	%	%
Mental illness	31.9	30.5	35.3	26.8	26.3	51.0	44.0
Physical illness	6.8	10.8	1.3	6.5	10.9	8.1	10.8
Remorse or fear of punishment	13.0	7.6	3.0	13.0	8.1	12.2	5.6
Alcoholism and other "vices"	11.6	11.1	7.0	14.0	12.9	2.5	5.4
Grief and passion	4.8	4.4	9.2	4.3	3.5	6.2	7.4
Financial reverses	11.7	11.3	8.1	13.8	13.1	3.9	5.5
Family strife	2.3	10.7	7.9	2.1	10.6	3.5	10.9
Dissatisfaction with life	6.3	4.9	2.7	7.0	5.2	4.1	4.0
No cause arrived at	11.6	8.7	25.5	12.5	9.4	8.5	6.4
	100.0	100.0	100.0	100.0	100.0	100.0	100.0

Recalculated from Wagner [636] on whose data both Durkheim and Masaryk drew, with rates derived from Masaryk [383]. Saxon causal data relate to 1847–1858; French causal data to 1856–1861; and Belgian ones to 1840–1849

Fig. 1.2 (p 14) illustrate. However, Halbwachs' other attempts to extend Durkheimian theory depended mainly on nineteenth century data, although his book [242] was published in 1930, and other followers such as Gibbs [213] have tended to ignore international comparisons in favor of studies within single societies. The most probable reason is that in comparison with the marked economic changes which have been taking place (and which Durkheim would have expected to affect suicide), the stability of most national suicide rates outside wartime during the present century did not appear to fit his theories as well, and hence did not have the appeal which the nineteenth century data did. To some readers this may appear all to the good, since we can then dispose of such purely sociological interpretations and return to a more psychiatric perspective; but the fact is that twentieth century data fit Durkheim's theories quite well, and we therefore need to be able to make allowances for the broad social forces which he discusses before we can recognize the other elements at work.

The most striking confirmation of one of Durkheim's categories, but one which has received little attention, concerns that category, the fatalistic, which he confined to a footnote on the grounds that it had "so little contemporary importance" [160, p 276 footnote], and which in consequence tends to be forgotten when his types are discussed. It is the suicide "of persons with futures pitilessly blocked and passions violently choked by oppressive discipline" (op cit). There have been few groups to which these words applied more justly than to the Jews under Nazi rule. In the previous chapter I stated that although Central European Jewry had exhibited an excess of manic-depressive psychosis during the first quarter of this century, I had come across no evidence that their rates for this disorder rose during their subsequent years of more open oppression. Their suicide rates did rise considerably, however. Dublin cites figures showing that the absolute number of suicides buried in the only Jewish burial ground in Berlin ran at an average of 64 per year from 1933 to 1937, jumped to an average of 132 between 1938 and 1941, and then reached 811 in 1942 although the number of Jews in the city must have been going down throughout this period [157, p 76]. In Vienna, the rate of suicide among the members of the *Israelitische Kultusgemeinde* jumped from the already high figure of 56 per 100 000 in 1937 to an average of 274 between 1938 and 1941, and then to 1192 per 100 000 in 1942 [356]. It is very possible that these figures reflect overreporting of the type mentioned in Chap. 2, and that some of the so-called suicides were murders, but this does not alter the overall picture and there can be no doubt that "fatalistic" is the label which best applies here. What had "so little contemporary importance" for Durkheim had very great importance for the next generation, and it cannot easily be maintained that the "main cause" of these acts was a form of mental disorder rather than the social realities. (In the nineteenth century the Jews had constituted a notable example of a people with low rates, on average.)

The other aspect of Durkheim's theory which more modern, comparative data on suicide permits us to test relates to the link between suicide and a relaxation of the social limits to ambition, something which can be regarded as an aspect of anomie but which could also be affecting what he called egoistic suicide, insofar as such relaxation is often accompanied by an increase in individualism. From his theory, one would predict that suicide would be higher in societies in which the opportunity for individual gain is both high and increasing than in societies where it is lower and/or is static. Furthermore, his text leads one to predict that such a difference would be greater in males than in females (since the former are more involved in the process of material gain than the latter) and in men of middle adult life rather than in those at the beginning or end of adult life, since it is among the former that striving for gain is greatest. I was surprised when preparing this chapter that I could not find any paper which had reported such a test of the theory with modern data on an international scale, but the task was not difficult to undertake and the results are shown in Fig. 7.2.

In this figure one sees the suicide rates for males aged 25-54 in all countries for which suicide data are summarized in the *World Health Statistics Annual* for 1964 (the year in which the greatest number of countries are brought together in a single suicide table), and these observed rates are compared with the rates expected on the basis of two simple indicators of economic development for each country. These indicators are the per capita GNP in 1965 and percentage increases in national GNP over an enclosing 8-year period, data which happened to have been brought together in the UN *Statistical Handbook* for the first time in 1967. The two economic indicators are not significantly related ($r = 0.14$), but the suicide rate shows a significant association with each of them separately ($r = 0.43$ and 0.42 respectively; $P < 0.02$)

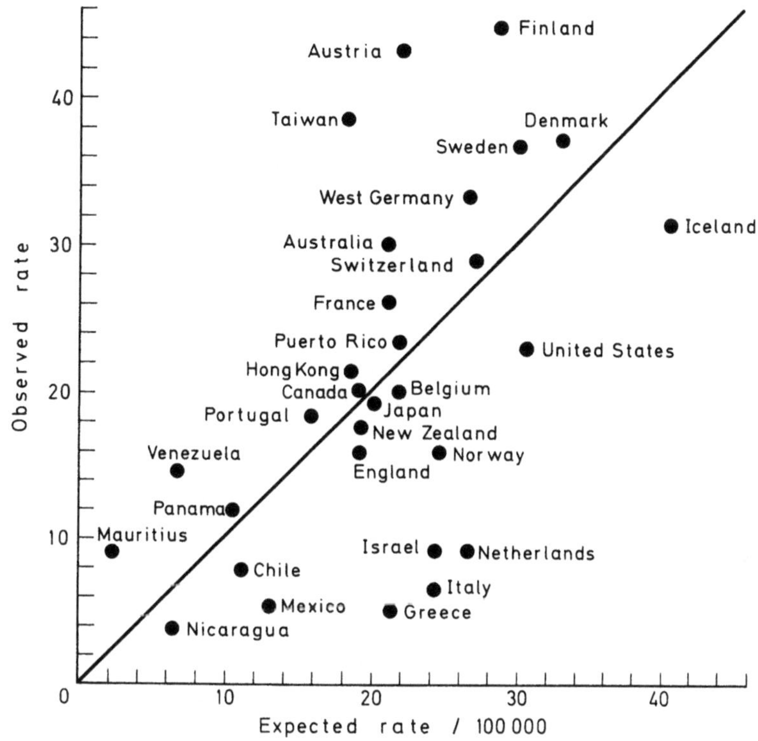

Fig. 7.2. Relationship of observed national suicide rates for males aged 25–54, to rates expected on the basis of a measure of economic expansion. Suicide data are from 1964; economic data are from 1959–1967. Expected rate calculated from the formula

$$E = 0.82\ (0.6x + 0.4y)^{1.1}$$

where x is rate predicted from increase in GNP over an 8-year period and y is that predicted from GNP in 1965.

and when they are combined by regression equation the correlation between the suicide rates and the joint economic measure is 0.56, meaning that 31% of the variance can nominally be accounted for on this basis.

3 Alternative Hypotheses Respecting International Variations

The foregoing correlations are in accordance with what Durkheim's theory would predict, but they do not thereby prove that theory; they merely confirm with twentieth century data the nineteenth century association between economic change and suicide on which the theory was based, and the same associations are capable of being explained in other ways. For instance, it could be argued that economic advancement depends on the ability to sublimate aggression, and that in the process of sublimating that aggression some of the latter is going to become internalized, i.e., to be turned against the self. In consequence, according to this argument, economic advancement can be expected to be associated with a decline in externally directed aggression (homicide, etc.) and an increase in the internally directed form, i.e., suicide, without any anomie being involved. Alternatively, it could be said that economic advancement is only possible through greater social complexity, and that increasing social complexity imposes increasing frustrations on the individual members of that society, with suicide being one of the unfortunate results of that frustration. But again, neither greater anomie nor greater individualism need be involved.

When one attempts to differentiate between these and similiar hypotheses on the basis of the quantitative measures available for comparing societies, the result is usually, as we have just seen, that associations which support one theory are almost equally able to be used in support of the others. This is because the available quantitative measures – the "hard" data – concern variables which are only a distant reflection of the factors being hypothesized; they do not provide direct estimates. An alternative approach to assessing the same hypotheses through comparative studies is to employ "softer" data which come closer to the factors believed to be at work. The use of "soft" data here may be needed because the hypothesized factor is an abstract – an "ideal type construct," in Max Weber's term – which is never going to be directly measurable; or it may be because although the phenomenon which one wishes to measure is concrete enough, the desired data are lacking. The former situation arises regardless of how rich the sources of data are; the latter arises particularly in underdeveloped societies which may have no pertinent records but which one may want to study precisely because they are underdeveloped.

A lack of records usually occurs when one attempts to assess the level of suicide in small, nonliterate societies, something which can be valuable as a means of testing a theory which has been developed on the basis of studies in complex literate societies only. For such nonliterate societies one may occasionally be able to have access to (and to trust) court records, as is illustrated in Bohannan's well-known book on African homicide [58] and in that by Elwin on the Maria of India [169]; but usually the anthropologist only has the remarks made by his informants on the subject, and the theoretician who wants to compare suicide and some other variable across a number of nonliterate societies has to make rather subjective judgements on the basis of what the field workers have written. Usually these judgements are checked by having other persons read the same material and estimate the level of suicide on an agreed analog scale, while remaining ignorant of each others' ratings and of the hypothesis being tested, something similar to having different judges make independent assessments of the same patients' histories or the same psychological test protocols.

The first attempt to apply the latter approach to suicide was probably that by Naroll [455], who took as his departure the work on frustration and aggression by Dollard et al. [154], and tested the hypothesis that suicide would be higher in cultures where individuals faced many frustrations (as assessed by a similar technique to that just described for suicide, but separately for 11 frustration indicators) than in cultures where the frustrations appeared slight. Covering over 150 texts on 58 cultural groups, he failed to detect any direct relationship, but discovered that there was a big difference between the picture when the assessed frustrations were those likely to be perceived as impersonal (e.g., famine and epidemics) and that when they were likely to be perceived as the work of man. Moreover, suicide appeared on this analysis to be related not to all types of man-produced frustration, but particularly to those in which the individual's links to his society were threatened or disrupted. That second impression was in clear harmony with Durkheim's conclusion that the suicide rate in more developed societies was inversely related to the degree of social integration; but the first impression goes beyond Durkheim and moves us from the purely social to a more psychological level, since what Naroll claims is that the suicidal impulse is only awakened when its victim can (rightly or wrongly) identify his frustrations with a particular individual. Moreover, although Naroll does not stress this point, it seems likely that this frustrating individual must be someone whom the victim knows relatively well – e.g., not a distant politician – and whom he might from a psychoanalytic viewpoint have been expected to at least partly internalize.

Naroll's basic material was reanalyzed in more systematic fashion by other researchers and his broad conclusions confirmed [323]; but his "thwarting-disorientation" hypothesis (an awkward term which has interfered with its wider use) has not been tested by other means. His suggestion that the suicide victim needs to identify his problems with a particular person in his environment is in harmony with some of the findings from analyses of suicide notes [545], but the latter source of information is not without bias and the point deserves further investigation.

At the same time as this study was being undertaken, another researcher was working on another hypothesis using sources and methods which overlapped Naroll's. Palmer took the observation that suicide and homicide are inversely correlated across United States cities [500], and asked whether the same inverse correlation existed among nonliterate peoples. He found that it did not. Rather, the two forms of aggression proved to a significant degree ($P = 0.02$) to be directly correlated [481], cultural groups in which the one was high tending to be those in which the other was high also. That positive association has since been shown to apply among more developed societies as well [526], and, what is of much more psychological interest, a link has been established between the combination of these two forms of personal aggression (but particularly suicide) and what national cultures teach regarding "need for power." Taking ratings from McClelland's [393] assessment of "need for achievement" and "need for power" as expressed in the children's stories in 16 countries around the year 1925, it was found that the "need for power" scores correlated significantly with the suicide rates in the same countries 25 years later [34, 526], although not 40 years later [34]. This correlation, in addition to being of interest for its own sake, helps explain why one can obtain a direct association between suicide and homicide when comparing across countries or cultures, but an inverse association when comparing social units within the same country or culture. In the first instance one is dealing with social pressures on the individual to strive for power, pressures which are likely to apply across a whole culture; in the second instance one is dealing with the facilities and models which are offered to the individual with respect to his striving for power, and which are liable to vary from one part of the country to another as well as from one social class to another.

These different cross-cultural studies enlarge our understanding of the social forces at work in certain common types of suicide, and they bring us closer to understanding the psychological factors at work than when we had only sociological arguments of Durkheim's type; but there is still a large gap between what can be gained from such broadly based but superficial approaches to suicide and what the psychiatrist seeks to know about the act. The studies just mentioned harmonize more than may appear at first sight, since a number of Naroll's indicators of "thwarting-disorientation" could also be used as indicators of "need for power," and the "need for power" measure used by McClelland and Palmer could be partially interpreted as an indicator of individualism, and hence inversely of social integration as well. Nevertheless, it still remains unclear on the basis of such data how an individual in a given society arrives at the suicidal act. For Comparative Psychiatry to throw light on this question requires that one turns from consideration of many societies to a consideration of only two or three at a time, going deeper into both the state of mind prior to suicide and the more subtle psychological traits in the culture.

4 Psychological and Psychoanalytic Viewpoints: Denmark, Norway, and Sweden

The main, almost the only, group of countries in which national patterns of suicide have been compared at the desired depth are Denmark, Norway, and Sweden. The comparison was prompted by the fact that Norway throughout this century had a suicide rate which is only half or less that of Denmark and Sweden, as we have seen (Fig. 7.1), and by the similarity of the rates of these other two despite the first being mainly agricultural and the second mainly industrial. The researchers seeking to probe the matter have been mainly American, but Scandinavian authorities have raised some questions regarding the validity of the apparent difference between Norway and the other two with respect to suicide, and these questions must be dealt with first.

It is known that in Norway, certification of suicide tends to be done by persons who might also be the local family doctors, while this is not the case in Denmark [136], and it is also known that when deaths attributed to accidents and to unknown causes are added to those attributed to suicide,Norway's rates become almost as high as those for the other two countries. This arouses the justifiable suspicion that Norway's rates are only low because of underreporting. However, it is not unreasonable to expect accidental death to be higher in Norway than in the other two countries, at least from the rural districts, because the difficulty of getting injured persons to hospital from the Norwegian countryside is much greater than in Denmark. Also, if underreporting were a major factor, one would expect the difference between the Norwegian and the other rates to be greatest in the countryside, where the certifying physician may often be the family doctor, and least in the urban centers where the two roles are usually separate, whereas there proves to be no such gradient [672]. Suicide in Oslo during the 1960s never exceeded 12 per 100 000 per annum, whereas the rates in Copenhagen and in Stockholm were never less than double and more usually were treble that figure [59].

A further suggestion as to why Norwegian suicide statistics should be lower than the others has been that a greater proportion of the population migrates overseas and may take the more suicide-prone with them. However, although the suicide rate of Norwegians in the United States is considerably higher than that in the homeland, the same is true for the Swedes, and the rate for Swedes in the United States is still 44% higher than that for the Norwegians there [533]. (Rates for Danish-born Americans were not available.) There seems no valid reason, therefore, to think that the difference between the Norwegian and the other two national suicide rates is spurious, and when one looks at these other two more closely one finds that they are not as similar as the overall figures might suggest. Danish female rates have run significantly higher than Swedish ones, except in the under-30 age groups, through most of this century, and Swedish male rates have run significantly higher than the Danish ones in the 40-60 age range, although closer in other age groups. In Denmark, in consequence, there have been roughly two male cases for every one female since 1920, while in Sweden the equivalent ratio is 3 to 1, but with more variation.

While that leaves the road free for an examination of the more psychological aspects of suicide and related matters in these three countries, it must be realized that any such examination has still to be quite indirect. Suicide is an almost unique subject for the psychological investigator, since by the time he learns of a case his subject is dead and hence inaccessible for interviewing or testing. Three out of four persons who commit suicide have never been under psychiatric care [673], so that those who have been cannot be considered representative of the majority. Those who attempt suicide or make a suicidal gesture but fail to complete the act are even less representative of those who complete it [590]; and any attempt to carry out what has been called a "psychological autopsy" by interviewing acquaintances is limited by the fact that these may feel guilty about the death and may assuage that guilt by distorting their memories. Interviewing parasuicides whose intent has been serious and whose survival was unexpected probably yields the most reliable results, but it is difficult to collect a sufficient number of such cases and to impose uniform criteria when working in different countries.

The first to attempt comparison of suicidal cases in Denmark, Sweden, and Norway was Herbert Hendin [256], who interviewed an average of 25 persons who had attempted suicide in each country and also interviewed small numbers of controls. Most of the patients were seen many times and the approach to them was psychoanalytically inspired, so that the material which they yielded was rich, but we are not given any evidence that they were uniformly serious in their suicide attempts and the clinical approach meant that the resultant interpretations are very subjective. Hendin went expecting to find differences in the modal characteristics of the suicide attempters in the three countries, and he found what he expected. He also went expecting to be able to link the suicide attempt to problems between the patients and their parents, particularly the mother, and this he also found himself able to achieve, whereas he had no particular expectations regarding the patients' religious conflicts or views on what it is reasonable to expect of life and he rarely found anything to report on these matters. Because of this nonobjective approach his findings have been criticized and they certainly need to be viewed critically, but there is no reason to think that they are less valid than the other often fruitful deductions which have been arrived at using other forms of psychoanalytically inspired approach.

Broadly, he found that in Denmark, suicide was particularly likely to be attempted subsequent to a rupture of dyadic emotional relationships of a dependency-giving and dependency-receiving nature, with considerable feeling of loss whether the patient had been the giver or the receiver. For this reason he suggests that an unconscious motive for the suicide is to be reunited in death with someone, such as a parent, with whom a previous dependency relationship existed. In Sweden the emotional state of the suicide attempters was less depressed and more anxious, and what precipitated the suicidal act seems to have been less a rupturing of relationships than a loss of self-esteem, so that it was a more private act and less a form of communication. In Norway the suicidal patients had more deviant backgrounds than those in the other two countries (as one would expect from suicide being rarer) and they were more likely to use suicide as a self-punishment for sin, an act which would lead to damnation rather than to reunion with a loved one. However, Hendin makes the further important point that the Norwegians whom he interviewed, suicidal or not, were more likely than the Swedes and Danes to vent their frustrations on others and hence to harbor less internalized aggression. Hendin attributes these differences largely to culturally based differences in the mother-child relationship, with Danish mothers being seen as encouraging dependency, Swedish ones as encouraging independence, and Norwegian ones taking the middle road but putting more emphasis on morality.

If for the present one takes these findings (and Hendin's other clinical observations) at face value, the difference between the Swedish and Norwegian modal patterns is in harmony with much of what has been discussed earlier, but the difference between the Danish patients and the others is not. The Swedish patients' self-condemnation for not having been sufficiently successful in their chosen roles or careers can be interpreted as arising from anomie (absence of guidelines as to how much success is sufficient) and/or from too great a "need for power." The greater emphasis of his Norwegian subjects, whether suicidal or not, on moral rules and on the moral right to react against someone who does one an injustice can be interpreted as evidence of greater social cohesion. However, his Danish subjects did not show signs of having expected too much of themselves and of having attempted suicide because of personal failure, even though the continued economic advancement of the Danes during this century and their position on Fig. 7.2 would lead one to expect considerable ambition.

Before one attempts to assess whether Hendin's findings are trustworthy or whether the sociological theories need modifying, it is preferable to turn to other sources of information and ask whether his observations are supported or not. In one important matter Hendin's findings do get support. The rate of clinical depression in Denmark has been estimated to be twice as high as in Norway and at least 50% higher than in Sweden [252]. Moreover, Danish students more frequently state that they "quite often" feel sad and depressed than Norwegian ones do (21% vs 13%), and they are more likely to feel that nothing can be done if they are in a highly unsatisfactory life situation (5% vs 0.6%) [182]. It appears quite plausible, therefore, that the Danish parasuicides should have a more depressive character than the

Swedish and Norwegian ones. Also supported by the comparison of Danish and Norwegian students [182] is Hendin's inference that Norwegians are less inclined to harbor resentment without reacting against the source of the frustration, and more likely to see suicide as a sin. However, when the personnel of a large international company with branches in all three countries were surveyed [264], individualistic traits were assessed to be no higher among the Swedes than among the other two peoples, and although Swedish students did more often state that their mothers tended to encourage competitiveness, the same was not true with respect to encouraging independence [57]. One must remember that with questionnaire surveys like those which have just been cited, the subjects are comparing themselves with other people of the same country and they are not being given internationally uniform criteria for what is meant by such a matter as "encouraging independence." Accordingly, an outsider like Hendin might perceive marked differences between Sweden and Norway with respect to parent-child relations, and these differences might not be apparent when subjects are giving, on questionnaires, their impressions of their own experiences as compared with those of their neighbors. Nevertheless, it has to be stated that the key differences which Hendin has claimed to exist between Swedes and Danes and to affect their patterns of suicide are unsupported by the results obtained by Block and Christiansen [57] from students or by Hofstede [264] from company personnel. There is some similarity between the picture which Hendin gives of Swedish suicide attempters, and the findings from the study of consummated suicide in Sweden by Rudestam [525]; but there are differences also, notably the high proportion (34%) of subjects who were in poor physical health (something Hendin scarcely mentions), the substantial number who were recorded as having said "nobody cares" about them (something which one might have expected from Hendin's Danish subjects rather than from his Swedish ones), and the fact that 56% had experienced a deterioration in relations with friends during the year prior to death. Rudestam compares his findings with some from Los Angeles, but unfortunately not with any from Norway or Denmark.

Drawing together the impressions from these various Scandinavian studies, it can be said that they give us a clearer idea of the psychological processes whereby social integration can protect against suicide, but not a clearer idea of how anomie and lack of social cohesion positively promote it. Compared with the other two peoples, the Norwegians more widely share the ideas that suicide is wrong, that neighbors will support someone in any attempt to speak out against injustices which he feels to be done to him, and that although independent striving is desirable, there are numerous social standards which all individuals should abide by. (The study of company personnel found the Norwegians to score very differently from the other two samples in assigning importance to rules, authority, and the search for absolute values [264].) In consequence, it could be expected that so deviant a solution as suicide would less often come into a Norwegian's mind, and that he would have greater faith in other answers to life's problems, including some in which neighbors could be expected to assist. On the other hand, the Danish and Swedish suicides do not seem to acquire any particular motive or momentum from the weakness of social norms or integration. In Hendin's Swedish cases the fact that society puts such weak limits on ambition may have contributed to their self-imposed demands having no ceiling, but it does not explain why these demands acquired such dominance, given the fact that these people had not been so successful earlier; while in his Danish cases we get no impression that such self-imposed demands were important.

Allowing for the fact that Rudestam's less clinical approach and the restriction of his study to consummated suicides yielded a much wider variety of clinical pictures and contributory factors than Hendin's method did, the most logical conclusion from the Scandinavian data is very similar to that which was arrived at from the nineteenth century data in Table 7.1, namely that anomie and lack of social integration contribute to a rise in suicide rates, if at all, by making a variety of different types of suicide more frequent and not by promoting any one particular type, whether it be labeled anomic or egoistic. The nearest we can get to seeing anomie as promoting rather than as simply failing to inhibit suicide, is by arguing that it is the pressure of insatiable desires which conduces to the act – regardless of whether these desires are for power, health, dependency, or something else – and that it is social norms which restrict our desires to what are satiable. But most people would see desires as being controlled quite as much by the concrete realities with which the ego must deal as by the norms which the social environment communicates, and in any case this argument does not help us to distinguish different categories of suicide which might need different preventive approaches. To identify such categories we need to turn to a more clinical approach, even though this does yield as neat a typology as the sociological approach did.

5 Suicide and Depression

Of the various types of suicide with which psychiatrists concern themselves, the most common is undoubtedly that associated with depression, and in some psychiatric texts one gets the impression that all other forms are rare or unimportant. Certainly, this is the form which psychiatrists most often come in contact with and most often have a chance to prevent, since the suicidal impulse usually loses strength when the depression is treated. From the standpoint of Comparative Psychiatry, one question which presents itself is whether the ratio of suicide to depression is fairly constant, so that societies with high levels of depression need to take extra precautions against suicide, or whether that relation shows marked sociocultural variation.

At first consideration the relationship seems fairly constant. We are accustomed to using the level of suicide as an indirect measure of the level of depression in a society (as formed part of the argument regarding the Malays in the previous chapter), and among the Scandinavians it was noted above that the Danes, who have many cases of depressive suicide, also had an estimated rate of depression double that of the Norwegians. More importantly, when patients with depression are followed up, it has been pointed out by several authors [516, 532] that approximately 15% of those who have died have done so by suicide, virtually regardless of the duration of the follow-up and the country in which the study took place.

This finding, if confirmed, could be valuable, both in assisting us to estimate what proportion of suicides in a given society are of the depressive type and, more importantly, in providing a base measure against which the effectiveness of suicide preven-

Table 7.2. Suicide risk in depressive patients, by country and by sex

	Germany [334]	Germany]546]	Sweden [591]	U.S. [497]	U.K. [572]
A. Suicides as % of deaths, both sexes	15.3%	13.4%	14.3%	16.1%	15.3%
B. Males only					
Cases	110	721	90	25	No
Deaths	92	204	14	25	distribu-
Suicides	23	27	6	7	tion
Suicides as % of deaths, males only	25%	13%	42%	28%	by
C. Females only					
Cases	231	1283	126	31	sex
Deaths	176	288	22	31	provided
Suicides	18	39	0	2	
Suicides as % of deaths, females only	10%	14%	0%	7%	

tion programs could be assessed. Unfortunately, however, the clustering around the 15% level seems on closer examination to have been the accidental result of different proportions of males and females in each sample. Table 7.2 presents, in the first row, the proportion of deaths due to suicide when no distinction is made by sex, and then, below, the proportions found within each sex separately. One sees that the risk of suicide in the males in these samples ranges from 13% to 42%, and among the females from 0% to 14%. Moreover, there appears to be a very different sex ratio regarding the risk of suicide in depressed patients in Sweden from those which hold in the other countries.

Returning from these relatively small samples of patients, with their correspondingly wide range of chance variation in rate, to national statistics, the evidence in favor of there being a consistent relationship between frequency of depression and frequency of suicide is no better. International comparisons of depression rates are difficult to achieve, for the reasons discussed in Chap. 6, but if we consider the rates of hospitalized depression indicated in Fig. 6.1 among immigrants to Britain, then we find that the rank order there is wholly different from the rank orders for suicide either of the homeland populations (insofar as the rates are given in the *Health Statistics Annuals*) or of other migrants from the same origins. Comparing the order in Fig. 6.1 with that in Fig. 1.1 gives the following picture for those groups that feature in both figures:

	Irish	*Poles*	*Rank order* *Americans*	*Italians*	*Germans*
Depression	1	2	3	4	5
Suicide	5	3	2	4	1

If it is argued that hospitalizations do not give an adequate reflection of the prevalence of depression in a population and that community survey data must be used, the result is no better. East Indians exhibited low levels of depression on community survey [114] as well as through hospitalizations in Britain, but they have above-average rates of suicide in all societies from which I have pertinent data. Mexicans exhibit, as Fig. 6.3 showed, an extremely high level of depressive symptoms or complaints when approached by community survey, but in the years for which its suicide statistics have been reported by the WHO, Mexico has had one of the lowest rates in the world.

There is a number of ways in which this lack of correlation can be explained. We can say that it is only in a few countries that most suicide is depressive, and that the differing proportions of nondepressive suicide in the others confuse the issue. Alternatively, we may say that before a relationship between suicide and depression can be assessed it would first be necessary to make allowance for social cohesion and anomie. However, if these were the principal reasons, we might still expect to get a more uniform relationship between the two variables than Table 7.2 indicates, and a third explanation is that allowance has to be made for more than one form of depression. In the two main reviews of suicide in Sub-Saharan Africans [58, 120], it is a striking fact that no case appears to have arisen from a state of endogenous depression, even though such depression exists in the reviewed peoples. The most probable explanation for this is that the depression was of the simple anhedonic type, deriving from biochemical and social origins but not including the ego-superego conflict which characterizes depression in most more individualistic societies. In theory, the simple, anhedonic type of depression should be able to lead to suicide if the person believes that he is never going to enjoy anything anymore [182], a state of mind which can quite easily develop during this condition; but in practice the person with such a depression rarely seems to be able to tap sufficient energy to take the final suicidal step, and as energy increases the depression is felt to be lifting. (Passive suicide by self-neglect is another matter, but in Africans it is more likely to be labeled "voodoo death" than suicide.) Where the anhedonia arouses an ego-superego conflict, on the other hand, psychoanalytic theory teaches that the suicidal act can be much more strongly cathected, either "from the standpoint of the superego [as] a turning of sadism against the person himself," or from the standpoint of the ego as ... "desperate attempts to enforce, at any cost, the cessation of the pressure of the superego" [183, p 400].

Such a theory could explain not just the apparent lack of depressive suicide in tribal Africans, but part of the rise in European rates of suicide during the seventeenth to nineteenth centuries. It was demonstrated in the previous chapter that guilt feelings only became a regular feature of depression in England in the seventeenth century, and had still not fully become so in the rest of western Europe by the time of the French Revolution. In this chapter it has been shown that suicide rates were probably quite low in most of Europe until the nineteenth century, but had risen earlier in England than elsewhere. It is possible to argue, therefore, that the rise in suicide rates followed, at a certain interval, the appearance of guilt feelings in depression, and was a reflection of the same psychodynamic change, as well as being a product of economic advancement and individuation. In fact, one could even say that these different elements belonged together, the economic advancement being achieved through the individuation, and the latter only becoming effective when there developed individual superegos of the type likely to produce both guilt feelings in depression and ego-superego conflicts liable to lead to suicide.

That is hypothesis. It should be possible to test it by comparing the incidence of suicide with the prevalence of guilt-associated depression in different societies, but unfortunately the latter information is not available. Until it is, we can only accept that the depression rate is not a good suicide indicator.

6 Revengeful, "Samsonic," and "Corrective" Suicide: Africa and New Britain

In some of Hendin's cases, he uncovers a desire to hurt other people through the suicide, and this is a feature which many other workers on suicide have recognized also. In its most obvious form it has been called "Samsonic" suicide, after the biblical hero who brought the temple down on himself and his tormentors. From the clinical viewpoint the subject's prior state is one of agitation or excitement rather than depression, although some desire for revenge can be recognized in certain depressed cases also. Some writers have seen the suicide as the expression of a rage against other people which the subject can for the present only vent on himself, since the hated persons are inaccessible to his attacks, but which seeks to do the maximum damage to these others also. The image is very different from that of anomic suicide, but closer to the one implied by Naroll in his "thwarting-disorientation" theory, and some psychoanalysts have argued that it is rage against a punitive superego (modeled after a harsh and rejecting or abandoning parent) which is behind even depressive suicide. Since "Samsonic" suicide is found in institutionalized forms in a number of societies, an examination of its characteristics in these societies may cast some light on its psychodynamics.

There are three main forms of revengeful or "Samsonic" suicide, ones which we may call the ghostly, the blood feud, and the corrective. The first of these derives logically from the belief which can be met in some primitive peoples that most sicknesses and other misfortunes are the work of malicious ghosts. In these peoples a person may commit suicide in a particular location or after particular ceremonies which it is thought will enable his ghost to have unusual power against his foes, and it can in a sense be seen as an extension of feuding into the supernatural realm, with the person who commits suicide having sometimes been a quite powerful member of his society, like Samson, and his goal being to attack his society's enemies. Jeffreys [279], who coined the label "Samsonic," cites instances of this type of suicide in the Herero of South Africa and some East African peoples, and similar traditions have been reported from other continents. We cannot say that the persons performing this type of suicide are suffering from a mental disorder if the belief in the potency of ghosts is still widely held in their societies, but where that belief has been largely abandoned, as in India, one may still meet the occasional case where the choice of method or of site suggests that the subject hoped that his ghost would be able to return and bother people; and in these instances it may be true to speak of a delusion, since most of the subject's neighbors would not think the same way. Some purer instances fall into Durkheim's category of the altruistic.

Suicide designed to produce or to perpetuate a blood feud is rarer than the ghostly revenge type, insofar as societies in which blood vendettas persist are rarer than those in which there persists some belief in the power of ghosts. In these cases the suicide is undertaken in such a way as to oblige one's family to vow the death of some member of the clan or family whom one conceives to have injured one; but it is to be noted that the revenge can be two edged, promising to bring pain not just to the enemy family which injured one, but to one's own family that failed to give one sufficient support, so that it cannot be called altruistic. I have come across individual histories of this from Albania, Sicily, and Corsica, but they do not seem to be common anywhere and when one looks for suicide histories in which the death has been so planned as to cause some other form of real and permanent hurt to another person, these are likewise difficult to find, something which is significant for the theory of suicidal rage. Much commoner, both in the institutionalized and the private form, is the suicide which seems intended to obtain only moderate punishment for the perceived culprit, and which I am calling the "corrective."

Institutionalized, "corrective" suicide is only found where the society has a belief in social justice and also believes that no sane person would commit suicide if he had not been mistreated or neglected. Jeffreys [279] quotes a law of one West African tribe as stating that: "If a man hangs himself in a Bamum village then the village head must give a slave to the king , 3,000 cowries to Tangwa (a court official) and 600 to his assistant. The reason that a slave is given to the king is because the man, being under the control of the village head, must have received some injury from him, otherwise the man would not have hanged himself"[279]. In a New Britain village where similar thinking is found, a father is quoted as saying "Why have you killed my child?" to the villagers when he heard that his daughter had committed suicide; and the other villagers agreed in treating the suicide as culpable murder and as requiring that a culprit – not just the suicide herself – be found [130]. Since the thinking behind that decision implies a moral viewpoint which may even encourage suicide, it invites our special attention.

New Britain has been estimated [269] to have a suicide rate considerably higher than that of neighboring Melanesian territories – 22 per 100 000 as compared with 0.7 per 100 000 for Papua New Guinea in general. It is unclear how far the view of suicide as culpable murder extends over the whole territory, since the earlier report [269] was by psychiatrists who did not have the same relationship with the local people that the anthropologists describing that attitude had, but it does seem fairly clear that the common precipitants of suicide throughout the territory were family conflict and shame, and that the views of many villagers were that the victim's family or acquaintances should have been able to find ways of sheltering him or her from that stress. In the case where the father said: "Why have you killed my child?", the background was a Romeo and Juliet type of situation which the girl had attempted to get corrected for some time without success [130]. After her suicide, the villagers found the boy's family guilty of having driven her to the act, condemned it publicly, and fined it a sum of money. Although that family eventually left the neighborhood, the punishment which it suffered – and which the girl presumably knew was likely to be all that they would suffer – was by no means commensurate with her death and hence one might think that this tradition was unimportant in motivating her suicide. However, she did not act on impulse, having been enquiring about ways of committing suicide for some weeks, and although she was suffering from the absence of her lover, whom his family had sent away, one gets the impression that she was also concerned about the injustice of his family's behavior in demanding an abnormally large dowry which her family could not pay. In this and in similar cases, therefore, the person committing suicide seems to be hoping to achieve some correction within his or her society, through the punishment inflicted on the other party, while not intending that that correction be of any personal benefit. In New Britain, as among the Bamum and in other societies where such institutionalized behavior exists, suicide thus seems to be socially accepted as one of the modes of social control, providing the weak with a drastic but still socially useful means of preventing the more powerful from abusing their powers. Amok, which was discussed in Chap. 5 (p 108) and is also a form of suicide, was in the nineteenth century a much more drastic but somewhat similiar method of restraining the powerful from abusing their power, and was also culturally accepted for this reason. Similar motives may be detected behind the outbreak of suicides by public burning in Western societies since the 1960s.

What these examples teach, I think, is that although some desire for revenge may exist in many suicide attempters, this is surprisingly rarely allowed the free rein which one would expect if it were true that the suicide were the result of uncontrollable rage which was venting itself on both the actor and the persons thwarting him. Much more commonly, even in the blood feud type of revengeful suicide, it is linked to an idea of justice, i.e., of morality. It would thus seem wrong (if one excludes amok) to think of this type of suicide as arising only from the suicide attempter being unable to vent his rage more directly on his thwarter. The superego, either in its individual form or in the form of the "clan conscience" referred to in Chap. 6, seems to play an important role in determining such suicides even in relatively "primitive" peoples. If a person hates someone so much that he seeks his destruction, it is not by the indirect route of suicide that this is attempted even by powerless persons; in such instances attempted murder comes first and the suicide is an afterthought. In the vast majority of suicides, whatever rage exists is still under considerable control, and one must consider that faulty thinking of the kinds which Neuringer [462] has explored in his long series of studies is of greater importance in these cases than the simple loss of ego control over anger.

7 Impulse Suicide in the Young: Samoans, Trukese, and Guyanese

The foregoing remarks were addressed to suicide which is premeditated at least to the extent that the site, method, or last communication has been chosen in such a way as to trouble particular persons or invite later social action. That an attack of rage should precipitate impulsive and unpremeditated suicide, however, is still a real possibility, and there are indications that in some countries there has been an increase in this type of suicide among young people during the 1970s. During that decade, the suicide rate in persons aged 15-24 rose in many countries although in other age groups it was tending to fall, and it seems probable that impulsive, unpremeditated suicide has contributed to that increase. (Another contributing element, in societies where suicide became rather casually talked about, is probably accidental death in persons experimenting with parasuicide.) What could be behind this rise in the major societies in which it has been recorded – United States, Germany, France, etc. – is still unclear, but something of the background to such a rise is known for two Pacific island territories, and the dynamics have been partly explored in East Indians.

The first of the Pacific territories is Western Samoa. In the past, suicide appears to have been rare there, with the cultural tradition and legends providing few guides or models to attract imitators. In the 1970s however, the police became disquieted by an upsurge of cases, and from data supplied me by the courts I was able to work out that although the rates remained very low in older men and in women, the males aged 15–24 had a rate of 65 per 100 000 population per annum in 1976 and 1977, higher than the equivalent in any country reporting to the WHO in these years and approximately four times the average male rates for the same age group in Australia and New Zealand. In a small country such a high rate over a brief period could have been due to one dramatic index case and a brief succession of imitators; and in fact something of this sort occurred in the autumn of 1976. (A similar high rate had briefly occurred in Taiwan some years earlier.) However, the rate continued high in subsequent years and the phenomenon appears to be more than just a passing episode. The main methods employed were hanging and gunshot, and the chief magistrate informed me that the suicides most often took place after a scolding from parents or other family members. (In the smaller American Samoa, the suicide rate appears also to have been above average, but with less focus on this age group. Young men from American Samoa found it relatively easy to leave home for Hawaii or California, whereas there were few comparable outlets for those in Western Samoa and Truk.)

The second Pacific territory so affected has been Truk in Micronesia. It has been estimated that throughout Micronesia in the mid-1970s, suicide in persons aged 15–24 was running at about 70 per 100 000 [257], or much higher in young males since suicide in females is relatively uncommon there. However, some other parts of Micronesia had for long had the reputation of producing relatively many suicides whereas Truk did not do this prior to the 1970s, and when the latter produced a rush of new young male suicides it gave rise to an extensive if unofficial enquiry. The outcome of this enquiry [257] suggests that the suicides were nearly all impulsive, with no prior indications of intent, and that as in Samoa they tended to be precipitated by a scolding from a parent or a minor quarrel with a family member. In the 1950s, when consummated suicide was infrequent but parasuicide more common, it was also noted that the more serious attempts always followed harsh or unkind words from a close relative [222]. The case histories from the '50s and the '70s indicate that there had usually been an impulse to attack an older family member more directly or strongly than custom permitted, that this impulse was restrained with difficulty, and that the residual anger was then turned on the self, sometimes with an indication that the act was an attack on the family as well. Thus, in one case the youth, after being rebuked by his aunt for quarreling with his mother "left the house with a look of almost hysterical desperation on his face; after picking up and dropping a steel bar he took a large stick and beat the side of the house a couple of times. Then he dropped the stick and ran quickly to the top of a fairly tall coconut tree ..." with the fairly obvious intention of throwing himself down from it [222, p 145].

There are two main questions raised by these increases in young male suicides in Samoa and Truk in the 1970s, namely why they happened at this particular time, and why the victims were not better able to restrain their impulses. Regarding the timing, the answer seems fairly simple and in accordance with the theory of anomie. in both territories, the 1960s had seen a considerable expansion of modern education, and families had been urged to get their young people educated on the grounds that the families themselves would benefit. Those that did so therefore had considerable expectations that with this education their sons would obtain salaried employment which would then result in the families reaping material advantages which their subsistance economy had not been able to pay for. But when the boys came to leave school they found few jobs available to them, and the families reproached them for not finding these jobs, not understanding the discrepancy between the economic realities with which their society was faced and the rosy predictions of the teachers from more developed countries. These young men thus bore the brunt of their society's economic discontent, and tradition dictated that when their elders spoke to them they should submit to whatever was said, without argument. (In Truk, although not in Samoa, it is also my impression that there has been an increase in schizophrenia within the same age cohort in recent years, something which would be in accordance with the "cultural double-bind" theory mentioned in Chap. 4.)

Why these young men were not able to handle their aggressive feelings less destructively is more difficult to infer. Psychiatric and more particularly psychoanalytic theory tends to link such outbursts to narcissism, i.e., to the excessive dependence of the ego on self-esteem and the collapse of ego control when that self-esteem is too sharply deflated [316]. However, one expects narcissism to arise particularly where children do not get the necessary feedback from their parents, and it has been demonstrated cross-culturally that narcissistic traits are inversely related to the maternal indulgence of male offspring [573]. In a number of respects, children in Samoa and in Truk are amply indulged. In the latter territory it is true that boys are indulged much less than girls (something which is related to matrilineal inheritance) so that at a relatively early age they are often sent out of the house to live in a shed at the back, and are then expected to spent most of their time with peer group gangs rather than with their mothers; but they get plenty attention in infancy and indulgence is not lacking. Since there is this indulgence, an alternative hypothesis could be simply that the young people of these territories are never taught to restrain impulses; but this alternative runs up against the fact that Samoan, and to a lesser extent Trukese, society puts great emphasis on propriety in the presence of elders, so that the youth are obliged to learn restraint.

A clue to the problem may lie in a report on parasuicide in East Indians in Guyana. East Indians have above-average frequencies of suicide in nearly all the sets of rates I possess, e.g., from South India, Sri Lanka, Singapore, South Africa, Mauritius, and Fiji. Moreover, Indian adolescents tested in Madras in the 1950s were significantly more likely to mention suicide and to avoid mention of homicide or assault, than were American adolescents when given a verbal projective test [560, 561]. Indian adolescent girls in Singapore were also much more prone to parasuicide than other girls there, as Fig. 2.3 illustrated, and Indian rates of consummated suicide tend to exceed world averages particularly in the 15-24 age group. For instance, in one part of Fiji, the East Indian suicide rate for women in that age range during the years 1962-1968 was 120 per 100 000, compared with only about 10 per 100 000 for Japan and most other countries [508]. In Guyana, suicide attempters of East Indian origin were compared with others of African origin, and were found not only to be considerably more numerous than the latter, proportionate to population, but to fall less often into the depressive category [391]. Rather, the Indian cases proved to have made their attempts impulsively, without apparent manipulative intent or premeditation, and apparently in the expectation of death, but with the idea that their death would hurt someone who had hurt them. The source of the impulse seems usually to have been loss of pride or self-esteem after rejection by a person to whom the attempter was attached, something which fits the narcissism theory mentioned above, but there was the further important fact that these patients could not allow themselves to express direct anger against the sort of person whose rejection hurt them. Using the local patois word "vex" to cover anger and other hostile feelings, patients would say: "If me vex, me walk away and cry." "I never show me vex even when me mommy beat me." "Me not angry, me so vex me could not talk." "Me no angry at her, me just feel so bad me took it" [391].

McCandless traces this difficulty in exteriorizing hostile feelings to the fact that in the Guyanese East Indian culture, children are encouraged to show a passive, compliant obedience toward those on whom they feel dependent and toward authority figures generally, while they are given no model of how to express anger acceptably. As in most other groups of East Indian origin, females are also encouraged to show only compliant obedience towards males, something in strong contrast to Caribbean Black traditions. Since the desired compliance depends so little on initiative and so much on waiting for the elders to show what is required, such children must depend on themselves for assessments of their own developmental progress, i.e., must become relatively narcissistic, but the fact that external rewards come most easily when expressions of hostility are completely suppressed adds a further element conducing to suicide. Finally, although expressions of hostility towards elders are suppressed in this culture, expressions of hostility by elders towards juniors (including children) are permitted free expression and McCandless's patients frequently reported that a parent had told them when younger "go kill yourself" or "go drink malathion," this being a poisonous insecticide in use in Guyana since 1960 [451].

In Truk and Samoa the small child is allowed much more spontaneity than is the case among the Guyanese East Indians, but a certain degree of narcissism in males seems to be encouraged and as the children grow older they get a strong training in respect for elders. In both territories it is almost unimaginable for a boy to raise his hand against his father, and it can occasion great shame to be reproached by one's father. Hence a similar suppression of hostility toward elders exists. I do not know whether "go kill yourself" is a remark made by East Indian parents toward children outside Guyana, but I have described elsewhere [422] how certain Indian beliefs in predestination and astrology lead some Singapore Indian children to be rejected almost from birth. McCandless adds the further interesting point that in the only mental hospital in Guyana, depression is a disorder significantly less often found in patients of East Indian than in those of African origin, thus further suggesting that depression is not a major factor in the former group's suicide attempts.

8 The Suicidal Gamble: Tikopia

As far as can be judged from the paper just cited, the Guyanese East Indian attempts at suicide were not undertaken for the purpose of changing the thwarting person's attitudes toward the one making the attempt, as is usually the case with true parasuicide; and the high rate of consummated suicide in that country, "between 43 to 75 suicides per 100 000 population" [391] also argues against this. However, it must be admitted that the attempters, on finding themselves still alive, would probably have hoped that their act would have modified the thwarting person's attitudes in their favor, and there are suicide attempts in which the attempter is neither clearly seeking his death nor clearly seeking to improve his social situation. Insofar as such persons are of a single mind at the time of the attempt, they can be inferred to be throwing themselves on the mercy of God or of persons whose attachment they doubt, implicitly saying: "If you save me and thus indicate that you care for me, then I want to live, but if you do not do so then I want to die." Such thinking is probably behind some suicide attempts in many countries, but there is one society in which it seems to have been particularly common and whose sociocultural background, therefore, might throw light on the etiology: the Tikopia.

The Tikopia are a Polynesian group living on a small island at the extreme northwesterly reach of the Polynesian culture region. The anthropologist Raymond Firth lived among them in the late 1920s and again in the early 1950s. On his second visit he compiled records of all adult deaths since his first visit, and discovered that the suicide rate averaged 53 per 100 000 man-years during that interval and affected the sexes about equally [193]. Six of these suicides were by hanging, 12 by swimming out to sea and 81 by going secretly to sea in a canoe without provisions and under such circumstances as made the chances of making landfall on another of the islands in that immense ocean very slight. However, the fact that most suicide attempts were by canoe is significant, since the other recognized method whereby the suicide attempter could escape death was through relatives or neighbors discovering the attempt and racing after the attempter before he was lost in the open sea. There was a tradition that when the father led the search, as was usual, and when his child was not found, he was likely to commit suicide the same way, not returning home from the search; and this would naturally increase the suicide rate. However, the records compiled by Firth indicate that few such secondary deaths occurred, whereas most of the original attempts were genuine.

Some of the suicides were clearly of the depressive type, as after the death of a loved relative; fatalistic, as in old persons with chronic illnesses; and altruistic, as when a father attempted suicide to persuade the gods to accept his own death in place of that of his sick son. However, the majority of cases occurred after a domestic quarrel or family scolding, so that "when it is known that for any reason a man has become angry, a watch is kept upon him. If he says he is going anywhere, a man follows to prevent him taking a canoe" [193, p 134]. This turning of violence in on the self does not seem to be due to the Tikopia being taught as children to suppress all outward manifestations of anger, or to parental neglect leading to excessive narcissism, since in his original description of these people [192] Firth gives abundant evidence that the children are shown much affection and much tolerance. The question arises, therefore, why this normally happy and peaceful people should turn so relatively easily to suicide, and a suicide of one particular type.

One factor is undoubtedly the belief that death at sea is a "good" death, better than death by disease, and another is the tradition that if a man strikes his father, he must immediately leave the island in a way likely to be suicidal. However, only a small minority of cases are directly linked to either teaching. A more important factor would seem to be that the culture teaches such strong interdependence that feelings which do not harmonize with that interdependence cause considerable emotional distress, and yet are quite likely to arise, due to the degree to which this people is crowded in on itself. The island is roughly circular, only about 1 mile in radius and with a considerable part of its center occupied by a lake or lagoon; yet its average population in the years referred to was 1500. The nearest small island is 70 miles across open sea and larger islands are much further. In consequence, this society has no room to expand, and not even a deserted area to which a person can withdraw to be alone for more than an hour or two when feeling irritable. When the inhabitants of another Pacific atoll, the famous or infamous Bikini, were forcibly displaced to one after another of a series of small islands [343], one of the major factors making these alternatives acceptable or unacceptable to them was whether it was possible to get away, even just far out to sea fishing, so that petty frictions could in this way be allowed to die down instead of being magnified to an extent that threatened the whole community. Among the Tikopia, various means had existed for keeping the population down, but the Christian missions interfered with some of these, the population grew, and the traditional balance was lost.

The most probable explanation for the high suicide rate among the Tikopia, therefore, is that they valued emotional harmony highly, found that harmony threatened by an increase of population with no increase in resources, and found any emotional disharmony so disturbing that they preferred not to live with it. The ocean offered an escape from that disharmony, and if family or neighbors raced behind one to retrieve one, then that provided a promise that they would make an effort to achieve harmony again, so that paddling out to sea with the chance that one would be retrieved was a way of resolving one's problems in one direction or the other. On such an island where both storms and drought could threaten starvation, and where it was often necessary to set out in rough seas to catch food, a risk-taking mentality was socially advantageous. It seems likely that the society encouraged or at least tolerated the suicidal behavior as being in the same risk-taking tradition and as being part of a general strategy of maintaining social harmony in the face of population pressure. Elsewhere in the world where suicidal gambles are taken, it is possible that one will find that the affected individuals have a similar background, although they probably have alternatives which the Tikopia did not have.

9 A Mutilating Gamble: Singapore Chinese

Where the suicidal gamble is taken in other societies, the commonest instrument is probably poison, often one which is well known to produce death, but not immediately. If these lethal poisons are neutralized in time, the victim's life is saved but he is quite likely to remain permanently handicapped, and the possibility arises that this permanent handicap is a recognized part of the gamble, and not necessarily an undesired part. The Tikopia, if my assumptions are correct, desired harmony rather than dependency; in that society everyone was interdependent. The Danish cases described by Hendin, however, probably valued dependency more than harmony and insofar as their suicidal attempts were gambles they were probably aimed at reestablishing the old dependency situation. In Singapore, in the 1950s, I came across an extreme example of this type of suicidal gamble.

The poison employed was caustic soda, something long available in the average household for laundry purposes but only coming into use for suicide in the late 1940s. By 1950 it accounted for 43% of suicidal deaths and 34% of the unsuccessful attempts recorded in the territory [417], extraordinarily high figures when one considers that caustic soda causes, and was known to cause, severe burning of the throat and esophagus, with either a slow and painful death or permanent disability if insufficient is taken. The users were mainly young Chinese women, and out of the 21 parasuicidal cases employing this method which I investigated, the major factor underlying its use appears to have been fear of desertion or abandonment by a spouse or parent. The most probable explanation for the choice of this method is that it served a double purpose, namely self-punishment and an assurance of continual dependency. Often, these patients had had unsatisfactory childhoods, with insufficient parental care, and they rushed or were pushed into unsatisfactory marriage or concubinage. By traditional Chinese standards most had to regard themselves as unsatisfactory partners, insofar as they were neither building up a stable family nor compensating for the male's defects, and they were likely to feel guilty for this reason. They had no parental family to which they could return, no individual skills with which they could feel self-sufficient (only the Cantonese women were at that time accustomed to seek individual employment outside the home, and these were not Cantonese), and the territory's social services were not such as would support them if they left their men. The suicidal attempt with caustic soda produced severe pain which probably helped assuage their guilt feelings; it resulted in their cases coming before the court where orders were likely to be made for their family situations to be supervised; and it placed them in a position of continuous dependency, since although local custom did not make much fuss about the desertion of a healthy family member, it strongly disapproved of the desertion of a crippled one. Two-fifths of these parasuicidal patients had had a psychosis, suggesting that their ability to choose between alternatives was likely to have been defective, and for the others also it is difficult to see this as a rational choice of action, regardless of how strong their reasons were for fearing abandonment.

10 Altruistic Suicide: Chinese and Eskimos

Having used the Singapore Chinese to illustrate a link between suicidal behavior and extreme dependency seeking, it seems appropriate to balance this by an illustration of clearly altruistic suicide which is linked to the same culture. When Durkheim described this type of suicide, the histories upon which he relied were scarcely good examples of altruistic thinking. Most of them concerned situations in which it was either decreed by tradition that someone should sacrifice himself whether he wanted to or not, or the act was undertaken impulsively, perhaps in battle. However, alongside the instances of suicidal gamble just cited from the Chinese, I came across fairly clear instances of privately chosen, nonimpulsive suicide of the altruistic type. The more frequent sort, of a type well known in Chinese literature, was where an elderly and disabled person felt himself to be a burden on his family, perhaps hindering them from moving to another location which offered better chances for the future. Some days after expressing concern about the family's future, the person would get up quietly in the middle of the night, go to a little-used part of the building and hang himself. However it was not only among the old that such behavior occurred. In one case the subject was a young married woman whose husband had died, leaving not just the children but his elderly and infirm parents in her care. The income which she could gain was barely sufficient to feed them and did not cover the medicine which the old people required, and so she drowned herself, leaving a note stating that her parents-in-law and children would have a better life if she were dead and if the territory's welfare department were then obliged to take them in charge, something which at that time was quite true.

Naturally, one can see both in this case and those of the older suicides other reasons besides the altruistic which might have led them to wish for death, but the evidence favored the altruistic motive being the dominant one. Only about 5% of suicides were attributable to this cause at that time, but the proportion had probably been greater earlier in the century. Today such behavior is unnecessary and has, I believe, died out.

The other contemporary people in which altruistic suicide was a cultural feature until about the 1950s but has disappeared since are the Eskimos. Although it is impossible to assess how frequent such acts were, there are many credible descriptions of Eskimos (not necessarily elderly) either walking out into the snow to die or asking someone to kill them, so that they would not be a burden on the clan, and in the 1950s related behavior was still occurring, although usually with a depressive or conflictual element involved as well as the altruistic one. In the 1960s, however, this pattern of behavior is reported to have disappeared even though the suicide rate increased greatly, [322] the reason for the double shift being not improved social conditions, as was the case with the Singapore Chinese, but social disintegration, something which will be discussed briefly below.

11 Parasuicide: Northwestern Amerindians and Scots

By parasuicide is meant behavior which simulates suicide but is not primarily meant to lead to death, although it may do so by accident. As Stengel showed in his original work on the subject [590], the commonest motive is probably to achieve a change in the actor's life situation, particularly in the attitude of his milieu toward him; and it is thus predominantly a form of social communication. Regardless of the society, it is a form most likely to be used by persons such as prisoners [284] who have too few other persuasive means of communication open to them, and those who, because of poor parenting, have poor skills at using the more conventional forms of expression. Since cultures vary considerably respecting the modes of communication which are the most likely to receive favorable attention, it can be expected that the cross-cultural variation in the incidence of parasuicide will be great. Thus, where members of a culture are hard on themselves and on their neighbors, communication by parasuicide runs the risk of being viewed with contempt rather than with sympathy and will therefore not often be resorted to, something which could explain the fact that Jamaica seems to have considerably less of this [258] than other English-speaking Caribbean territories (of which Guyana may represent the opposite extreme), since the Jamaicans are usually regarded as being a tougher people than these others.

Such cultural differences in attitudes towards the parasuicidal communication can make quite a difference to the risk of accidental death or injury, since if that attitude is unfavorable the actor may have to use more extreme methods than if it is favorable. However, from a theoretical angle the most instructive cross-cultural differences are not the ones which depend on receptivity to the intended communication, but those which indicate differences of intent or differences in abnormality of thinking. To illustrate these latter differences I have taken illustrations from the northwest United States and from Scotland.

In the northwest United States certain Amerindian peoples have for long had the reputation of having high suicide rates, high parasuicide rates, or both. Table 7.3 illustrates their high parasuicide rate in the city of Seattle around 1950. (There were only 666 Indians there in 1950, which explains why rates for consummated suicide have not been calculated.) In the mid-1960s, as was mentioned above, these high rates spread to the Eskimos to the north of them, the consummated suicide rate almost doubling each year for a time [322]. The consummated suicides occurred

Table 7.3. Suicide and parasuicide in Seattle, 1948–1952; by ethnic group and sex [542]

Ethnic group	Suicide		Parasuicide	
	M	F	M	F
White	31.1	10.2	34.9	52.9
Black	14.4	4.4	26.3	122.8
Indian	a	a	290.7	621.1
Japanese	19.6[a]	a	26.1[a]	14.7[a]
Chinese	1.5[a]	a	23.1[a]	a

[a]Less than 5 cases

mainly in young adult males and in association with alcohol, while the parasuicides occurred mainly in adolescent girls, often in association with separation from their original community for higher schooling. Thus, at the only Bureau of Indian Affairs boarding school situated in this region, there were 30 suicidal attempts from among a population of less than 900 during 8 months of 1969–1970 [566], and another report suggests that such attempts were occurring at a rate of two per week for a time [248]. In the 1960s, these attempts seemed to occur mainly among certain Amerindian groups, but in the 1970s it was the Eskimos who produced the most cases.

The histories behind these suicidal gestures were of a familiar type. If the adolescents were living with their families, the parasuicide would be precipitated by a quarrel or by recent tension [591]; if they were in boarding school it would be precipitated by a sense of isolation and apparent lack of other means of expression. The actors always proved to have a poor self-image, and at school the gesture had some aspects of an abasement to the more powerful people around them, an abasement which seems to echo that shown by nonhuman primates to more powerful members of their bands. But there were features which are more specific to that cultural setting. In the first place, although parasuicide tends generally to be found among persons stemming from broken or "problem" families, and outside the boarding school it tended here to occur mainly in Amerindians who had been displaced from their original communities to towns such as Seattle, the boarding school cases tended to have come not from the communities most affected by modern changes, but from those which were the most traditional, small, and isolated [248]. Secondly, as illustrated in the title of Jean Briggs' book *Never in Anger; Portrait of an Eskimo Family* [69], many Eskimo subcultures and some neighboring Amerindian ones provide children with no acceptable way of expressing strong emotion, any such expression being treated not by scolding but by virtual ostracism. Accordingly, when the adolescent girls came to the boarding school and were in the grip of strong feelings of isolation, impotence, fear of authority, or hatred of those who had sent them there, their upbringing blocked them from using any of the normal North American channels of expressing these feelings. (The boys at the same school had the male model of acting out under the influence of alcohol, and this was a serious problem there also.) Harvey et al. [248] make the interesting suggestion that the suicide attempts were the modern equivalent of the culture-specific *piblotoq* syndrome formerly exhibited by Eskimo women, a syndrome somewhat similar to possession syndromes elsewhere, except that the behavior was much less structured and no belief in spirit possession was attached. Fortunately, these adolescents were relatively susceptible to sociopsychiatric intervention, a story similar to that which proved true in Malaysian boarding schools with their outbreaks of epidemic hysteria [611], and by the mid-1970s these school parasuicides had virtually ceased [248].

The same cannot be said of attempts at preventing parasuicide in the second group we are considering, the Edinburgh Scots. After a Regional Poisoning Treatment Centre was established there at the beginning of the 1960s, the parasuicide rate increased steadily by about 10% each year until the mid-1970s, and for the age group 15–20 it rose from below 300 per 100 000 in 1962 to almost 500 for males and 1000 for females by 1974 [11, 265]. Moreover, attempts at preventing "repeaters" by providing sociopsychiatric support failed [108]. The characteristics of these Edinburgh cases have a familiar ring. They derive predominantly from overcrowded inner-city districts, have been disproportionately involved in divorce and separation, have a disproportionate amount of contact with the police and courts, and either they in person or their children had relatively often to be "taken into care" by the welfare services [492]. The most marked of all associations, however, was with persistent truancy, 68% of the parasuicides having had this characteristic as compared with only 0.2% of Edinburgh children in general [492], something which seems symbolic of a refusal to learn conventional modes of communication.

In contrast to the Indian and Eskimo youth discussed above, these Edinburgh young people had suffered no displacement from familiar neighborhoods; they had not been prevented from expressing their feelings when children; they were not trapped in schools, families or prisons; they had relatively rich access to social welfare services and when special arrangements for social welfare support were offered them experimentally, they made regular contact with these although without reducing their parasuicide behavior [108]. When given psychiatric assessment, most of them fell into the category of "character disorder" whose main features were "chronic interpersonal difficulties, plaintiveness and arousal of antipathy in those who treat them" [492]! It does not appear that their suicidal gestures were motivated by the desire to effect a change of attitude in particular persons, and although it seems somewhat more likely that there was a desire to effect a change of attitude on the part of society in general, this is not something which was supported by what they said when they were provided with special social casework. Accordingly, the social component of the parasuicidal behavior seems low, and one is forced to consider that this type of parasuicide has a purely private meaning for most of them, not that of a gamble with death, since their methods were not drastic and the Regional Poisoning Treatment Centre assured them of excellent care, but something more like a drug "high," relieving boredom. (It is significant that many of the repeaters showed dependency on alcohol or drugs [108].)

If that interpretation is true, we must then see parasuicide as taking its place for these people as one among various ways – rioting [78], drug taking, gang fights, etc. – of getting rid of emotional energy which has become detached from the effort of satisfying the basic needs of life, now taken care of by society, and has not become attached to the pursuit of any higher goal, since no such pursuit had been learned; and that means that the psychiatric problem is very different from that in the other forms of parasuicide. In the commoner forms the patients must be taught better skills at relating with others, while society may have to be taught to remove barriers to the attainment of needs; but in this form of parasuicide the patients may need to be taught how to develop attainable needs.

12 Conclusions

The main lessons which this brief survey of suicide across time and place has to offer are twofold. On the one hand we see, as is well known, that suicidal behavior can arise from a wide variety of psychological states and motives so that is is of little value for either the psychiatrist or the sociologist to think of it as a single entity. On the other hand we see that although there is this variety, there are certain common social factors which increase the probability of suicide (and parasuicide) occurring, factors which operate almost regardless of the type of suicide which the psychological state predisposes to. Of these common factors the most important is lack of social integration. There are a few exceptions to this rule, instances where individuals kill themselves for the sake of society and are the more likely to do so if they are fully integrated, as among the Eskimos in earlier times. Also, where social integration may reduce the search for private alternatives to suicide, as with the German Jews in 1938. But "hard cases make bad law." Durkheim distinguished between the loosening of social ties which results from certain rules becoming out of balance (anomie) and that which results from greater individualism (egoism); but in history the two have often gone together and in specific cases of suicide it is usually difficult to say which type of loosening has been mainly at work. The term anomie can be applied to most of the social situations in which we have found suicide increasing, but the individual cases often fit his "egoistic" category better. Since social integration can be of different types and at different levels (as for instance when people have close kinship but poor neighborhood ties, or vice versa) it ought theoretically to be possible to state which types of integration are most important for preventing suicide, but I have been unable to derive any such rules from this review. (Ireland, with its extremely low suicide rate despite the intrafamilial tensions described in other chapters here, and the German Democratic Republic with an unusually high rate despite its strong integration at the national level, would make good test cases for any rules of this sort.)

Shifting to the more personal, intrapsychic level, a different type of common factor which one can detect underlying many forms of suicide is the availability of psychic energy for aggressive purposes. Although depression is so often associated with suicide in modern psychiatric studies, comparisons over time and involving less developed societies suggest that simple anhedonic depression does not conduce to suicide; only when one can infer that some degree of ego-superego conflict is also present is suicide to be expected. Naroll's discovery of an association between culturally indoctrinated need for power (as distinct from need for achievement) and the prevalence of suicide in nonliterate peoples points in the same direction, and it is a striking fact that when a people's emotional energy has to be largely absorbed in finding their daily food, suicide is rare. Cora Dubois remarks repeatedly on the rarety of suicide among the Alorese [158], despite the fact that their lives were not only miserable, but poorly socially integrated. The Amerindian peoples in whom suicide has been highest, on the other hand, have been those who put the highest value on power, and the Samoans and Trukese also put a high value on this. It seems possible that where need for achievement and need for power are sufficiently distinguished (and in many societies they are not) this is a factor that affects both the risk of suicide and, as will be discussed in the next chapter, the risk of alcohol dependency.

Despite these common factors, however, it is the variety of types of suicide which is the most important lesson for the psychiatrist from this review, since the different types imply different preventive and treatment strategies. The impulsive suicide of the Guyanese East Indian and the planned suicide of the Chinese elder may both stem in some way from a sense of loss and of uselessness, but their prevention demands very different policies; and with parasuicide the same applies. Working only in a single society it can be easy to gear preventive efforts to a particular type of suicide, probably but not necessarily the most common, but when one views the variety revealed through international comparisons the need to evolve a useful typology and to cater the different types can be better appreciated.

Chapter 8

Disorders Associated With Alcohol and Other Drugs

There are no forms of mental disorder for which comparative studies hold more promise than those to be dealt with in this chapter, and none for which as much comparative work has been undertaken. However, the practical value of these numerous comparisons has yet to be demonstrated, and as one reads through the relevant literature one is frequently uncertain whether it is psychopathology or not which is being discussed. In part this uncertainty derives from technical difficulties and the consequent use of indirect measures, but mainly it derives from the ambiguity of the terms customarily employed in the field. There is an almost deliberate obfuscation regarding (a) what should be considered pathological and what normal; (b) where the boundaries between the social, the psychological, and the somatic lie, in this area; and (c) how far the indicated drug is a primary cause or only an auxiliary factor. In this book we are concerned with psychopathology and its etiology, but much of the pertinent literature does not differentiate these from other disturbing aspects of drug use, more particularly alcohol use. Before international and cross-cultural comparisons can be properly dealt with, therefore, some demarcation of boundaries and clarification of terminology is necessary.

The main problem has been the ambiguity of the terms which dominate the pertinent literature – alcoholism, alcohol abuse, drug abuse, problem drinking, and drug dependency. When introduced by Magnus Huss in the 1850s, " alcoholism" carried partly a medical but largely a moral implication. It referred to those observed states which were associated with heavy drinking and which middle class European society disapproved of, this disapproval being by no means clear cut but varying with the observer, the observed, and the situation. In the 1950s the "disease concept" of alcoholism was promoted, largely for the purpose of removing the moral stigma and encouraging persons to seek treatment, but although Jellinek [280] made a valiant effort to clarify the matter and distinguish different syndromes, alcoholism has remained an umbrella term under which all sorts of percepts and concepts are thrust. There is really little more justification for regarding alcoholic dependency and alcoholic pancreatitis as aspects of a single disease than there is for regarding traumatic epilepsy and a sprained wrist in this fashion when the latter both happen to be produced through the agency of an automobile accident. Respecting conditions associated with other drugs the situation is somewhat better, insofar as drug dependency is in theory a clear-cut psychic or somatic state "characterized by behavioral and other responses that always include a compulsion to take the drug on a continuous or periodic basis in order to experience its psychic effects, and sometimes to avoid the discomfort of its absence" [675]. However, this apparent clarity only lasts until we ask ourselves what is meant by "compulsion"; and the terms "drug dependency" and "drug abuse" are frequently applied in instances where the individuals have made no statements that they feel under compulsion to pursue the drug against their own free will.

In this book we are concerned with psychopathology, and I believe it important to maintain as clear a distinction as possible between this and social pathology or somatic pathology even though they overlap, since the psychiatrist can claim no special competence in these latter fields. For this reason, imprecise terms such as alcoholism and drug abuse will as far as possible be avoided in this chapter, even though they have occasionally been used in previous ones, and an effort will be made to focus on distinct syndromes rather than on drug-associated psychopathology as an assumed entity. Before coming to the question of the distribution of these syndromes across nations and cultures, however, it is desirable to consider in some detail the "normal" use of alcohol and other drugs in different societies, and the possibility of racial differences in susceptibility to their psychological action.

1 Drug Preferences: India and Elsewhere

There would be no drug-associated psychopathology in the present sense if men were not attracted to drugs. Why they should be so attracted either to a specific drug or to drugs in general is a complex matter largely beyond our scope, but since some psychopathology may be merely the extreme expression of the needs which push normal men towards such drugs, variations in these needs or at least in "normal" drug usage are also our concern. International and cross-cultural comparisons of drug preferences may cast some light on these needs, bearing in mind that availability, cost, marketing, and legislation may make the spontaneous preferences difficult to discern.

Few of the drugs in nonmedical use are immediately attractive to the naive subject and many produce some initial discomfort – think of a child's first reactions to beer, tobacco, and intravenous injections. If genetic or racial factors influenced the degree of such discomfort, this could significantly affect preference. Racial differences have been demonstrated in the effects produced by a number of drugs, mainly purely medical ones [164], and alcohol is one of these. Wolff [667] has shown that Japanese, Koreans, and Taiwanese experience more face-flushing, sensation of heat in the stomach, tachycardia, dizziness, and somnolence than Americans of European ancestry when individuals with similar prior experience of the drug are given matched doses. Accordingly, it might be expected that the former peoples would less readily develop a taste for strong drink than the latter, if some other drug giving some of the same advantages were available. This conclusion accords with historic fact, the Orientals having been in general less interested in alcohol than in other drugs, when compared with Europeans. However, Wolff also explored the same question with North American (Cree) Indians [668] and obtained the same differences vis-à-vis persons of European origin, something which fits the racial hypothesis but conflicts with what we know about the attractiveness of alcohol to this people. Moreover, although there is evidence that alcohol is metabolized less rapidly by Indians and Eskimos than by Caucasians, allowing for diet and familiarity with the drug [184], the former are not content with smaller amounts of alcohol than the latter, as might be expected on the basis of the drug being able to affect the brain for longer, but are heavier drinkers. Therefore, racial factors would appear to play only a small part in determining acceptance of alcohol, or the quantity consumed.

Cultural factors clearly play much more of a role, as demonstrated by the intense objections which some Mohammedan societies direct against alcohol and Christian ones against cannabis. However, the declared reasons for one culture attacking the use of a particular drug do not cast much light on why another facilitates that use, and there may also be important reasons which each culture is hiding from itself. Rather than compare societies in terms of their official stances in this matter, therefore, it would seem more promising to look at the factors which appear to determine group preferences when access to several drugs is relatively equal, and also to look for situations where preferences change.

The classic paper on group differences in preferences for different drugs is that by Carstairs on alcohol, cannabis, and opium in North India [90]. He showed that when the first two were equally available, alcohol was the favorite of the aristocratic Rajputs and cannabis that of the other-worldly Brahmins while opium, when previously available, had been the choice of the ordinary soldier and laborer. Nominally, these people of one race also all belong to one culture, but they adhered to considerably different belief systems, the Brahmins relating man to God and emphasizing the conquest of worldly needs, the Rajputs theoretically guarding the Brahmins from attack bur more basically valuing courage and action, and the lower castes most strongly concerned with survival. The Brahmins condemned alcohol largely because it was seen as tying the individual to the present world and interfering with detachment from worldly desires, while they favored cannabis because it facilitated that detachment and sometimes also facilitated supernatural experiences. The Rajputs condemned neither cannabis nor opium, but preferred alcohol since it facilitated action and in particular aggressiveness. The lower castes used cannabis as a means of escape from their daily burdens and as a facilitator of social intercourse [107]; but when it was available opium was still further preferred in conditions of danger and misery, since it provided more euphoria and anesthesia.

The reasons for these preferences harmonize well but not completely with what we know about the reasons discovered in other societies. The Rajput's preference for alcohol is based on reasons very similar to those attributed to the Caucasian and Amerindian groups studied by McClelland and his colleagues in their wide-ranging study of normal drinking [394], but not to those found in Italian youths. Among Americans, the drug usually seems important for providing confidence or a sense of power (perhaps spurious) in readiness for action, but the Italian subjects of Jessor et al. [282] tended to turn to it after an activity had been successfully completed rather than beforehand, and there are a number of Amerindian and other peoples among whom serious drinking seems to be directed at attaining unconsciousness, perhaps in the hope of effecting communion with the ancestors. The withdrawal from the world which is implied in the Brahmins' use of cannabis has an echo in the use of the same drug by some North African cultures, e.g., Moroccan [48], and by parts of the counter-culture movement in the United States during the late 1960s [300]; but there are other societies in which it is turned to for relaxation only, and its employment by the original "Assassins" was apparently to increase aggressiveness. The Indian soldiers' former use of opium is very similar to that exhibited by Chinese laborers in South China, Southeast Asia, and the American Pacific seaboard between 1850 and 1940, insofar as those persons who had the hardest life were the most prone to use the drug, particularly when they were away from their families (as the Indian soldiers were) and still felt an obligation to earn money for these families [348]. (Opium was not employed by lower class Chinese for other than medicinal purposes prior to the social upheaval caused by the invasion of European traders [653].) However, European use of opium in the nineteenth century and of heroin in the twentieth century does not have any such association.

In India itself, as just noted, the peasant and laborer have tended to use cannabis rather than alcohol even in states where the latter is legally produced. However, one of the shifts in preference deserving our attention is that when such people migrated to other countries, e.g., to Trinidad [40] or Singapore [306], they shifted their allegiance from the first to the second of these drugs even though the other was also available, that shift being greatest in territories where the traditional Indian village structure had not been reproduced and least in those such as Fiji and Mauritius where it had been. The most probable explanation for this is that the migration has opened up opportunities for advancement within this world, while reducing the other-worldly aspects of Indian culture, but at the same time had called on the individual to exhibit personal mastery rather than to participate in a communal advance; and the need for a sense of personal mastery is one to which alcohol appears to cater [394]. A similar shift has been observed among the overseas Chinese, with the traditional use of opiates almost disappearing by the late 1960s, both in the United States [32] and Singapore [348], and with a marked rise in consumption of alcohol at least in the latter. (Singapore is alleged to have the biggest per capita consumption of brandy in the world [306].)

Regarding reverse shifts, i.e., from alcohol to cannabis, opiates or some other drug, there was one example in Japan just after the Second World War when an amphetamine stimulant ("philopon") became much more popular among the youth than alcohol, but that may have been merely because pharmaceutical companies dumped enormous amounts of it on the black market at prices lower than alcohol [70], and not because there was a more basic sociocultural reason. Whether there was a real shift among North American and European youth away from alcohol towards cannabis and opiates in the 1960s and 1970s is more doubtful, the main evidence suggesting that it was merely a broadening of the drug spectrum. However, we have one clear and very dramatic example of the massive although temporary adoption of a nonalcoholic drug in an alcohol-using population, namely in the United States forces in Vietnam. It has been estimated that 43% of troops used heroin at least once and 29% used it regularly [515], although both alcohol and cannabis remained easily available and although heroin was recognized to reduce efficiency and increase risk to life, quite apart from disciplinary punishment. We know now, thanks to the excellent report just cited, that the switch was only temporary, that the resultant psychological dependency was very much less than had been feared, and that heavy prior use of alcohol predisposed to taking heroin rather than interfering with the latter as Indian experience might have suggested. However, when one examines the results in detail one finds that what was remarked above regarding the probable reasons for preferring one drug to another are supported rather than refuted here. The opiate was employed to enable the individual to survive an unpleasant experience of limited duration in which personal mastery did not add much to survival chances and did not promise much in the way of longer-term rewards. Those soldiers who looked forward to an army career after their Vietnam stint was finished turned much less to heroin than those who saw that stint as a disconnected, externally imposed episode in their lives, and it was in this group that did not take heroin regularly that heavy drinking was most likely to develop or persist [515].

All the foregoing examples have dealt with peoples who were using drugs quite extensively in nonmedical fashion, but what about those that seem to have preferred none at all? Anthropological reports suggest that these are not so rare, but the information is usually not really satisfactory, since it is frequently unclear whether the people knew of any drugs which could serve in this fashion or did not know of any, and it is also sometimes unclear how representative the studied sample had been in space and time. The Amerindians of the northeast and northwest seaboards were apparently using no drugs at the time the Europeans arrived, although more southerly tribes were, and when first introduced to alcohol they were not particularly either enthusiastic or upset about it [364]. It was only really after the Europeans had seriously disturbed their traditional life-styles that they began to clamor for liquor and suffered so much social disturbance under its influence. In more recent times the main instance known to me in which a major culture remained for a long time relatively unattracted to nonmedical drug use, despite being exposed to the latter, concerns the Malays. Although definitely acquainted with opium, cannabis, and alcohol through the Chinese, Indians, and Europeans who settled among them, the average villagers in Malaysia and Indonesia used them all very rarely (although they did take to tobacco), and the same was true even of most Malays in Singapore until the late 1960s, although they had become a relatively powerless minority in the latter territory considerably earlier. The fact that they were Moslem undoubtedly contributed to their resistance to alcohol but does not seem a sufficient explanation, and there are plenty Moslem peoples using other types of drugs. In the late 1960s, however, Malay youth in Singapore began to use cannabis, and in the mid-1970s they suddenly became heavy users of heroin, featuring proportionately much more frequently in the abundant arrests for that use than the Chinese Singaporeans who had previously been assumed to be the most opiate prone. Little information has been released at the time of writing concerning this serious heroin epidemic in Singapore, and the reasons for the younger Malays' receptivity of the drug can thus only be conjectured. However, it is known that Singapore Malay society put a much higher value on emotional and interpersonal rewards than on those relating to possessions or power [151], and it is possible that the forced transfer of many Malay families out of village-like enclaves into tall apartment buildings among neighbors of other cultures may have interfered with these emotional rewards. If that were the case it could be expected that a drug which provides euphoria would have greater attractions for them than drugs which provide an other-worldly feeling or a sense of power.

Although there are religious movements which have switched their members from taking drugs to taking no drugs, and although there are many instances of national consumption of a drug being reduced, as will be noted later, there is no nation or whole culture known to me which has spontaneously preferred no drugs after having used some. The nearest example to the abandonment of some drug without increasing use of another which comes to mind is the relative cessation of coca chewing by the inhabitants of the Andes when they join the Peruvian army, which disapproves of this habit, and move down to the coastal plains [190]. However, there is reason to think that the attraction of the coca-leaf alkaloids (which have an effect quite different from cocaine) may be based on physiological as well as psychological factors, since they increase the availability of oxygen at high altitudes [60]; and this effect is not needed on the coast.

2 Consumption Levels and Drunkenness: Primitive Cultures

While the foregoing examples have shown that national and cultural preferences for particular drugs can cast light on the psychological needs and stresses that may motivate their use, that use need not imply that these stresses are present, and the level of consumption may be so low that very little pathology ensues. It must be remembered that over many centuries wine was consumed in preference to water in Europe, even by children, because it was safer, less likely to be contaminated by cholera and typhoid, and possessed a weak bactericidal action. Similarly, opium and cannabis were used in many societies for their medicinal action in the body rather than for their psychological effects, while coca, which had once been thought to be taken for psychological reasons alone, has now been shown to have the valuable physiological action just mentioned. Given the additional fact that in many societies there is only one drug readily available, therefore, comparing preferences is likely to have less practical importance than comparing consumption levels and styles. However, what is meant by these last-named terms can vary considerably, and some definitions are much more pertinent to psychopathology than others.

In comparing societies, what is usually meant by consumption level is the mean per capita consumption per year, either for the total population or for total adults. In recent years there has been a strong effort to get governments to pay attention to this measure, with the argument that the rate of alcoholism is closely linked to the mean level of consumption since the heavy drinker tends to establish a consumption limit for himself which is higher than but still linked to the consumption of his neighbors. This holds quite well for countries with a unified culture when one year is compared with another and when "alcoholism" is estimated on the basis of the mortality from liver cirrhosis [436]. It may also hold for a drug like heroin in societies where only a tiny, already disturbed, fraction of the population uses it and where a doubling of amount imported can be reflected by a sharp jump in reported pathology among that tiny fraction. But the argument becomes much less valid when one is comparing countries with different consumption styles or even when one is studying a single country in which cultural attitudes towards the relevant drug markedly differ, if *psycho*pathology is the focus. I knew a Moslem state where the averaged per capita consumption of alcohol was minuscule but where the drug was associated with considerable social and psychological disorder, since it was used almost exclusively by the military who were also the de facto rulers. Within the latter group the per capita consumption was high, with resultant psychopathology, and since the daily decisions of a single one of these heavy drinkers could affect thousands of persons, this pathology or even a simple impairment of judgment was very serious.

Attempting to assess the percentage of the population that consumes more than a nominal amount of the drug, and then estimating the average annual consumption by those using the drug, may be more useful, particularly in predicting the level of demand for treatment services, than estimating the national per capita consumption level. However, even this more precise approach can yield very deceptive results if the society's modal style of consumption is changing, as I have seen in some Pacific territories where drug-associated disorders were decreasing as consumption rose and increasing as it fell [436]. Also, such an approach can usually tell one only a very little about the etiology of the drug-associated psychopathology or point towards preventive actions other than restricting access to the drug. To find clues to etiology in international or cross-cultural comparisons one has to look not so much at per capita consumption as at the prevalence of drug-associated disturbance – i.e., at drunkenness in the case of alcohol – even though estimates of the latter are usually much rougher than the per capita consumption estimates, and may combine very different types of pathology under one head, while failing to include less apparent pathology.

For reasons that have relatively little to do with psychopathology per se, social scientists have shown an unusual interest in comparing drinking patterns in different societies and cultures. Perhaps because the data are not so readily and so widely available, they have not undertaken this with respect to other drugs, and their comparisons have mostly related to so-called primitive peoples, thus having a reduced significance for the countries in which most psychiatrists work. The general question underlying these social science studies is whether drunkenness and apparent loss of self-control represent a failure by the society to cater satisfactorily to its members, or whether they represent institutionalized methods of interaction and social control. Unfortunately, in the original descriptions of community life from which the data for these studies derive, there are many different meanings given to the terms drunkenness and heavy drinking, and there has usually not been much effort to distinguish pathology from what the observer finds objectionable or incomprehensible. Nevertheless, there is much of interest to psychiatry and psychology to be learnt from this work, not least in the method whereby societies are ranked or rated in terms of some social variable and then in terms of the measure of pathology.

The two basic collections of data [29, 268] for this type of assessment of the social correlates of alcohol use drew on reports about 57 and 139 societies respectively, and most of the subsequent studies have depended on the same collections, using different social measures. Since the original descriptions by anthropologists, missionaries, etc., did not report on all the aspects of life that other researchers would like to know about, most of the comparisons have had to be made on smaller subsamples but still represent a wide range. The earliest study [268] posed the hypothesis that drunkenness is linked to anxiety, with uncertainty of food supplies (which was much more easily inferred from the anthropological reports than more subjective measures are) being assumed to be a major potential source of anxiety. This hypothesis is recognized today as having been too simple, both with respect to its anxiety indicators and its unitary approach to drunkenness. Later work [536] has yielded moderate support for the basic idea, but one has the familiar problem of deciding between cause and effect, since a child with violently drunk parents may be expected to grow up with anxieties, and these may be what lead him to seek escape in drink. Just as not all individuals showing evidence of anxiety drink excessively, however, so not all communities with good reasons for being anxious show this trait, and it is clear that the anxiety factor by itself is insufficient.

Later hypotheses tested in the same way have concerned themselves with factors operating in infancy and childhood – particularly ones which seem likely to give rise to a conflict regarding dependency – or factors relating to social structure. Numerous, so-called significant, associations have been reported and it seems frequently to have been forgotten that if one is exploring multiple variables, the fact that something should happen less than one time in 20 (i.e., $P < 0.05$) may be a poor criterion, quite apart from the fact that the eager researcher can innocently word his other criteria in such a way as to favor his hypothesis. Table 8.1 summarizes

Table 8.1. Sociocultural correlates of marked communal drunkenness in primitive peoples

Stage mainly affected		Sociocultural variable	No. of societies	r	P
Infancy	1.	High frequency of crying observed [35]	13	0.77	0.01
	2.	Low ceremonialism centered on child [35]	38	0.42	0.01
	3.	Late introduction of new foods [35]	23	0.59	0.01
Later childhood	4.	Absence of pressure to conform and obey [188]	20	(z = 2.76)	0.01
	5.	Indulgence by adults [188]	25	0.81	0.01
	6.	High achievement anxiety shown [35]	54	0.35	0.01
Adulthood	7.	Absence of clear kinship organization [188]	55	0.67	0.01
	8.	Absence of social class distinctions [536]	(22–57)[a]	0.56	0.005
	9.	Low social complexity [536]	(22–57)[a]	0.63	0.005
	10.	Not patrilocal residence [188]	55	0.67	0.01
	11.	Emotional interdependence not encouraged [29]	45	0.38	0.01
	12.	Instrumental dependence not encouraged [29]	45	0.48	0.01

Only variables associated with marked communal drunkeness at beyond the 0.01 level are shown. Method of assessing r is usually by means of the phi-coefficient.
[a]Exact number of societies for this calculation not stated, but within the indicated range

the major associations between level of reported drunkenness and level of some other variable, ones which had a chance probability of less than 0.01 and which therefore ask to be taken seriously. Keeping in mind that these variables have been defined on the basis of certain hypotheses and do not spring "naturally" from the data, they nevertheless give support for certain theories. The three variables relating to infancy all suggest that marked drunkenness is more frequent in communities in which the infant receives relatively little attention than in societies in which he receives much. Variables 4 and 5, when taken by themselves, suggest that absence of demands on children conduces to drunkenness, but variable 6 appears to point in the opposite direction, insofar as one would only expect children to show high achievement anxiety if their society were urging them to achieve or were otherwise indicating that achievement was necessary. A resolution of that contradiction, however, appears when one looks at variables 11 and 12 and remembers that achievement pressures can be either in the direction of group effort and conformity, or in the direction of individual effort and rivalry. These variables, and to a lesser extent variable 10, suggest that it is need for *individual* achievement which is associated woth drunkenness rather than anxiety to achieve in cooperation with one's fellows, and the remaining variables (7–9) suggest that this is most likely to occur when the society is poorly structured and each man must fend for himself.

These associations thus give some support for the dependency-conflict theory of alcoholism which was promoted by the McCords [395] on the basis of a follow-up of United States children and which is linked to psychoanalytic theories of oral deprivation [314]; but they give still stronger support to theories concerned with social support, anomie, and individual power needs. Taking all 12 variables together, the impression is that drunkenness is most liable to occur when the society is weakly structured and provides individuals with few rules, when oral deprivation occurs in infancy, and when emphasis is placed on private, individual achievement. A later addition to the picture has been to realize that drunkenness of a relatively non-pathological kind tends to occur or even be encouraged when the drinking is fully socially integrated [654], for instance at ceremonials. However, before one can accept these findings as pointers to etiology, it must be remembered that the communities surveyed were all in "primitive" cultures and often disturbed by the impact of larger civilizations. One would therefore like to know how far the same associations apply when the society is more complex and when there has been less disturbance from colonizing powers.

Regarding whether the same associations were likely to have applied prior to the colonial impact, the most convincing answers come from an analysis which has been made not on the basis of direct, contemporary, observation but on the basis of the content of folk tales [394], since such tales tend to relate to events or attitudes of a former time. Forty-four geographically dispersed collections of folk tales were used: little support could be found in them for the oral deprivation and simple anxiety theories; but support did come through quite strongly for the importance of social structure and communality. This study concludes that "Sober societies... are better organized, hierarchical, solidary, often agricultural and settled communities which give wide and strong support to a man and which stress inhibition and respect. Societies which do not provide a man with this solid support apparently often put him in a situation of conflict, where he wants or is expected to be assertive and yet must be obedient." [394, p 70]

When one comes to large, complex societies the validity of such inferences is more difficult to assess, in part because there are various and competing ways of assessing drunkenness, in part because different sections of the same society can present very different pictures, and in part because it is less easy to compare one complex society with another as respects social variables such as those listed in Table 8.1. For instance, public drunkenness is more frequent in Copenhagen than in Helsinki, but arrests for drunkenness are much more frequent in the latter than in the former capital [77], and it is difficult to assess whether this difference should be attributed entirely to the attitude of the police or to the degree and type of drunkenness exhibited. Admissions to alcoholism treatment centers tend to derive from a wholly different social stratum than admissions to police cells for drunkenness do, and the factors referred to in Table 8.1 such as pressure to obey adults can also vary greatly from one social class to another within the same society. For these reasons it appears better to drop the broad concept of "drunkenness" at this point, and consider more specific categories of alcohol- and drug-associated disorder.

3 Chronic Somatic and Social Disorders

Although our main interest here is with psychopathology, it was pointed out earlier that the concepts of alcoholism and drug abuse have customarily been employed in such a way as to avoid clear distinctions between the social, psychological and somatic types of pathology, and even between what is pathological and not pathological. Admittedly, the subject is not simple, in part because divisions between the somatic, psychic, and social are at base artificial, but also because the relations are particularly complex in this instance, Figure 8.1 represents an attempt to clarify

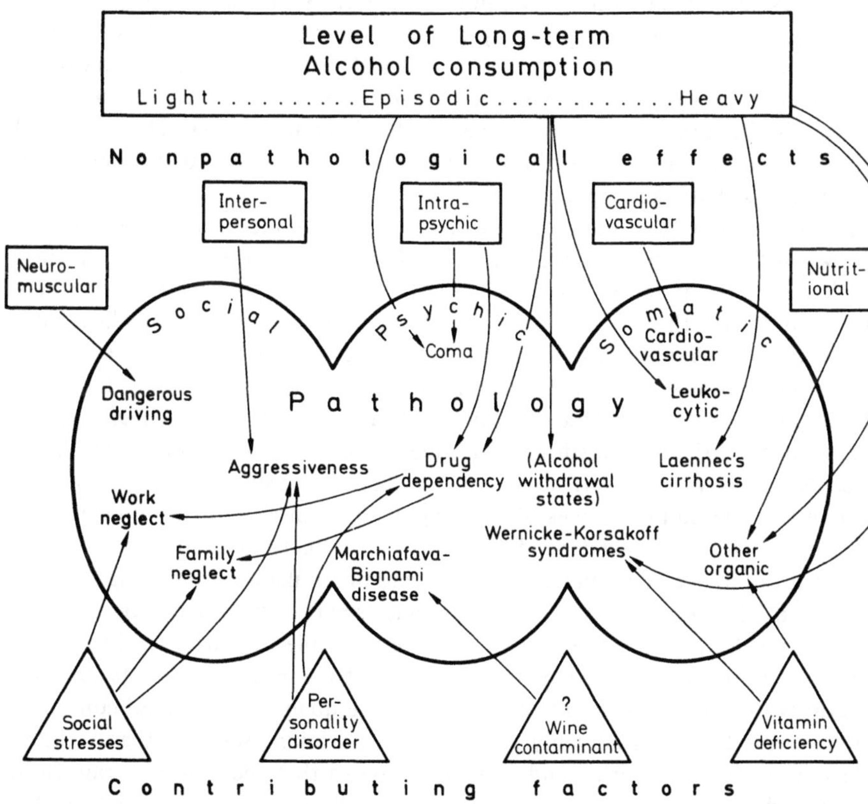

Fig. 8.1. Components of "alcoholism"

for my own benefit these relationships as respects alcohol-associated pathology, and it may be of slight help to the reader despite its complexity. Psychiatry's concern is most directly with the elements inside the central oval, while other conditions included under the term "alcoholism" are shown in the ovals to the left and right, with arrows suggesting causal relationships. Because of the looseness of customary thinking on this subject, it appears desirable to consider the international and cross-cultural distributions of these somatic and social conditions before going on to deal with what I regard as true psychopathology.

What is normally considered to be the most accurate international indicator of alcohol-associated pathology is the mortality rate from liver cirrhosis, and even when one rejects the idea of "alcoholism" as a unitary disease, this indicator can be quite instructive when properly interpreted. For the psychiatrist, the key point about Laennec's cirrhosis is that it is quite treatable and reversible when caught reasonably early, provided the patient accepts to cut down (not necessarily stop) his drinking. On the other hand, the condition usually leads to death, often within 5 years, if heavy drinking is maintained. Only perhaps a quarter of persistently heavy drinkers ever get the condition, in part because some of them die before it develops but mainly because some develop unusually efficient means of detoxifying the alcohol and protecting the liver cells from damage. Cirrhosis will also not usually develop if the drinking, although heavy, is episodic, allowing the liver cells a chance to recover between times; and on the other hand, not all cirrhosis occurs in alcohol users, most younger cases of this disorder probably arising from another cause. Nevertheless, death from liver cirrhosis after the age of 40 will usually mean that, unless the requisite medical care is not available, the patient has refused or has been unable to cut down his drinking sufficiently to permit his liver to recover. Thus, national mortality rates from Laennec's cirrhosis can be taken as a measure of alcohol dependency as both a somatic and a psychological state.

Figure 8.2 presents the mortality rates from liver cirrhosis in the age range 45–64, i.e., when the cirrhosis is most likely to be of the Laennec type, for 53 countries. Although the facts are fairly familiar, it is still worthwhile pointing out that there are eight countries with male rates of over 100 as contrasted with eight whose rates are below 20, a vast range considering that this is a condition within man's control. The eight highest-ranking countries are nearly all wine-drinking while the eight lowest-rate ones, with the possible exception of Israel, are not, and this might suggest that there is a particular constituent in wine, apart from the alcohol, which encourages dependency. However, no such constituent has ever been found, and it is therefore either the national styles of drinking in the high and low rate societies or their attitudes toward fighting dependency which seem likely to be to blame.

The main difference between wine-drinking and other alcohol-consuming societies is well known. The former tend to regard the wine as part of their daily nourishment, to be taken regularly (but not exclusively) at meals, while the latter tend to regard alcohol as an aid to recreation, mostly consumed outside mealtimes and its use varying greatly with mood. One result of this is that the quantity of alcohol consumed per capita tends to be considerably greater in wine-drinking societies than in those that depend on beer or spirits, and it is often argued that the mortality rate from Laennec's cirrhosis and from other aspects of alcoholism is a simple function of the

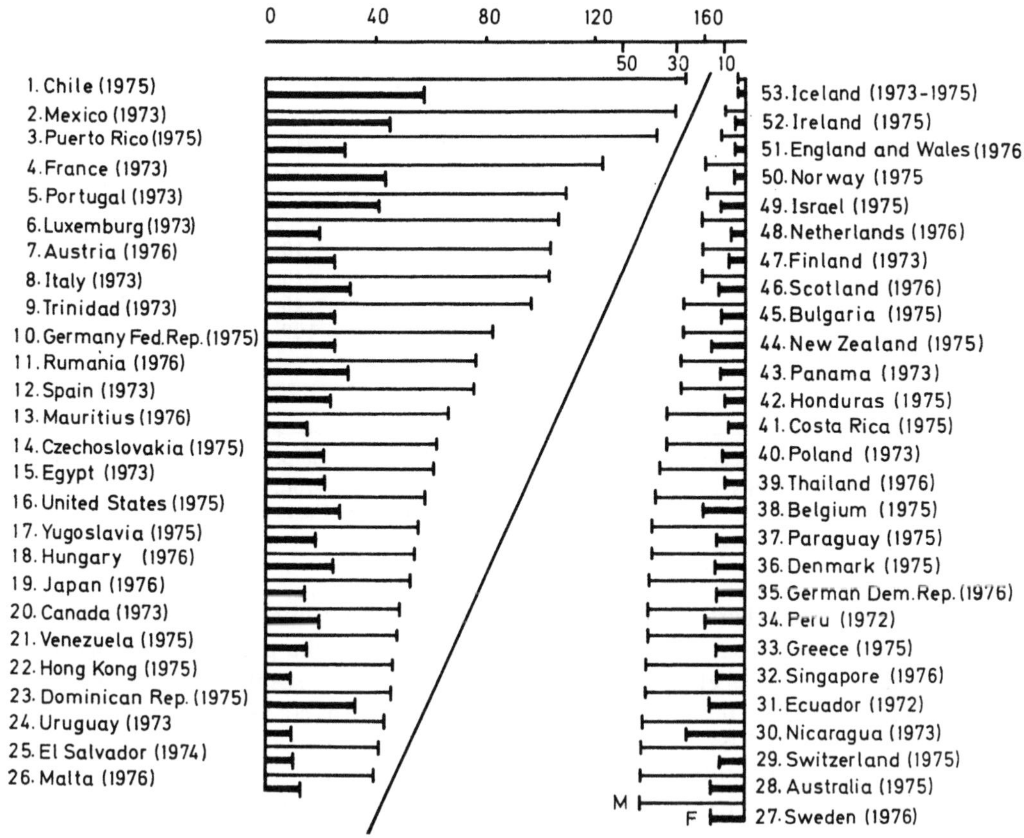

Fig. 8.2. Mortality from liver cirrhosis per 100 000 aged 45–64, by sex, in 53 countries [676]

amount of alcohol consumed. Certainly there is a high correlation between the rates shown in Fig. 8.2 and national consumption rates, and it has also been argued that with wine the cirrhosis develops insidiously, causing irreversible damage before the victim realizes that he has to reduce his drinking. However, there is evidence that the latter is not the whole explanation. Two illustrations will suffice.

In Hawaii, there are marked differences in the degree to which the various subcultures have recourse to alcohol, and this is reflected in the degree to which they have recourse to alcoholism detoxification units, Asians making the least use of both, and Caucasians the most. This is shown in Table 8.2, but what is also shown is that the Portugese-origin group, who come from a wine-drinking background, produce a type of alcoholic who needs to come back time after time, despite being warned to stop, while the spirit and beer-drinking "Other Caucasians," although more often needing some detoxification, appear more able to reduce the need for that over time. Such a picture could result from the chronic drunkards of the other subcultures avoiding the detoxification service after their first visits, while the Portugese-origin group did not, but my own impressions in Hawaii were that the Portugese-origin group had been taught that wine (or alcohol) was a necessary food, and could not contemplate its absence.

Table 8.2. Culture and recidivism at an alcoholism detoxification unit in Hawaii. Recalculated from Bickerton [54]

Cultural origin	Percentage distribution of population	Percentage distribution of patients	Frequency of visits proportionate to population			
			1	2–5	6–19	20+
Chinese	3.9	0.9 (6)	23		0	0
Filipino	7.9	2.3 (16)	29		0	0
Hawaiian	17.2	8.0 (54)	10	20	12	5
Japanese	26.8	5.7 (39)	10	6	2	3
Portuguese	4.0	7.4 (50)	46	33	54	54
Other Caucasian	29.0	71.8 (489)	109	89	42	7
Others (incl. Black)	11.2	3.9 (27)	(not given)			
Totals	100.0	100.0 (681)				

Proportionate frequency of visits is calculated by multiplying the percentage distribution across admission categories by the percentage strength of cultural group in the patient group and dividing by the latter's percentage strength in the population. Figures in brackets indicate numbers of patients studied.

The second illustration concerns a comparison of patients with Laennec's cirrhosis in two Amerindian tribes [329]. When Hopi and Navaho population samples were screened for cases of this condition and the identified patients then followed up, it was found that 10 out of 25 Hopi cirrhotics had died as compared with 17 out of 91 Navaho ($P < 0.005$). The probable reasons for this difference will be discussed below, but for the present it can be inferred that dependency on alcohol is not an automatic result of having consumed a certain amount of the drug over a certain length of time, and not simply a matter of the body's ability to detoxify the drug either, but is a state of mind which depends considerably on social background.

4 Drug Dependency: Amerindians and United States Forces in Vietnam

The idea of drug dependency being something which can be submitted to or can successfully be fought is even clearer with respect to the opiates, which at one time were supposed to establish a virtually irresistible grip on those that got into their power. The highly important study of repatriated heroin users from the United States forces in Vietnam has proved that belief to be quite untrue, and since the full report on that study [515] is not easy to find it seems worthwhile mentioning its findings in some detail here. These findings are based on 900 interviews carried out with a stratified sample drawn from the roughly 13 000 men who had returned to the United States from Vietnam in September 1971, at a time when heroin use among the forces was at its height. These interviews were undertaken between 8 and 12 months after the return, great efforts being made to trace each person in the sample and then persuade him to cooperate, with the result that 95.5% were found and interviewed. Forty-three percent of the sample had, while in Vietnam, used narcotics (opiates), and 29% had done this regularly, i.e., more than ten times in total and more than once per week. At the time of return to the United States,

10.5% were estimated to have had urines positive for illicit drugs, and of those detected as drug-positive at that point in time, more than three-quarters exhibited three or more signs of drug dependency. However, at time of interview, only 2% of the total, or 8% of those who were drug positive on return, stated that they were still using drugs, and various checks, plus the care used in the interviews, makes it likely that this was a true picture. Hence, almost 90% of those who were showing signs of drug dependence at time of return to the United States (when most of them were discharged to civilian life) had apparently stopped taking the drug and had shaken off the symptoms of dependency within the following year. Switching to other drugs had occurred in some cases, and 12% of those who had used narcotics in Vietnam stated that they thought that they were suffering from drug-caused problems at the time of interview. There was a considerably greater likelihood of the heroin use continuing if the interviewee had already used it before going to Vietnam, and if he had taken it by injection rather than by the more normal routes while in that country, but both these facts suggest that the latter individuals were unusually drug prone.

The report just cited does not go into the probable reasons why so many of these men were able to shake off their dependency so seemingly easily, but we can get at that problem from another angle by returning to the Hopi and Navaho cirrhosis patients and considering other studies of recidivism in alcoholics. Regarding the Hopi and Navaho cases, what the researchers found was a substantial difference in communal attitudes towards drunkenness [329]. The Navaho expected some acting-out in association with alcohol in their younger men and tolerated that, but also expected that the older ones would exhibit self-control; and many quite heavy drinkers among the Navaho stopped drinking completely when they reached a certain age or status, being respected for this by their fellows. Among the Hopi, acting-out with or without alcohol was strongly disapproved of, the habitual drunkard was ostracized or exiled, and there were no effective social mechanisms, old or new, for reincorporating a reformed drunkard and providing him with social rewards which would make up for the loss of what alcohol gave. A similar picture has been found in a very different setting, the city of Montreal, among peoples of different European backgrounds. French-Canadian alcoholics proved to show considerably less recidivism and deterioration than those of British Protestant origin [460], and when the attitudes of the general public were explored with respect to drunkenness and alcohol consumption it was found that the French-Canadian public were definitely the more supportive and tolerant [459], while still encouraging a reduction in consumption. (French Canada is a beer-drinking rather than a wine-drinking society.)

For the psychiatrist, therefore, evidence of drug dependency and of the more chronic accompanying somatic disorders need not indicate any mental disorder in the customary sense, but do indicate a state of mind which it should be possible to change if the patient's social situation is favorable enough. Civilian life in the United States offered sufficient rewards of both a short-term and a long-term nature for the rewards of heroin use and the discomforts of heroin withdrawal to be resistible. Many older Navaho drinkers also apparently found the rewards accorded an elder who exhibits self-control to be greater than those provided by alcohol and were able to stop or greatly reduce their drinking. The social rejection which the average Anglo-

Canadian and Hopi drunkard encounters, however, is such as to make life without alcohol seem often much poorer than what the alcohol itself can provide, and for many of the latter the only social contacts which they have are with other heavy drinkers. Finally, although the Portuguese-origin drinker in Hawaii is not likely to suffer rejection from his fellows, he is not likely to encounter any aid in stopping or substantially reducing his drinking either. Rather, he is going to be expected to drink alongside his fellows, and wine is likely to be available wherever he goes within his own circle, whether at home or at the club.

5 Social and Acute Somatic Disorders

Somatic pathology can arise not just from repeated but from a single ingestion of one of the drugs we are considering here, and it can even lead to death. CNS functions can be depressed by massive doses of these drugs just as they can by a massive dose of ether or chloroform, and other functions can also be interfered with, notably by alcohol on the leukocytic defense against infection. Insofar as these effects are accidental they concern psychiatry only slightly, and the same is true of death or injury from accidents while under the influence of some drug. However, it must be borne in mind that in many cases these "accidents" are not undesired, but are the expression of an urge toward suicide or excessive risk taking, both of which will usually indicate some psychopathology. In some northern Amerindian peoples it is well known that death from exposure or pneumonia has been due to the individual avoiding the protection of his fellows after drinking and wandering off to collapse in the snow or in a ditch, deaths from related causes being so frequent in some communities that relatively few adults over the age of 40 remain. Overdoses of other drugs in urban subcultures may have a similar basis; but what needs to be realized is that the psychological factors predisposing to suicide may be quite different from those which have promoted the use of the relevant drug. It is a relatively frequent mistake to assume that treating the depressive state which has led to a suicidal attempt will remove the alcohol or drug dependency which accompanied that attempt, so that the latter need not be given specific attention.

Acute social disturbances in association with alcohol or another drug are also states which need to be divided into those implying and those not implying some psychopathology, since it is a waste of the psychiatrist's time to attempt treating someone whose drug-associated actions are approved by his culture or subculture, and it is usually a misdiagnosis to allege in such cases that the cause lies with the individual rather than with the society. In many societies there is a general belief that alcohol (or occasionally another drug) makes men violent or removes inhibitions to violence. For that reason, violence after consumption of alcohol is often excused when the same violence without the alcohol would not be, and the same is true of acts or remarks which offend custom and morality. This belief has a valuable social function, insofar as it permits the limited expression of hostility or other feelings without incurring the retaliation that would normally be expected if the acts or remarks had been assumed to be made "by intent," but also without the individual having to be labeled insane. It has been argued that this potentially offending behavior has to be learnt [364], and it is certainly true that in most societies in which this occurs it assumes certain sterotypic forms. However, it is also true that such behavior is much more likely to arise in some circumstances than in others, whether modeled on observed behavior or not, and the commonest such circumstance is when a whole society or section of society is made to feel impotent after previously having been taught to value and pursue power.

In virtually all parts of the world, at some time or another, people have gone through such a phase, but the power frustration is usually felt much more strongly by males than by females – which is one of the factors leading to the sex differences observable in Fig. 8.2 – and it is usually felt less by a peasantry, whose rewards arise partly from diligence and partly from luck, than by a hunting society which depends on individual strength and prowess, or by an urban one which depends partly on the domination of men by other men. The power frustration has been felt most markedly by conquered or colonized societies, and alcohol-abuse has often for this reason been described as a curse which the White man has brought to the rest of the world. The accusation is not without justice, but it has not needed to be the White who does the conquering, since the same behavior has been described among the aborigines of Taiwan [511] under the domination of the Chinese or Japanese. Conversely, when alcohol was introduced to North America without the White newcomers yet being seen as a threat, the Amerindians did not abuse it [364].

When such frustrations develop, attacking the conquering or colonizing power is quickly discovered to threaten the very existence of the society, so that it usually cannot be permitted, and allowing individuals to take out their frustrations by attacking their own community members or themselves in systematic or revenge-inviting fashion threatens the social structure as well. If temporary escape valves for the frustrated aggression can be established, however, the social structure may survive or at least adapt, and the myth of diminished responsibility under the influence of alcohol or another drug is one of the commonest ways in which such an escape valve is provided. In recent years one of the regions in which alcohol is performing such a function is Micronesia [369], where young men act out not so much against foreign colonists as against their own rulers who are attempting to apply foreign codes of law and custom and are communicating to their young people expectations which cannot be met. Most of the acting-out exhibited under the influence of alcohol in the latter circumstances permits the men to escape from unmanageable situations without loss of prestige, and this behavior is very common in the Micronesians who are sent overseas for study without having been sufficiently prepared to compete academically there. Only a token amount of alcohol is needed to precipitate the behavior, which may start before the drug could have reached the brain, and a similar picture can be encountered in women whose culture prohibits the expression of sexual feelings but who begin to make sexual advances after only a few sips of beer [245]. Among the people who act out in such a fashion there may be, of course, individuals who are mentally disturbed, but that fact should usually be assessed or established on the basis of evidence other than this particular type of behavior, since most of these actors are not cases for a psychiatrist.

In some peoples it has been observed that such a drug-associated escape valve is needed only for a limited period, certainly less than one generation when circumstances are favorable. In others, history records it to have lasted much longer. Among the latter the phenomenon may still be socially useful and the actors socially integrated, as for instance when the drunk man acts the court fool during certain fetes in Mexico and is permitted to voice truths which would otherwise be suppressed. More commonly, however, the behavior serves no social purpose, the actors are poorly integrated, and the drug-associated behavior is only one aspect of a deeper psychopathology which requires psychiatric attention. Certain northern Amerindian peoples exhibit this problem and a comparison of those in which it is most marked with those in which it is much less throws light on the underlying psychodynamics. Before we consider the latter, however, we need to examine what types of psychopathology are drug-associated.

6 Drug-Associated Psychopathology

With drug-associated disorders, data regarding patients coming into care are less satisfactory for the purpose of international comparison than is true of most other forms of psychopathology. Regarding drugs other than alcohol, one epidemiological review has noted that "the literature on drug use morbidity and mortality was particularly unsatisfactory. The authors suspect that the majority of toxic or psychotic reactions caused by illegal drugs are not reported to the authorities and, of those reported, only a few find their way into the literature" [406, p 311]. Regarding alcohol, the problem has not been concealment so much as the confusion of labels and services. In one health administration, alcoholic psychoses will reach the psychiatric services but all other forms of alcoholic psychopathology will be referred to a special service which does not differentiate them from conditions like cirrhosis or pancreatitis; in a second, cases without psychosis will be admitted to psychiatric hospital because other medical institutions will not accept them, but in order to get them into that hospital they are labeled psychotic even though they are not; in a third administration all alcohol-associated disorders, psychotic or not, are treated in the same special institution and the psychiatric service records show no admissions of such disorders at all.

For these reasons, we will in this section have to depend mainly on (a) cross-cultural comparisons within single medical administrations; and (b) a few outstanding examples of national groups with unusually high or unusually low rates.

Table 8.3 presents comparative data on different groups of immigrants or descendants of immigrants admitted to New York and Canadian mental hospitals. As with all such data relating to immigrant groups, one has to think of the possible effect of migrational strains and selection, and also of a possibly distorted age structure. Nevertheless, there are certain consistencies across the whole table, namely the high Irish-origin rates, very low rates for Jews, and comparatively low rates for Italian and Russian/Ukrainian-origin groups, thus indicating that the relationship between culture and alcohol-associated psychopathology is relatively long lasting. The high Irish and low Italian rates here are just the reverse of what was shown in Fig. 8.2, and the position of the "Other British" is also very different here from what it was in that figure, thus indicating that cirrhosis data are quite unsatisfactory as predictors of psychopathology, and vice versa.

Table 8.3. Psychiatric admissions for alcoholic psychosis and alcoholism: various United States and Canadian subcultures at different periods

Origin	New York 1911 Foreign-born [498][a]	New York 1929–31 Foreign-born [373][a]	New York 1929–31 U.S.-born [373][a b]	Canada 1961 Foreign-born[d]	Canada 1961 Canadian-born[d]
Italian	2	4.8	0.3	0	2.0
French	16			3.0	3.5
German	11	3.8	5.0	0.2	1.2
Dutch				0.3	1.1
Jewish			(0.6)[c]	0	0
Scandinavian	16	7.8	3.6	1.9	2.3
Russian/Ukrainian	1			1.3	1.8
Polish				1.5	0.4
Black			15.1		
Indian/Eskimo					2.2
Gt. Britain (a) Irish	34	25.6	12.7	(6.3)[g]	
Gt. Britain (b) Other	18	4.3	5.1	(2.5)[g]	

[a]Rates per 100 000 total population, not age-standardized.
[b]"Native Whites of foreign parentage", i.e. second generation; except for Blacks.
[c]Generation of immigration not specified; data for 1939–41 [374].
[d]Own data; rates per 100 000 aged 15+, standardized for age and provincial distribution.
[e]British-origin of Roman Catholic affiliation, it being known that this group came largely from Ireland.

In such admission data for so-called alcoholic psychosis and alcoholism, quite a variety of conditions are included, not necessarily under their proper labels. For instance, in Malzberg's statistics all are labeled psychotic, which was not true. It is hopeless, with such country-wide or state-wide data, to attempt to distinguish categories more precisely, since even when more detailed labels are employed in the hospital records, they are not used consistently. In consequence we are usually unable to say whether, for instance, the excess of French-origin admissions over German-origin ones in the above table relates mainly to delirium tremens, to coma states, or to simple alcohol-dependency. However, from the clinical literature one can gather general impressions regarding the sociocultural factors underlying the different syndromes, and these are worth summarizing.

In most psychiatric inpatient services, the commonest forms of alcohol-associated psychopathology (ignoring schizophrenia-with-alcoholism and similar conditions) are delirium tremens and hallucinosis. In Fig. 8.1 these do not appear as such, but rather under the title of "withdrawal states," which has been placed in brackets to remind us that it is usually not the consumption of alcohol but its withdrawal which precipitates the disturbance. (The term is also made to overlap the somatic pathology area, since such withdrawal states can sometimes have somatic symptoms such as tremor, with a clear sensorium.) The sociocultural factors which seem most likely to affect the appearance of this rather than another form of psychopathology are drinking style and education. Style of drinking is important insofar as withdrawal states occur more often in "continuous" than in "episodic" drinkers [186], but less often in those "continuous" drinkers who space their drinks or are accustomed to make them last some time, as is true in most European wine-drinking countries, than in those following no such custom. Education, as in the acute reactive psychoses of Chap. 5, appears to diminish the likelihood of hallucinations occurring, although it cannot prevent them. In the United States, Black patients with an alcohol withdrawal psychosis are more likely than White patients to get hallucinations [236], most probably for this reason, but one of the most highly educated of recent English novelists, Evelyn Waugh, has left us a thinly disguised description of his own alcoholic hallucinations [644]. Poverty is obviously going to affect the risk of this form of psychosis, also, since such psychosis is more likely to happen when the drinker cannot afford to buy more drink, something which is important in parts of South America, than when money is more widely available. Restriction of the hours of sale of alcohol, as in Australia where this psychosis is relatively common, may influence national rates, and distance from a source of alcohol, as in the Canadian north or central Australia, is another environmental factor.

A lesser form of alcohol withdrawal syndrome is alcoholic convulsions ("rum fits"). I have found this unusually frequent in Melanesians, specifically in New Caledonia [436], but the reason is unclear. In the United States it is commoner in Whites than in Blacks [236].

After the withdrawal syndromes, the commonest form of alcohol-associated psychopathology met in psychiatric inpatient services is probably marked intoxication with resultant or threatened coma. Acute alcoholic intoxication, of course, is not usually something which is brought for psychiatric care at all, and even when hospitalization is provided this may be in a general emergency ward rather than a psychiatric one. When there is mild fever and some clouding of the sensorium after the initial effects should have worn off, however, the psychiatric ward may receive the case, although this varies very much from country to country so that treated incidence may not adequately reflect true incidence. Coma is relatively commoner in societies where a major goal of alcohol consumption is to lose consciousness rather than simply to enjoy the sense of power or sociability which the drug can provide in lesser doses. There are tribes in which it is customary for individuals not to drink alcohol at all until they have accumulated a sufficient amount to ensure that the whole drinking coterie will lose consciousness, this choice of goal sometimes being based on the belief that at such times one can make contact with one's ancestors. Usually such drinking has few aftereffects, but in Alaska's native peoples it can be a serious problem, due in part to the extreme weather conditions and in part to self-neglect. Repeated drinking to unconsciousness can be expected to produce some chronic brain damage, but whether this becomes a problem depends on the level of mental effort customarily demanded in that society or social stratum. In Argentina we were able to demonstrate that regular use of coca over many years produces brain damage [443], but found also that the deficit was unimportant in the users' daily lives, those who showed such damage on psychological testing being just as good workers, husbands, etc., as those who did not, and suffering no more distress. On the other hand, brain damage from excessive alcohol use can be felt as severely disturbing to people who put high value on their mental competence, such as

European company executives, and a secondary psychosis or severe neurosis may result.

Marchiafava-Bignami disease is a relatively rare condition with a very strong selectivity for certain societies, notably Italy where it was first described, but the key factor is thought to be a constituent or contaminant of red wine, not the alcohol itself or any more social factor. Neuropsychiatric disorders resulting from the contamination of alcoholic drinks by methyl alcohol, glycol, etc., can be more than just exceptional accidents in some disorganized societies, but not where either the traditional social structure or government administration is sound.

Korsakoff's psychosis, or the "Wernicke-Korsakoff group of syndromes" as is the more approved classification today, is mainly the result of a dietary deficiency which can occur in the absence of alcohol but usually appears as the result of neglect of diet during heavy drinking. For that reason it is to be expected mainly in societies in which alcohol abuse is associated with self-hatred and hence with self-neglect or perhaps the idea of drinking oneself to death. It may also be found in relative excess in those populations where food is difficult to obtain and near-starvation conditions are exacerbated by spending money on drink. Unfortunately, the condition is not usually distinguished from other types of alcoholic psychosis in national statistics and I do not have satisfactory, comparative data on its distribution relative to other alcoholic psychoses or, what could be still more instructive, on the ratio of Korsakoff to Wernicke syndromes in different societies.

Dependency on alcohol has already been discussed when considering the risk of dying from alcoholic cirrhosis, and of recidivism at detoxification clinics. The sociocultural setting is highly important here, as I tried to indicate, and further aspects of the question are best examined by taking up the other main approach mentioned earlier, i.e., considering a few cultures with particularly high and particularly low rates.

7 Vulnerable and Resistant Cultures: Irish, Apache, Jewish, and Chinese

In the general literature on alcoholism, the two peoples who are most commonly contrasted are the Irish and the Jews. As could be seen in Table 8.3, official rates of alcohol-associated psychopathology have been consistently high for the first and low for the second over several decades, and their respective reputations in this matter go much further back. Thus, death from alcoholism was thrice as high among the Irish born as among other urban groups in the eastern United States during the 1880s, and European psychiatrists had at about the same period been commenting on the low rates of alcoholic psychosis among Austrian and German Jews [569]. Of course, it is theoretically possible that the official sources of data are biased, for reasons discussed in Chap. 2, but when one looks at other types of investigation similar results appear. Thus, when Americans who had been investigated as children were followed up in adult life, those of Irish origin proved to have developed the most signs of alcoholism and those of Jewish origin the least, as Table 8.4 shows. Regarding peoples of non-European origin, those which have attracted most attention by reason of their abundance of alcohol-associated problems are certain Amer-

Table 8.4. Alcoholism in Americans with behavior problems followed from childhood to adulthood: by subculture

Subculture	Cambridge-Somerville Massachusetts [395]		St. Louis Missouri [517]	
	N	Alcoholic	N	Alcoholic
Jewish	a		15	20%
Italian	86	6%	a	
Other Latin	47	6%	33	33%
East European	14	14%	a	
British West Indies	17	6%	a	
German	a		64	31%
Irish	13	38%	28	46%
Other West European	41	17%	a	
"Old" or "Native" American	141	19%	78	31%

The Cambridge-Somerville study concerned "pre-delinquent" children for whom a special (but largely unsuccessful) program aimed at preventing delinquency was established in the 1930s. The St. Louis study concerned children referred to a psychiatric clinic for behavior problems during the 1920s. These samples were then followed up in the 1950s and 1960s. The diagnosis of "alcoholic" was established for the first on the basis of official records and membership of AA only; for the second it could also have been established on the basis of statements by the subject himself, or his family.

[a]Too few subjects in initial sample to be treated separately

indian tribes, while a group often coupled with the Jews as having unusually few such problems are the Chinese. It must be emphasized that these four are not alone in showing extremely high or extremely low rates of alcohol-associated psychopathology, and others such as the Finns and Italians could also be chosen. However, the former are the ones on which we have the most information of pertinence to this chapter and hence they are the ones which are best suited for comparison here. It is on the high-rate pair that we will mainly concentrate, but the cultural similarities and differences between them and the two others can be instructive.

Regarding similarities the main point to note, although one which is often forgotten, is that all four have been disadvantaged minorities in the societies with which we are concerned. In the United States during the past 100 years, each of these four groups has been despised and has had to struggle against prejudice, in three of the four with considerable material success in the long run. Earlier in history, the Jews, the Irish, and Amerindians also suffered persecution by greater powers, and the pogroms conducted against the Chinese in Southeast Asia during the present century have been as bad as many experienced by the Jews in Europe. Therefore, although domination by a larger power is often, as was noted earlier, followed by the dominated peoples taking recourse to drink, the Chinese and Jews provide clear exceptions to that rule, and hence we cannot say that it is merely because they have been dominated and persecuted that the Irish and Amerindians have turned to misusing alcohol.

A second similarity is that all four groups are interested in acquiring power, i.e., they are not peoples who have submitted to domination passively as is the case with some small agricultural cultures in which alcohol use is low. Among the Amerindian tribes, as will be touched on below, there have been some that have taken this posture, but the ones with which we will be mainly concerned have not. It could have been that the highly vulnerable pair of cultures we are considering at the moment had stronger power needs while the highly resistant pair had not, following McClelland's power-need theory [394]; but the rapid social advance of Jews and Chinese in any society in which they establish themselves suggests that they do seek power over their own situations, although such power may be less crude than that which is sought by some other peoples. Hence a difference in level of power need would also seem unlikely to explain the difference in vulnerablility to alcohol.

Turning to differences, these are so numerous that one must be selective, but a couple of elementary points may be worthwhile making before we focus more closely on the culture and history of the highly vulnerable peoples. The Jews and Chinese stand out as representing two of the oldest, most persistent and in some ways most successful cultures in the world, and when one makes other comparisons such as between Italians and Finns, Brahminic Indians and Gonds, English and Scots, Provençaux and Bretons, one usually finds that membership of a long and rich cultural tradition is linked to less alcohol-associated psychopathology than membership of one in which the literary (and hence cultural) history is shorter. The simple inference from this is that the former group have had more time to learn, and better means to communicate, methods of handling the types of problem which might otherwise call for recourse to alcohol. A second difference is in the valuing of physical strength and aggressiveness. Chinese family-centered culture taught that it was more virtuous to run away from danger and hence save one's life for the purpose of serving one's family, than to risk that life on a point of principle or to avenge an insult. Jewish belligerence is of very recent origin, and I well remember the scorn which some of the Palestine-born Jews directed at the concentration camp survivors in 1949 because the latter had not attempted to kill their enemies.The Amerindian tribes with which we are mainly concerned, on the other hand, put high value on personal bravery and aggressiveness, and although one part of Irish culture has put considerable emphasis on the need to avoid confrontation, particularly since Ireland became overcrowded, another part, from the ancient legends to the present-day I.R.A., has lauded aggressiveness, particularly against odds and in disregard of personal safety. In societies in which aggression was formerly condoned or valued but in which a relatively abundant use of alcohol did not seem to bring much psychopathology in its train, such as the Japanese and Sicilian, it often seems to have been the case that attack by stealth or cunning was valued as much as or more than open confrontation.

Turning now to the individual cultures, it is natural to ask whether the *Irish* vulnerability to alcohol-associated psychopathology has anything to do with their vulnerability to schizophrenia, as discussed in Chap. 4. At a superficial level this is probably the case insofar as what is diagnosed as alcoholic paranoia may sometimes be schizophrenia, and vice versa [30]. Also, the readiness of the Irish schizophrenic to be hospitalized is in recent years being copied by the alcoholic, admission rates having mounted greatly both in the Republic and in Northern Ireland without much other evidence of an increase in alcoholic psychopathology. However, the geographic and occupational distributions of schizophrenia in the Republic are almost the reverse of those for alcoholism [638], since the latter is commoner in the urban east than the rural southwest, and commoner also among white-collar groups than in farm laborers. As well, whereas the incidence of schizophrenia tends to decline when the Irish move into a more mixed society, the incidence of alcoholism does not [429]. When the Irish are compared with the Jews, as is traditionally done, emphasis is placed on the fact that the latter use drink in a ritual fashion, associating it with solemn events, whereas the Irish use it to increase sociability and relaxation [31, 221, 577]. However, if the comparison is instead made with the Chinese, this difference does not apply. The Chinese do not associate alcohol with solemnity, whereas they do use it to increase sociability, and it is very definitely something which they associate with relaxation, as numerous classic poems indicate. What the Jews, the Chinese, and to a lesser extent the Italians have in common in their attitudes to alcohol, is that drink is associated with the attainment of success and the relaxation which is earned by that attainment. The Purim festival, when Jews are most encouraged to drink [577], celebrates the triumph over Haman and, in times of misfortune, perhaps the fact that the people have survived another year. Among the Chinese it is the person who has retired after a successful life who is most encouraged to drink. Among the Italians, Jessor has noted that drinking tends to be at the conclusion of a stressful experience rather than in preparation for it [282]. In contrast, although a drink will certainly be taken to celebrate success among the nonabstinent Irish, it is even more likely to be taken in preparation for action (even if that act be no more than approaching a girl for a dance) or as compensation for a sense of failure. The same is roughly true of "Old American" approaches to drinking, some Amerindian ones, and perhaps most Scandinavian.

The fact that the Irish use alcohol in preparation for action or to increase sociability, however, still does not explain why there should be so much resultant psychopathology. Nor does it explain the strong ambivalence which the Irish people as a whole have toward the drug, an ambivalence which resulted in 60% of the population being sworn to abstinence during the 1840s. The theory which comes closest to explaining that ambivalence is the "dependency-conflict" theory of the McCords [395], as adapted by Barry [35] and some others. The argument here is that this type of alcohol-associated pathology is rooted in an ambivalence toward dependency in general, of which dependency on a drug is but one aspect. Anthropologists have described the ambivalent way in which Irish children, particularly male children, are treated in early childhood by their mothers, and the ambivalence which these males then direct toward their mothers, toward women in general, and toward situations of dependency [407, 73]. That ambivalence toward dependency can make the enjoyment of alcohol a guilt-inducing experience, and a Dublin psychiatrist has therefore written that "many social drinkers have the next morning experienced feelings of dejection and guilt brought about by their intemperance the night before" [122], feelings which tempt the drinker to drink again for solace, creating a vicious circle. In this view, therefore, a large part of the psychopathology which is linked to alcohol among the Irish is really based on conflictual dependency needs rather than power needs, with one of the ways of resolving the dependency conflict being to accept the label of alcoholic patient, someone who has a right to be cared for by the medical services.

That theory seems able to explain much of the psychopathology which alcohol brings in its wake in this people, but it does not explain the quarrelsomeness which Irish drinkers often show, a quarrelsomeness which is also found in most Amerindian alcohol abusers. According to McClelland [394], a switch from feeling a sense of power *on behalf of* others to a feeling of power *against* these others is a normal progression as more alcohol is consumed, and it is the quantity consumed which is the key factor. However, there are peoples such as the Chinese and Bavarians in whom further drinking simply increases sociability until consciousness is lost. The most probable theory attempting to explain the Irish drinker's increasing quarrelsomeness is that a distrust of, or hostility toward, other males is induced in childhood as an aspect of sibling rivalry, and that it is this which comes to the fore as the initial alcohol-induced euphoria passes away. In the anthropological sources cited earlier, we are told how difficult it is for the western Irishmen to cooperate with others [73], and a major reason for this may be that the mother's ambivalence toward her children provokes rivalry between them. Scheper-Hughes has described how mothers in west Ireland society tend to select a favorite son and then to nag the other children into the impossible task of taking her favor from him [539].

With the *Amerindian*, provoked sibling rivalry seems a less likely explanation, but distrust of other men as a result of their disadvantaged status is undoubtedly a factor among those who live outside reservations, (Brody's description of the "skid row" Indian behavior in northwest Canada [72] is very similar to descriptions of the Irish equivalent,) and in some tribes the cultural tradition seems a major factor. Taking United States Indians and Eskimos as a whole, their mortality rate from alcoholism, alcoholic psychosis, and cirrhosis-with-mention-of-alcohol was 39.2 in 1969, as compared with a rate of 7.5 for the total populations in the 24 states having reservations in them [457], a fivefold difference. If deaths attributed to accident, exposure, or infection but also associated with alcohol had been added to each rate, the gap would have been much greater, and such rates would still be only a partial reflection of the treated morbidity, far less of the unrecorded alcohol-abuse. In one reservation with a total population of about 1200, there were 61 arrests for drunkenness in a single month, and "the actual incidence of drunkenness is probably ten times greater than the court records" [66]. Moreover, the homicide rate among the Indian and Eskimo population within the age range 15–44 is over six times that for the corresponding United States White population [457], and much of this homicide (73% of that in the Navaho [349]) is associated with alcohol. Since this homicide is not directed against the White oppressor, nor undertaken for gain, and not in revenge for persecution by the murdered person, it must be considered an expression of mental as well as of social pathology, and in tribes where alcohol is used sparingly these various types of pathology are much less common. Hence the association with the drug is definite.

The frequency of psychological and social pathology associated with alcohol varies widely among the various Amerindian tribes and there is no space here to go into this variance properly. Merely as an illustration, Table 8.5 gives the homicide

Table 8.5. Homicide rates for selected Amerindian tribes at two points in time

	1880s	*1960s*
Pueblo and Hopi	1.9	6.0
Navaho	5.9	5.3
Sioux	16.3	
Shoshone	73.5	
Apache	141.5	72.0

Recalculated from Levy and Kunitz [349], p. 99, to which the reader should refer for information regarding original sources and representativeness of data. Rates per 100 000 total population per annum.

rates at two points in time for selected tribes, the homicide being usually associated with alcohol as has just been noted. All authorities on the problem agree that the degree to which a tribal or band council can control and guide its members is the major factor in determining whether alcohol-associated psychopathology will be abundant or rare. Such pathology is usually more frequent among Indians living outside of the reservations than in them, and it may take the form of cirrhosis rather than psychosis in people such as the Hopi who value self-control, as was indicated when discussing the first-named condition earlier. The rate of psychopathology does not just depend on the degree to which the community elders exercise control, however; the value orientations and childrearing practices of each tribe seem also to play an important role.

To assess that role it is convenient to take the extreme case of the Apache, who have the highest homicide rate in Table 8.5 and of whom it was quoted that unrecorded drunkenness is ten times that of the high, recorded rate. The Apache are a tribe related to the Navaho who had remained nomadic at the time when the Navaho themselves came under the influence of the more southern Zuni and developed stable settlements. During the second half of the nineteenth century they had fought fiercely against the United States Army, and their enforced pacification was more brutal than what many other tribes experienced. They greatly valued hardiness and cunning in both sexes and in the prepacification period boys between the ages of 8 and 12 had to undergo many trials of endurance and courage, their passage into manhood often involving stealing a horse from outsiders [66]. In earlier childhood they were indulged and succored, so that neither dependency ambivalence nor sibling rivalry would seem likely to derive from that stage, but the matrilocal structure of their families and inheritance system placed young males under considerable strain and their belief system promoted distrust of others in two ways. In the first place, shamanistic power was conceived as being able to divert misfortune from one person to another rather than to absolutely prevent it, and the person onto whom it was diverted often had to be an intimate of the shaman, so that "no old person or shaman, no matter how beloved, was to be trusted" [66, p 53]. Secondly, their boys were taught that women had teeth in their vaginas – the famous *vagina dentata* myth – so that women were likewise to be feared rather than trusted.

In the past, the tensions induced by such a belief system could be not merely released but exploited through aggression against outsiders, and the young men could bolster through feats of war and bravery a self-image which was otherwise weakened by the need to subordinate themselves to their wives' relatives. However, even at that time, before stronger alcoholic drinks were imported, quarrels during the drinking of a weak corn-beer were frequent and the use of peyote, which was able to promote a sense of unity in tribes to the south of them, could not dispel their mutual distrust. Today their young men still have the heroic legends as models, and personal power is still highly valued, but aggression against outsiders is now self-defeating and the tribe has not yet learnt to sublimate this aggressiveness in a commercial, missionary, or other more productive form. If one now thinks of the Jews and Chinese, then one can say not merely that these have learnt to sublimate aggressive drives into commercial and professional activity, but that they are probably the world's most successful peoples at doing so. With the Irish, particularly those overseas, aggressive drives have also been often quite successfully sublimated through politics and occupations such as that of policeman, but the opportunities for this type of sublimation are fewer and more likely to require daily reassurance regarding personal power, hence making alcohol more attractive.

8 Prevention and Treatment Responses: Salish and Trinidad Indians

The Apache group's behavior can be taken, as was indicated, as the extreme example of a maladaptive, alcohol-linked, response to culture change. Nearly all other Amerindian tribes have some trouble with alcohol and some resentment against White domination which gains expression through the alcohol, but there are among them examples of relatively successful adaption to the White society and there are also efforts being made to exploit local cultural resources as a defense or treatment. Among the Apaches's neighbors, the Navaho, it has been shown that those residing in or near the White-dominated county town have less problem handling alcohol than those who are less acculturated [349], and we have also seen in this tribe that their traditional culture enables their older men to cease alcohol consumption entirely if they remain on the reservation, although they may have been drinking quite heavily when younger. Among the northwest-coast Amerindians, a combination of modern and traditional approaches, namely of Alcoholics Anonymous and certain Shaker Church procedures, has recently been developed. This fact, i.e., the apparent need for a support and treatment service different from the standard Alcoholics Anonymous approach, brings us to the question of how far nationality and culture influences the effectiveness of the various available treatments for alcohol and drug abuse.

There is little evidence of a cultural factor in the results from intensive treatments for alcoholic and drug psychoses such as delirium tremens, once one makes allowance for the degree to which the patient has allowed himself to deteriorate before seeking aid. When one comes to treatments for alcohol- and drug-dependency, on the other hand, there is much international and cross-cultural variation in populations, and there is reason to think that at least part of this is due to variations in treatment effectiveness. For alcohol dependency, the three main treatments offered today are psychotherapy, aversion treatment (disulfiram, etc.), and referral to Alcoholics Anonymous (AA). A quick review of the literature on disulfiram [86] suggests that this drug, although developed in Scandinavia, has become relatively popular in French- and Spanish-speaking countries but has not made much headway in Germany, where the success rates with it are lower than average, and had had very mixed success in the United States. Obviously, its results are going to depend on the types of patient chosen and criteria of success, and are going to be better when the patient has no psychopathology and merely wants something to help him protect his liver than when he is neurotic or high amibvalent about dependency in general, including dependency on the disulfiram and his physician. Nevertheless, international differences in response to aversion treatment probably exist even when these factors are allowed for. Regarding psychotherapy, knowledge of the patient's cultural background is always important, regardless of the disorder, but in alcohol dependency there is the additional question of the patient's ambivalence toward feeling dependent on the therapist, something which gives rise to the "alcoholic game" [51] in the United States and which may be much less common in some other societies. However, the most interesting international variations in alcoholism therapy concern Alcoholics Anonymous.

Alcoholics Anonymous was developed in the United States for what was mainly an urban middle-class membership which valued privacy and had conflicts regarding dependency. The need for privacy was catered to by the anonymity (using only first names and strongly limiting record-keeping), while dependency conflicts were reduced by (a) insisting that it is not the alcoholic himself or any other man who is responsible for the disorder and the mastering of it, but some God in comparison with whom it is easy for the most power-sensitive person to admit his impotence; and (b) eliminating status differences between the helped and the helpers. The other aspects of the program – public confession, group support, absence of recrimination, and emphasis on positive aspects of daily life – can be transplanted to almost any other society, but the anonymity and absence of status differentials become untenable in small communities and the effort at alleviating the dependency conflict becomes of little relevance in societies in which interdependence is a more highly stressed virtue than independence. One result of this is that although AA has branches in almost every country and although the idea of getting ex-alcoholics to help current alcoholics is probably valid everywhere, the model has had a very limited success in some parts of the world and a great success in others. For instance, in Japan a more conventional type of abstinence movement predominates, and local forms of either psychotherapy or religious support seem preferred [602].

One of the groups of peoples in which AA has achieved relatively little success is the Amerindian, at least part of the reason being that it is too identified with Anglo-American culture. However, among the Coast Salish of British Columbia, the movement has in modified form achieved considerable success. In this modification the anonymity is abandoned, mixtures of White and Indian alcoholics are avoided, members of the families of the alcoholics are often present at the branch meetings, and time is devoted to group problems such as the Indian-White relationship which AA meetings usually do not examine [283]. Also, although traditional healing ceremonies are not directly incorporated, there is a link to these in some of the activities. The importance of these changes is that they treat the alcohol problem as communal rather than personal, they tie in with the movement toward an Indian cultural renaissance, and they permit the expression of justifiable resentments against White society, resentments which would have had to simmer unexpressed in a mixed White-Indian AA meeting. More success is undoubtedly being achieved among Amerindians with this approach than with the traditional AA groups, but there are no comparative data by which to assess whether this success is greater or less than what orthodox AA is achieving on its own home ground.

The other main location where the AA approach has been taken up and modified to suit another culture is not one in which there was a feeling of resentment towards or rejection of an Anglo-American institution, or where a return to older local traditions is being attempted, but rather one in which the United States origin of the movement is exploited in a positive sense. In Trinidad, the AA approach had first been introduced by a member of the White elite and initially had as little success as in many other Third World countries. Then, quite suddenly, the idea was taken up not, as expected, by the relatively anomic urban population but by the relatively coherent, East-Indian sugar plantation proletariat, so that in a few years there were 42 AA groups for a population of less than 400 000. In this proletariat, the main social affiliation for younger males, apart from the family, was with some street-corner-type gang in which the paying of drinks by individual members in rotation was important. This drinking habit promoted alcohol dependency, and some of the stronger members of such gangs realized as they grew older that this dependency was frustrating economic advancement. They therefore sought help from an alcoholism treatment unit, were introduced to AA, grasped the latter's potential as a social power base, and returned to their villages to recruit their former gangmates into AA branches. These branches differ from the original model not merely in the abandonment of anonymity and the active recruitment of members (AA customarily avoids active recruitment, waiting until individual alcoholics feel sufficiently in need of aid), but through having the membership virtually closed to persons outside the original gang and its associates, and through emphasizing modernization or westernization as a means to personal advancement [19]. The AA branches in Trinidad function not just as a brake on personal deterioration and a means of regaining former status, as is mostly the case elsewhere,but as a means of social advancement both for individual members and for the branch as a whole. Hence I have been told by a leading Caribbean psychiatrist that he has known people in search of political advancement in their villages to feign alcoholism in order to be able to join the AA branch!

Regarding international and cross-cultural variations in the choice and success of treatments for disorders associated with drugs other than alcohol, it is my impression that the main factors are the attitude of the local law enforcement agency and the cost of the drug, matters which are outside the scope of this chapter. Much of the information which we have on this subject derives from treatment settings into which patients have been driven by the law or by the scarcity of the drug on the market place, and these patients tend to present a very different psychiatric picture from that which is met when patients seek help by reason of drug-induced psychopathology or a personal decision to become abstinent. In the United States there are substantial differences in the results claimed for certain treatments with different subcultures, but these seem much more related to social class and relative disadvantagement than to cultural factors.

9 Conclusion

At the beginning of this chapter it was remarked that with the drug-associated disorders the boundaries between the social, psychic, and somatic, plus those between the normal and pathological, are so confused as to amount almost to deliberate obfuscation. If all that is placed under the umbrella term "alcoholism" had been left undifferentiated, it would have been very difficult to derive any meaningful results from international comparisons. Once the different states are distinguished along the lines proposed in Fig. 8.1, however, international and cross-cultural comparisons do become capable of casting light on the subject, as I hope this chapter has been able to show.

Broadly, what the comparisons presented here suggest is that when psychopathology develops through alcohol or drug abuse, it is a side effect of men's efforts at responding to certain types of social demands and pressures. Cannabis was known as a medicinal drug in many parts of the world for centuries, but it appears only to have been abused when men have been encouraged to seek otherworldly gratifications on top of the social and material ones which this world provides. Alcohol has been used, mostly in moderation, by large numbers of people for centuries also, but it seems to acquire a strong association with psychopathology as distinct from somatic pathology only when individuals find themselves called upon to measure up to some ideal image which is beyond their reach – so that they seek the spurious sense of power that the drug gives – or when they find current social conditions so unpleasant that they prefer a supposed union with the ancestors or a disguised suicide. The opiates, used medicinally for so long in Asia, only became widely abused when it became realized that they could assist the individual to withstand pains or fears which he was prepared to undergo for the sake of longer-term or more communal (family) benefits; and it seems likely that coca, with its derivative cocaine, was used by the Amerindians for the same purpose.

These points are clearer when one makes international comparisons than when one considers only single cases or single societies. When comparing individuals it is difficult to distinguish between those instances where what the drug represents or offers is an essential element in the pathological process, and those instances where its use is incidental to a pathological process which would have developed without it. When considering the picture in a single societey at a single point in time, one tends to recognize the situational difficulties which may "drive a person to drink," but not the society-wide expectations which make these difficulties permanent burdens rather than just problems to be avoided. Sometimes, as with anomie and suicide, alcohol-associated psychopathology may be induced more by the removal of social limits to individual striving than by direct social expectations regarding striving, and it is possible that international rates of suicide would imitate rates of alcohol-associated psychopathology (if we were able to measure the latter) although other factors would prevent that correlation from being strong. However, the amount of drug-associated psychopathology would probably be small if the social pressure for individuals to measure up to certain cultural models was absent, or if society also taught effective and available ways of matching these models.

Two further lessons can be drawn from what this chapter has reviewed. The first is that drug dependency can usually be overcome when the individual sees sufficient rewards to his efforts, but that for many people ordinary social life does not provide these sufficient rewards, and the motive for cure is absent. This is probably true with other forms of psychopathology as well, and one of the questions which must be asked regarding the course of schizophrenia in different societies is whether the schizophrenic patient's picture of life after recovery is such as to encourage him to abandon his sick role. The second is that effective treatment of the drug-associated disorders must incorporate either means of attaining the goals for which the drug was used in the first place, or something like a religious conversion whereby these culturally-based goals are abandoned and new ones put in their place. One of the problems in attempting to treat alcohol dependency in North American and some other societies is that the patient has quite probably turned to alcohol in an effort to persuade himself that he is "as good as any other man" (as the culture has taught him to think), while the seeking of help from a therapist can be taken as admitting that the therapist is a "better" man than he is.

Chapter 9 Psychosomatic Disorders

In previous chapters, some attention was usually paid to what is meant by the diagnostic label under discussion, with perhaps a brief history of the term. In the present chapter I have no intention of exploring the various meanings which the term "psychosomatic" has carried, or developing any argument as to why certain diseases should be included under this title and others not. The Cartesian divorce of psyche from soma which Western medicine took over after the sixteenth century is being questioned from all sides, and although the attempt to distinguish illness (what the patient experiences) from disease (the underlying pathology) [178] has been used by some in defense of this division, there is abundant modern evidence of psychological factors being associated with what would at one time have been considered to be purely somatic disease. For instance, youthful attitudes toward parents have been shown to be related to the risk of cancer in middle age [614]. It is still appropriate to pay particular attention to those diseases – for instance, the seven chosen by the Chicago psychoanalytic school for their study of psychosomatic specificity [13] – which have in the past been thought to possess the strongest psychological components, but it has for long been apparent that we cannot treat them as completely separate entities or assume that each has a specific relationship to a different psychological factor. The risk of ischemic heart disease is increased by the presence of hypertension and (separately) of diabetes, and all three are made more likely and/or dangerous by the presence of obesity. However, the psychological factors most directly associated with hypertension are different from those most directly associated with obesity and diabetes, and neither set of factors shows much overlap with the type A behavior pattern with which ischemic heart disease is principally linked in the minds of today's researchers.

For these reasons I have no intention of taking up in turn each of the diseases customarily considered psychosomatic, and then seeking out examples of unusually high, unusually low, or relatively atypical occurrences for it, along the lines followed in some of the previous chapters. Too often, the unusual character of the disease in a particular people would prove either to be explainable on the basis of a purely physical factor, or to be insufficiently investigated for us to assign that character to any etiological element. Something will be said about the broad factors affecting the world distribution of some of the diseases, and reference will be made to some cross-cultural comparisons involving psychological assessments, but attention will mainly be paid to changes of incidence occurring within specific peoples, changes which either do not seem to be explainable on the basis of purely physical agents or which can be theoretically linked to psychological ones.

1 Gastrointestinal Disorders: Somatic Factors

Psychoanalytic theory concerned with the oral and anal stages of early childhood initially found an apparently easy target in the noninfectious gastrointestinal disorders, peptic ulcer and anorexia nervosa suggesting obvious connections to oral conflicts, and ulcerative colitis and some forms of constipation to anal ones. If the psychiatrist is not to make a fool of himself in this field by proposing theories for which he can as yet demonstrate little objective support, however, he needs first to show that he knows what other factors are considered to be influencing the risk of such disorders, and that he has taken them into consideration when assessing the part which psychological factors also play.

The first such other factor, and one which is more easily identified at the international level than in smaller samples, is the genetic or racial one. Both ulcerative colitis and regional ileitis (Crohn's disease) occur significantly more often in Ashkenazim than in non-Jews or Sephardic Jews within the same society [216], and hence the proportion of Jews in experimental and control groups needs to be kept in mind in clinical research. In East Africa, duodenal ulcer more often affects the Nilotic peoples than the Bantu living in neighboring areas and existing on roughly the same diet [620]. In Indonesia and Malaysia, appendicitis occurs much more often in the Chinese than in the Malays living within the same urban areas and using virtually the same food [201]. In India, peptic ulcer appears to occur much less often in the Pun- from the northwest than in either the darker Dravidians in the south or the more Indochinese Assamese in the northeast, an experienced physician claiming never to have encountered the condition among Punjabi living in Assam although they comprised 8% of the local population and although 4% of Assamese hospitalizations were for this condition [370]. In each of these instances, of course, there are cultural differences as well as racial ones, and it is possible that the supposedly genetic factors are really cultural ones, but the evidence does not at present favor such a belief and it is safer to assume that a racial factor has to be allowed for, although not necessarily one of primary importance. The prevalence of ulcerative colitis in the Ashkenazim of Tel Aviv is reported to be considerably lower than that in the American Jews [216], and when the Bantu, who have a high resistance to duodenal ulcer in rural settings, move to the cities, their rates increase considerably [514, 550].

A second influence to be kept in mind is diet. It is well known that diverticulosis of the colon occurs more frequently in peoples consuming low-fiber foods than in peoples consuming high-fiber ones [480]; and the same is probable respecting colonic cancer [80]. The distribution of peptic ulcer in Africa and India, after broad racial divisions are allowed for, appears to vary with the degree to which cereals are refined [370, 620], the less-refined forms possessing more vegetable protein which may act as a buffer against the peptic acid. In addition to conventional diet, however, it is probable that allowance needs also to be made for other consumables. The rate of peptic ulcer in Samoa [366] is much higher than that in the New Zealand Maori although they are of the same race and although the Maori probably eat the more refined cereals, the most probable reason for this (in my opinion) being the Samoans' use of the mildly hallucinogenic and sedative drink, kava, which can be a stomach irritant. In Peru, similarly, the rate of peptic ulcer in the Andean peoples is higher than that among the peoples of the coastal plains [128], and a probable explanation for this (again, in my own opinion) is that the coca leaves which the former chew have to be taken along with an alkali, something likely to stimulate peptic acid production.

In these last instances it is possible to argue that the main factors underlying the differences in vulnerability to peptic ulcer must be psychocultural, i.e., must rest with whatever psychological factors made these drugs attractive to these peoples, an argument which could equally be applied to lung cancer and whatever induces people to smoke cigarettes. However, the connection between mental state and gastrointestinal pathology here is relatively accidental and uninstructive, and if one seeks to be reminded of such distant connections it is better to take the question of the possible relationship between perforated peptic ulcer and clothing in western Europe during the nineteenth century, since the mentality which underlay the clothing fashion could be regarded as somewhat pathological.

2 Perforated Peptic Ulcer: Nineteenth Century Europe

Acute perforation of a peptic ulcer is a phenomenon whose history can be traced with relative confidence, since the onset is very dramatic, the symptoms very characteristic, and the outcome (prior to modern surgery) was usually death within a few hours or days. Nevertheless, in the first important paper on the subject, the Frenchman Gerard [211] was able to bring together in 1803 only eight cases from the medical literature of the previous 50 years, half of the cases carcinomatous. This suggests strongly that in the eighteenth century, such acute perforations were little known despite the extreme abuse of alcohol in some countries during the latter half of that century. In the nineteenth century, cases seem to have remained rare until 1830, when an Edinburgh surgeon was able to report on five cases personally treated, four of them in women, and by the 1840s numerous cases in young women were being reported from other parts of western Europe. (I am depending on Jennings' [281] admirable history of the condition, here.) By 1857 a review paper was able to count 234 cases, and the age and sex distribution of these, something which is shown in the first diagram in Fig. 9.1, confirmed a general impression, namely that the condition was mainly affecting women in their twenties. Until the end of the century and beyond, the ratio of female to male cases remained at between 2 and 3 to 1 throughout most of western Europe [281], with only young women being seriously at risk, as illustrated in the second diagram in this figure, even though male rates were beginning to catch up with the female rates in Britain by the turn of the century, something which will be discussed below. However, it was reported that not a single case in a young woman had been seen in Moscow over a 10-year period [109], and my own reading of the American literature suggests that the condition was rarely met there also, Mayo indicating fairly clearly [388] that he was not acquainted with it, despite his wide surgical experience.

The surgeons of the time had no agreed explanation for the sex difference. Gilles de la Tourette claimed that a third of his own sample of 18 patients suffered from hysteria and another substantial proportion from alcoholism [217], but he was

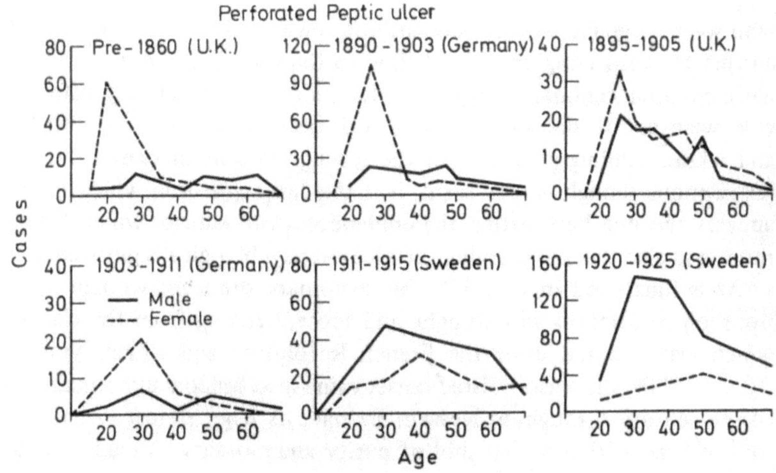

Fig. 9.1. Shifts in the sex ratios of cases of perforated ulcer reaching European hospitals in the nineteenth and early twentieth centuries. Data derived from Jennings [281] and Murphy [437]

thought to use these diagnoses too loosely. Some authors blamed the taking of laudanum (an opium preparation) as a sedative and others the taking of vinegar as an aid to slimming. In the early period it had been noted that the female patients seemed to have been suffering from some disturbance of uterine functioning and later analyses showed that the condition was considerably commoner in women who had not commenced childbearing than in those who had had a child or, in particular,

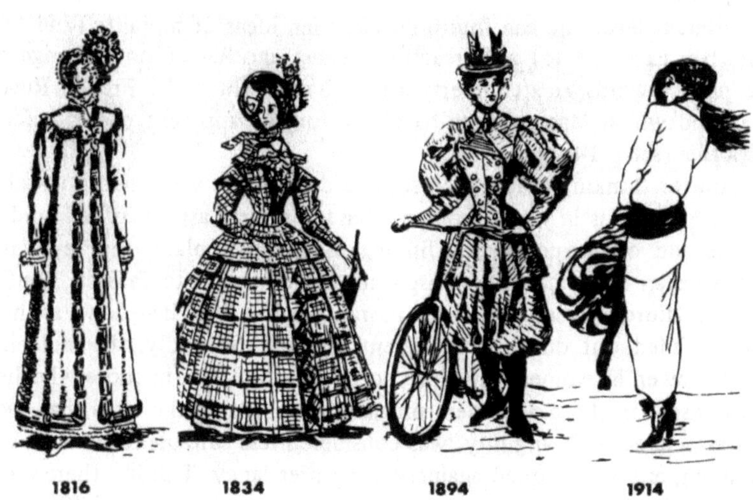

Fig. 9.2. The reign of the tight corset in European female dress during the nineteenth century. The first and last illustrations show the styles immediately before and after that reign; the two middle drawings show variations in between (redrawn from fashion plates of the periods) [437]

who were pregnant. A very few authors towards the end of the period blamed tight corsets for restricting the blood flow to the bowel, and one author associated that with external trauma, noting that the condition particularly affected dressmakers who were apt to dress in relatively high fashion, in harmony with their customers, and whose bending posture over the sewing machine increased the corset's pressure [6]. Curious though it may seem, it is this last suggestion which in retrospect today appears the one best fitting the epidemiological features which I have just summarized, and also the one carrying the greatest psychological significance.

As is illustrated in Fig. 9.2, the customary dress for women at the time of the Bourbon restoration was straight and loose, deriving from the classic Grecian style which was adopted after the French Revolution and which symbolized freedom. By the 1830s, the wasp-waisted corset came into fashion and remained so for the rest of the century throughout western Europe, its reign almost exactly coinciding with that of Queen Victoria, symbol of purity and morality. A reading of texts from that time indicates fairly clearly that the corset was an instrument of that morality, an important aid in restraining the expression of the sexual impulses which women, particularly young women, were then thought scarcely to be able to control on their own. Yet, as with most devices designed to inhibit powerful impulses, it is equally clear that it was turned into an instrument of that suppressed sexuality, since the more a young woman tightened this cage around herself, the more her breasts and buttocks became prominent, particularly when the bustle was also used.

The corset was not, of course, an invention of the Victorian era; it had been used by the upper classes in previous centuries. However, it was only with the industrialization of clothing manufacture from the 1820s onwards that what had been an upper class fashion became available to, and adopted by, women of all classes. This constituted a cultural change no less important than, say, the replacement of locally made tools by imported factory-made ones in the Pacific islands during the present century. At a different level one can interpret Victorian ideas of morality (and the dress style that they gave rise to) as a reaction against another cultural change of that time, the push towards greater liberty and equality which the French Revolution ushered in and which Masaryk was to blame for the apparent rise in suicide and mental disorder (see p 149).

My reason for thinking that the corset and dress styles were instrumental in producing the perforations in young women is based on three aspects of the epidemiological picture and one experimental finding. In the first place, the "epidemic" of perforations began soon after the wasp-waist style came into fashion, confined itself to western Europe where Victorian morality ruled, and died down as the use of tight corsets faded out during the present century. Secondly, the incidence was considerably lower in women who had borne children than in those who had not, and almost absent in those who were pregnant, thus fitting the facts that the wasp-waist was associated with virginity, was considered less suitable for women who had borne children, and was warned against during pregnancy. Thirdly, there was a marked seasonal swing in the incidence of perforations in women aged 15-30, as Jennings [281] has shown, with the winter rates two to three times the summer ones; yet there was no such swing in the incidence in men and in older women. In winter, the fashionable woman wore not just a corset but a mass of heavy clothing (one husband weighed what his wife proposed to wear for dinner and found it to total 50 pounds) whereas in the summer the extra pressure on the abdomen was much less and one frequently read of women loosening their corsets in this season, the fewer additional layers of clothing making this easier to effect. The experimental finding is that peptic ulcers can be induced in a variety of laboratory animals by both physical restraint (tying down) and reducing cage size without direct tying down, the vulnerability being increased by superimposing emotional stress [8].

It may be argued that even if the mechanism which I am hypothesizing were a fact, it is not one which we would normally think of as psychosomatic, since the crucial element was external. However, alcohol is also an external agent, and psychiatry is not the less interested in its effects. Also, it seems likely that the excessive tightening of corsets by a relatively small proportion of their wearers happened particularly in the presence of strong conflicts regarding sexuality, since the extra tightening and more elaborate clothing served simultaneously to restrict the body and emphasize sexual identity. Medical men at the beginning of the present century recognized the existence of a *maladie du corset* [251] causing distortion of abdominal organs, and psychoanalytic theory later suggested that the corset might represent a displacement of "muscle eroticism" [197], a concept I find difficult to grasp, but in both instances it was a general tendency that was being referred to, whereas the present hypothesis relates to a much smaller number of women, but ones who usually died as a result of their habit.

3 Duodenal Ulcer in Males: Twentieth Century Western Societies

As was noted above, the nineteenth century "epidemic" of peptic ulcer perforations in young women was confined to western Europe and does not seem to have extended to the United States where Victorian ideas about the protection of women held only limited sway. Around the turn of the century, however, a new "epidemic" of peptic ulcer began, this time in males and on both sides of the Atlantic, but not particularly associated with perforations. This new wave of peptic ulcers, although much written about, has never been adequately explained, because although there initially appeared to be a close parallel between the increasing consumption of cigarettes (mainly by males) and the increasing rate of peptic ulcer, the consumption of cigarettes continued to rise when the male ulcer rate dropped, and female cases have not risen in line with the increase in their smoking. Certain features of this male "epidemic" point to the cause being primarily psychological and related to another culture change which Western society has undergone.

The shift from an excess of female to an excess of male cases of perforating peptic ulcer at the beginning of the present century is illustrated in the last two diagrams in Fig. 9.1. However, the type of ulcer which aroused concern between the two World Wars was not that producing acute perforations but a more chronic form, and to get a better picture of the historic changes in this it is better to turn to national mortality statistics. These still do not properly reflect the extent of the epidemic, since only a minority of persons suffering from peptic ulcer die from it, but they are more trustworthy than most morbidity data, since there can be marked differences

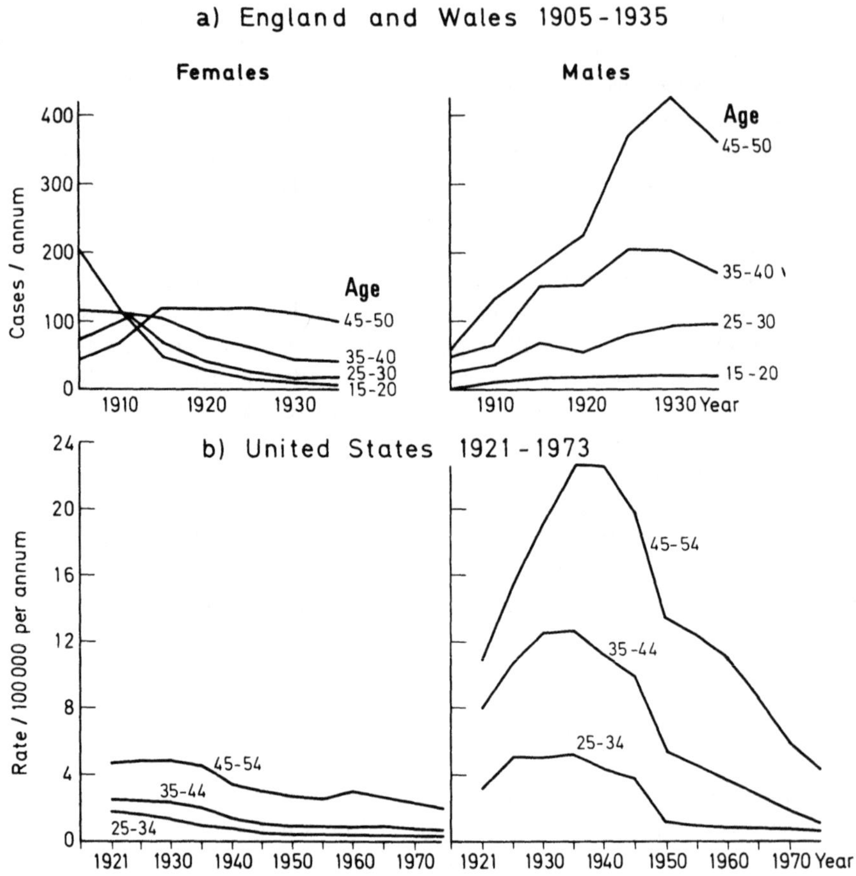

Fig. 9.3. Comparative mortality from peptic ulcer for selected age groups in males and in females. **a** England and Wales, 1905–1935. **b** United States, 1921–1972. British curves are redrawn from Jennings [281]; United States curves are calculated from various official sources [456, 625, 626]. Jennings gives only numbers of cases, not rates, since these were sufficient for his purpose, and conversion of his data into rates did not seem necessary for my own purposes, since the population-at-risk was relatively stable.

in the proportion of peptic ulcer patients coming into care. Fig. 9.3 presents mortality data from England and the United States, the first enabling us to see how the male rates at the beginning of the century were lower than the female ones but overtook them to reach a peak in the 1930s, while the second enables us to see that a similar peak occurred in the United States and was then followed by a continuous fall in rates. In both countries X-rays and other technical advances led to some shifts in what was regarded as evidence for a death from peptic ulcer during these years, but not sufficient to seriously affect the chronological comparisons. In both countries, also, the treatment of ulcer and its complications improved over the period so that the death rates do not necessarily parallel the prevalence rates, but there is ample evidence that prevalence in males did fall sharply after the 1930s in these countries, while the prevalence in females is not usually considered to have fallen, resulting in a marked reduction in the ratio of male to female cases coming into care [504, 642].

There are no known changes in diet, drink, tobacco, or any other external agent which took place over approximately the same years in these societies and which affected men much more than women. However, in 1962 Susser and Stein [599] pointed out that the ulcer mortality curves in Britain peaked at later dates for older men than for younger men so that, for instance, the curve for those aged 15-24 peaked between 1920 and 1929 while that for those aged 45-54 peaked between the years 1940 and 1949. They suggested (a) that the vulnerability to peptic ulcer over this period must have been linked to birth cohort rather than to year of death; and (b) that the change was probably related to the stresses of urbanization and eventual adjustment to urbanization. As Fig. 9.3 indicates, the peak of the curve for older men occurred later than that for younger men in the United States as well as in Britain, thus supporting the cohort hypothesis; and the urbanization hypothesis has received some support from the findings regarding rural and urban Bantu mentioned earlier [514, 550]. However, it is difficult to see why urbanization stresses should relate to birth cohorts rather than to, say, the total adult population over a given period; why in Britain the epidemic should only have appeared in the twentieth century when the worst impact of urbanization is usually considered to have been much earlier; and why only males should have been affected. When one finds the incidence of some disease being linked to birth cohort, it is to the perinatal period which one customarily looks for an explanation, asking if there were any changes likely to have affected the mothers' health at that time, or changes affecting infant care which could have effects extending into adult life. When one asks these questions respecting the cohort born around the beginning of the century or a little earlier, one discovers that infant care did in fact undergo considerable changes about this time, changes which might be relevant.

In the first half of the nineteenth century, if the mother either could not produce enough milk herself of preferred not to feed her infant, the normal solution in all classes in Europe and the United States was the "wet nurse." As the century progressed, wet nurses became both less available and less accepted for moral reasons, the latter attitude being particularly strong in Scotland [657], although Paris was still sending up to 5000 infants a year to the countryside for wet-nursing in the 1870s [600]. Replacing the wet nurse in popularity came "hygienic" artificial feeding, with numerous "patent" formulae for powdered milk – 27 proprietary brands in Britain by 1883 [657] – and with the sterilization of bottles, nipples, and milk being widely taught. This switch to the bottle and the spoon might of itself have induced a certain degree of the "oral conflict" which psychoanalytic writers [12] have viewed as underlying the development of the "peptic ulcer personality," but it seems scarcely sufficient to explain the marked increase in ulcers in the ensuing generations and it certainly would not seem able to explain the male preponderance in that increase. To account for this male preponderance I have given some thought to the fact that the male infants might have been sucking on lead toy soldiers while female infants were sucking on rag dolls; but I can find no clinical or laboratory link between early lead absorption and later ulcer, and there was another shift in infant

Table 9.1. Childrearing advice on certain topics provided by American women's journals at 10-year intervals from 1890 to 1948. Adapted from Stendler [589]

	1890	*1900*	*1910*	*1920*	*1930*	*1940*	*1948*
Number of articles analyzed	53	78	62	65	49	59	66
	%	%	%	%	%	%	%
Infant feeding to be given:							
(a) Informally	100	78	23	0	0	0	0
(b) Strict schedule	0	22	77	100	75	33	0
(c) On demand	0	0	0	0	25	66	100
	%	%	%	%	%	%	%
Character to be promoted by:							
(a) Good home models	61	53	30	12	14	5	3
(b) Disciplining	18	14	34	34	38	28	2
(c) Other methods	21	33	36	54	48	67	95

The journals surveyed were *Ladie's Home Journal, Woman's Home Companion*, and *Good Housekeeping*.

handling practices around the same time which fits theories of the "peptic ulcer personality" quite well and also accounts for the sex difference.

In 1890 women's journals were still advising their United States readers that "loving, petting and indulgences will not hurt a child if at the same time he is taught to be unselfish and obedient" (quoted by Stendler [589]). Within 10 years that view had been largely abandoned by journals in the United States and in western Europe, as an increasing emphasis was placed on the conditioning of children from their first weeks on to learn adult rules, a teaching which then lasted several decades, as Table 9.1 summarizes. This era, which has been labeled that of the "mechanical baby" [43], was partly an outgrowth of the new enthusiasm for scientific methods in everything, and in part an aftermath of the fear of "degeneracy" to which I referred in Chap. 5. Children – but particularly boys – had to be made tough and thus be able to resist degeneracy. As part of this new attitude mothers were taught "never to give a child what it cries for" and "Babies under six months should never be played with" (quoted from a popular child-care manual of the time, by Beekman [43]). As a further way of avoiding degeneracy, children in Anglo-Saxon societies were then taught quite early to reject dependency feelings and, as Table 9.1 also shows, this teaching was increasingly seen as being effected through disciplining rather than through the provision of the good models which the nineteenth century had thought appropriate.

The feeding by the clock and the teaching of mothers to ignore their infants' cries probably produced many more emotional conflicts (eventually internalized) around feeding than the switch to artificial feeding alone had done, but both these behaviors probably applied almost as much to girls as to boys. What did not apply nearly as much to girls as to boys, particularly as they approached adulthood, was the emphasis on independence. Western society of that time did not want women to become too self-sufficient, and through most of the twentieth century it has indulged or encouraged the desire of women to return to dependency on others – their spouses – while it has rejected and condemned any desire by men to regain dependency for themselves in similar fashion. Alexander states that in the peptic ulcer personality, "the wish to remain in the dependent infantile situation – to be loved and cared for – was in conflict with the adult ego's pride and aspiration for independence, accomplishment and self-sufficiency" [12, p 102]. He thus makes it clear that for him, peptic ulcer is as much the result of the dependency-independence conflict as it is of a conflict regarding oral gratification, although he exhibits a cultural bias in assuming that a desire for independence is more natural or innate than a desire for interdependence, a point on which Asian psychiatrists such as Neki [461] are challenging their Western colleagues. The pressures towards independence on the Western male, and the conflicts to which that may give rise, are culturally based, with the cultural pressures having been particularly strong during the first half of the twentieth century, and are not nearly as strong on women. When there are also oral conflicts, one would on this theory expect the two factors to combine to produce peptic ulcers, which would not appear if one or the other factor were absent. In women it has been the dependecy conflict which has been relatively absent; in men before and after the "mechanical baby" period it was the oral aspect that was absent.

This hypothesis is difficult to prove now that the epidemic is over, and it can be argued that the ulcer patients treated by Alexander and his colleagues could have been very different from those dying of the condition, so that the Chicago observations are irrelevant. However, a partial test of the hypothesis can be obtained from international mortality rates, since the "mechanical baby" doctrine affected some countries more than others. It was mentioned earlier that France clung to the wet-nurse tradition after it had been largely dropped by Anglo-Saxon societies, and anyone who has seen the series of films on the feeding and bathing of infants in different cultures with which Margaret Mead collaborated in the 1950s [397] must be aware of the much greater emphasis given to feeding and the mouth in France than in North America, so that one would expect the "mechanical baby" doctrine to have less impact in the former country. Another culture in which emphasis on oral gratifications is well known to have persisted is the Jewish, hundreds of novels having described the Jewish mother's urging of food on her offspring. The Scots, in contrast, were noted above to have rejected the wet-nurse tradition earlier than the English, for moral reasons, and are known to have had a relatively puritanical attitude toward childrearing, so that this hypothesis would predict them to have not merely a higher ulcer mortality rate than the French and Jews, but probably than the English as well. Finally, from what was noted regarding the different Scandinavian cultures in Chap. 7, it seems probable that the Swedes have put more emphasis on individual independence (as opposed to interdependence) than the Norwegians, and possibly also than the Danes, so that in these peoples the hypothesis would predict the Swedes to have the highest ulcer rate and the Norwegians the lowest.

Table 9.2 provides peptic ulcer mortality rates from 19 societies at a time when these rates were still relatively high, data for combined gastric and duodenal ulcer being given as well as for duodenal alone, since countries varied in the precision with which the distinction between the two types was made. We see that, as predicted,

Table 9.2. Annual age-standardized rates of death from peptic ulcer in 19 societies in 1954–1955, by sex, in rank order

	Deaths per 100 000, age-standardized				Rank order
	Duodenal and gastric ulcer		Duodenal ulcer only		Duodenal and gastric ulcer
	M	F	M	F	male rates only
Scotland	16.36	4.05	10.43	1.59	1
England and Wales	13.98	3.66	7.47	1.42	2
Irish Republic	11.63	3.09	4.13	0.82	3
Northern Ireland	10.91	2.63	5.84	0.56	4
Australia	10.60	2.86	4.25	0.80	5
New Zealand	10.39	3.28	5.49	1.40	6
Sweden	9.54	3.12	4.39	1.11	7
Austria	9.24	3.18	3.95	0.99	8
Italy	8.81	1.57	3.91	0.51	9
German Fed. Rep.	8.78	1.66	2.67	0.37	10
United States (Whites)	8.29	1.98	4.40	0.91	11
Finland	8.08	1.52	1.58	0.16	12
Switzerland	7.65	3.18	2.45	0.85	13
Netherlands	7.50	1.99	3.79	0.66	14
Denmark	7.42	2.64	2.23	0.48	15
Canada	7.37	1.71	3.90	0.74	16
Israel	4.99	1.56	3.19	0.72	17
Norway	4.62	1.68	1.74	0.36	18
France	4.00	0.69	0.56	0.07	19

From Segi et al. [551], combining their Tables II and III. The original tables included data on Japanese and on American Blacks, data which have been omitted here because of the greater probability of racial factors entering into play.

France and Israel are among those with the lowest rates, while Scotland has the highest, significantly higher on the male side than the rates for England. The Swedish rate is at least twice that of the Norwegian, as expected, with the Danish rate falling in between. Finally, it can be seen that all these expected differences prove to be much stronger on the male side than on the female, which is also what the hypothesis would predict. The only feature of the table which does not quite accord with my expectations is the rate for United States Whites. On the basis of the promotion of the "mechanical baby" doctrine by United States women's journals, it might have been expected that the United States ulcer mortality rate would be higher (compared to other countries) than shown, but the multicultural background of that population might also have led to the doctrine being less accepted than in more culturally uniform societies such as England and New Zealand.

4 "Organ Specificity" and Cerebrovascular Ischemia: Japanese

In what has just been presented regarding a possible association between peptic ulcer and sociocultural influences, the psychophysiological mechanisms whereby these influences are supposed to operate were largely ignored, since the question of such mechanisms has been the subject of considerable debate. The more simple psychoanalytic theories assumed that a disturbance of emotions which had been associated in childhood with a particular organ would lead to a disturbance in the way that organ was used in adult life and thence in certain instances to disease of that organ, something which has been called "organ specificity." However, it was early realized that matters were much more complicated, with nonpsychological factors having to be taken into account, and there also arose various theories of general psychosocial stress, something which would increase vulnerability to a wide range of psychological and psychosomatic disorders and not be specifically linked to particular organs. The best-known attempt to assess the relative validity of these two points of view was that undertaken by the Chicago school of psychoanalysis in the 1950s and 1960s. Lengthy personal histories were taken of patients with different types of psychosomatic disease and, after extraneous clues had been removed, psychoanalysts were asked to judge "blind" which of the seven diseases chosen for that study the patient had suffered from [13]. The analysts' judgments were considerably better than chance and than the judgments of internists given the same information, but still over a third of the patients were placed in a wrong category, suggesting that there must be nonspecific factors at work as well as specific ones. Returning to the material of the present chapter, the "mechanical baby" regime and its association with independence ambivalence appear to have had a specific relationship to peptic ulcer, insofar as none of the other major psychosomatic diseases increased and then decreased in harmony with the ulcer epidemic. However, there are other types of international comparison which favor the theory that psychological influences on psychosomatic diseases are nonspecific, and these now deserve our attention.

The international study which addressed itself most directly to the question was that by Rudin in 1968 [526]. Being impressed by McClelland's earlier demonstration of a rank-order correlation between economic development over a quarter century and the degree to which achievement was mentioned in the children's stories of 22 countries at the start of the period [393], Rudin asked himself whether this economic development might have been at the expense of mental health; and he set out to test the possibility. Taking the death rates from peptic ulcer and from hypertension in 1952 as partial indicators of mental health (and thereby implying a common, nonspecific factor) he compared the rank order as respects the achievement motive in children's stories in 1925, and demonstrated a statistically significant correlation, something which he proceeded to theorize from. Unfortunately for Rudin, other researchers discovered that mortality data were available for the six countries out of the original 22 that he had dropped from his analysis, and when they repeated his calculations with all 22 countries for other years they could find no significant association between the achievement motive rankings and rankings for mortality from psychosomatic disorder [34]. In place of that, they obtained a significant association between national rates of economic growth and peptic ulcer mortality alone (something which fitted Rudin's more general thesis), and in pursuing a very different type of hypothesis they uncovered a possible relationship between hypertension mortality rates and national industrial consumption of zinc and cadmium.

Since the association between national peptic ulcer mortality rates and economic development harmonizes quite well with the relationship of the former to independence and striving which was mentioned in the previous section, and since hypertension mortality rates did not significantly correlate with the economic development measure, these international findings can be taken as supporting the organ specificity theory rather than the reverse. However, at the same time as Rudin was undertaking his somewhat elementary analysis (there was no standardization for age or sex, and no birth cohort analysis such as might have been expected of a study focusing on children's stories in a particular year) a more experienced researcher was uncovering a most striking and puzzling international association between ulcer mortality and mortality from a very different condition, cerebrovascular accident (c.v.a.), something which reopens the door to the possibility of a nonspecific influence being at work.

Table 9.3. Correlations between causes of death in 28 countries [593]

Cause of death	Peptic ulcer		Cerebrovascular lesions	
	M	F	M	F
Peptic ulcer	–	–	+0.848	+0.757
Hypertensive heart disease and hypertension	+0.330	+0.065	+0.124	- 0.149
Cirrhosis of liver	+0.190	+0.136	+0.283	+0.009
All causes	+0.494	+0.243	+0.314	+0.235

Based on age-standardized rates for 1960–1961.

Table 9.3 presents the correlation coefficients obtained by this other researcher, Stocks, when comparing the age-standardized rates of mortality from selected disorders across 28 countries around the year 1960 [593]. The coefficients of 0.85 on the male side and 0.76 on the female are high even for comparisons between diseases with a manifestly linked pathogenesis, and they are extraordinary to find between diseases usually thought to be unrelated; but the reliability of the association is backed by the author's high reputation. One extraneous, nonetiological, explanation for the association could have been that the variance in each rate depended on the numbers of persons dying from other diseases before the peak ages for ulcer and c.v.a. mortality were reached, such a contingency being most obvious when developed and underdeveloped countries are compared. However, Stocks' 28 countries were all relatively developed ones, and if that explanation were valid we would have expected high correlations between the two diseases and the other noninfectious ones in Table 9.3, which is not the case. Other extraneous explanations similarly and some etiological association between the two diseases therefore appears highly probable, this explanation being more likely to fit the nonspecificity theory than the organ specificity one since such different organs have been affected.

As far as I am aware, no one has offered an explanation for Stocks' surprising finding or even undertaken more elaborate analyses of related data. From almost any angle it poses problems, since although there was this marked association between the two causes of death across countries at a given point in time, there appears to have been no such association between them when one studies either a single country or several, across time. Also, insofar as c.v.a. is linked to psychosomatic theory, this is usually via hypertension, leading us to expect a strong international association between c.v.a. and hypertensive mortality, whereas Table 9.3 shows that that association is much weaker than the one we have just been discussing. Nevertheless, a more thorough search of the literature uncovers facts which enable us to make somewhat more sense of Stocks' findings, and to build new hypotheses from them.

The first point which a closer look at c.v.a. uncovers is a historical change in the incidence of one form which, although not closely paralleling the peptic ulcer curve during this century, at least makes an association between the two more plausible. As is well known, c.v.a.s are of two main types, hemorrhagic and thrombotic or ischemic. Mortality statistics usually do not distinguish these accurately, since if death is sudden the differentiation may only be possible through autopsy, but it has been shown that in Britain the ratio of cerebral thrombosis to cerebral hemorrhage recorded at autopsy increased from about 0.4/1 in the 1920s to 1.3/1 in the 1950s [681]. Given that the overall age-standardized mortality from c.v.a. remained relatively stable over these years, this indicates that there was an increase in *ischemic* (thrombotic) c.v.a. roughly paralleling the increase in peptic ulcer mortality in Britain over those years, particularly if we think in terms of birth cohorts and allow for the fact that c.v.a. deaths usually occur at a later age than ulcer ones. Since neither the c.v.a. mortality rate nor the ratio of the ischemic to the hemorrhagic forms has since declined substantially, it would obviously be wrong to assume that the social factors affecting peptic ulcer have equally been affecting c.v.a. in Britain during this century. Nevertheless, if one recalls the known relationship between cerebral and coronary atherosclerosis, and then the increase in coronary mortality which occured as ulcer mortality was declining, the possibility of a common factor having influenced both peptic ulcer and ischemic c.v.a. between 1920 and 1960 is definitely increased.

The second point of interest here is that although no British researcher appears to have followed up Stocks' findings by investigating possible relations between cerebrovascular and gastrointestinal disease at the clinical of laboratory level, such studies were undertaken independently by researchers in Japan, where there is an additional incentive for investigating the question, since the Japanese have probably the world's highest mortality rates for both peptic ulcer and c.v.a. I had not mentioned the Japanese when discussing peptic ulcer earlier, since I did not want to have to discuss racial and dietary factors at that stage, but this people become highly pertinent now that we are considering relations between vulnerability to ulcer and vulnerability to c.v.a. The Japanese researchers just mentioned carried out gastroendoscopic examinations of patients who had recently suffered a c.v.a., and they discovered acute gastric ulcers in 6%, multiple erosions in 5%, and gastric mucosal changes such as might precede ulcer in 52% [311]. Moreover, an increase in urinary catecholamines was discovered in all those showing gastric changes but not in the rest, and the mortality rate was 40% in those with gastric changes as against 10% for the rest. It appears reasonable to assume, therefore, that localized cerebral ischemia, which can be both transient and "silent," may contribute significantly to the development of ulcers in this people.

Gastroendoscopic studies of c.v.a. patients in Western peoples have not to my knowledge been undertaken, and there is also to my knowledge no answer yet to the question whether racial and dietary factors are contributing to the high Japanese peptic ulcer rate. However, there is strong evidence to the effect that Japanese Americans have a considerably lower rate of c.v.a. than people in Japan [286], so that it seems unlikely that the high c.v.a. mortality rate in the latter country is due to a racial factor. The high Japanese rate for peptic ulcer may be quite independent of their high rate for c.v.a., and even if the two are not independent, the factor linking them could be purely somatic, e.g., dietary. However, there is no reason to exclude the possibility of it being psychological, and the next step in this line of thought would seem to be to enquire whether what we may call the "peptic ulcer personality" and the "c.v.a. personality" have anything in common that is likely to be found more often among the Japanese than in peoples with lower ulcer and c.v.a. rates.

Personality studies of c.v.a. victims are very few, and insofar as the psychosomatic literature does make reference to this subject it tends to treat the c.v.a. subjects as a subgroup of the hypertensive ones, whereas it seems likely in view of the shifting ratio of cerebral ischemia to cerebral hemorrhage [681] that it is the ischemic form we should be paying more attention to. However, there is one major (American) study of the personality of patients recently affected by an ischemic c.v.a. [9] and this claims that the modal personality of the group is considerably different from that of hypertensive patients. In place of a need to suppress anger or an anxiety about failing to cope which tend to characterize the hypertensive patient (see next section), the ischemic c.v.a. patients are reported to exhibit much more of a conflict over dependency. Out of 32 male patients having recently suffered from an ischemic c.v.a., 26 expressed a sense of personal weakness or failure (something which is different from the hypertensive's fear of being unable to cope), 11 showed resentment at not having been taken care of by their wives or nurses as they wanted to be, and 13 reported feelings of shame. Yet nearly all also put considerable emphasis on the importance of individual responsibility. This study was in no way "blind," and it needs replicating before we can build confidently on its findings, but there appear to be considerable similarities (which the authors do not mention) between the conflict over independence and responsibility which these ischemic c.v.a. patients are reported to exhibit, and the dependence/independence conflict which ulcer patients have frequently been stated to show.

That study was of American patients, as were most of the ones concerning the "peptic ulcer personality" with which it was implicitly being compared, and it gives us no cross-cultural comparisons with the Japanese such as we might like in view of the high c.v.a. and ulcer mortality rates in the latter. However, there is one feature in the description of the c.v.a. patients which is considerably more often found in psychiatric and psychoanalytic descriptions of Japanese patients than in descriptions of Western patients falling into other categories. That is the reported feeling of shame in 40% of the cases. In Western psychiatric literature shame is something reported mainly in female neurotics [351] and occasionally in peptic ulcer patients, but very rarely in association with other disorders in males. In Japan, shame is an important, "normal," emotion, as Benedict described in her *The Chrysanthemum and the Sword* [49]; and in exaggerated form it is also an important psychiatric symptom, as we will realize when discussing phobias in the next chapter, this symptom being clearly linked to a special form of dependency conflict. The American c.v.a. patients are reported to have been made ashamed by having to reveal their dependency desires openly and then to have them not gratified, something which implied that other people did not think these desires justified. This is very similar to what is reported in Japanese neurotics [153]. Accordingly, there would seem to be a psychopathological factor – the dependency conflict – which is to be found associated with the two diseases whose rates correlate so highly at the international level, and which is also relatively common in the people with the highest rates for these two diseases in combination.

That is as far as these data appear to be able to take us. Stocks' international comparisons revealed an association between two diseases which had not previously been seriously thought of as being associated (unless perhaps in Japan), and a case has been made for suspecting both of them to be linked in some way to dependency conflicts. If the links with dependency conflict are validated, this would support neither the organ-specificity theory nor the idea of a completely nonspecific stress but rather would suggest something in between these, a mental tendency predisposing to certain psychosomatic diseases but not to others. If this same tendency proves to be an important etiological factor in Japanese peptic ulcer, that will call for a rethinking of the psychoanalytic theory on this disorder, since Japanese mothers are relatively generous in their feeding and handling of their infants [99]; but that fact does not exclude a dependency need from being symbolized as a need for food, and in consequence an overstimulation of the stomach.

5 Hypertension: Tokelauans, Samuru, and Zulu

In addition to the association between peptic and c.v.a. mortality, Table 9.3 has two other features which some may find surprising. One of these – namely that hypertensive and c.v.a. mortality rates bear no significant relationship to each other despite the known fact that hypertensives are up to four times more likely than other people to get a c.v.a. [584] – had been reported earlier [3] and has probably a nosological explanation. Death tends to be attributed to hypertensive disease only after the heart and major blood vessels have become manifestly hypertrophied. Fatal cerebral hemorrhage, on the other hand, is somewhat more likely to occur before the vessels have become manifestly hypertrophied. Fatal cerebral hemorrhage, on the other hand, is somewhat more likely to occur before the vessel walls have been reinforced, and when the cerebral vessels can be burst during a sudden rise in blood pressure. Moreover, as we have already noted, fatal c.v.a.s have increasingly been found to be due to thrombosis without hypertension rather than to hemorrhage with hypertension. The other feature of Table 9.3 which deserves discussion, however, is of greater psychiatric interest. This is the weak but significant positive correlation between ulcer and hypertensive mortality in males, an association which had earlier been more marked ($r = 0.54; P = 0.02$) [584].

At one conceptual level it is relatively easy to imagine why peptic ulcer and hypertension might tend to affect the same people. Both can be conceived of as "effort" disorders, or alternatively as results of struggling against frustrations, and experiences which frustrate covert dependency needs could result in raised blood pressure as well as increased gastric motility or secretion. However, reports from Israel [401] and Czechoslovakia [263] indicate that the two disorders bear an *inverse* relationship to each other in clinic populations; classical psychosomatic texts describe the "hypertensive personality" as very different from the "ulcer personality"; and the Japanese whom we have seen to have unusually high mortality rates from ulcer and c.v.a. do not have particularly high blood pressure levels or hypertensive mortality rates [250]. I therefore think it better to examine the possible psychosocial factors contributing to hypertension in some detail before attempting to explain why national ulcer and hypertensive mortality rates should correlate.

The commonest theory linking hypertension to emotional stress is that blood pressure rises when the person perceives a threat or challenge in the environment and readies himself for action to meet it. However, it has been suggested that the more basic factor is not the threat but the psychological readiness to react with anger to situations which other persons might not view as a threat at all [535]; or that it is not so much anger as the need to suppress it [669]; or that it is neither anger proneness nor its suppression, but the idea that one might not be able to cope [647]. Each of these theories has been related to hypertension as a disorder in the living person, not to death from hypertensive heart disease which is what Table 9.3 refers to; and these two conditions are not necessarily the same. I will therefore turn away from mortality data for the present, and review instead such international and cross-cultural data regarding blood pressure levels in representative population samples, as may be able to cast light on psychosocial factors.

The two most widely known and fully established facts about the international distribution of hypertension are that the American Black suffers much more from it than the White, and that many preliterate tropical peoples suffer from it hardly at all as long as they remain in their traditional settings. The first of these points is usually attributed to a racial (genetic) factor, perhaps linked to an ability to live under conditions of low sodium availability [235], since the excess Black vulnerability – a hypertensive mortality in males six to seven times higher than that in Whites, during the 1960s – applies almost regardless of weight, age, district, and education. However, there is loose agreement that genetic factors, when specifically investigated, can account for only about a third of the variation in blood pressure levels [409], and the blood pressure of Blacks outside the United States seems considerably lower than inside it, as Fig. 9.4 shows, although some of this difference may come from the measurement techniques. Therefore, although a racial factor may be operating it is surely doing so only in conjunction with other types of factor, probably including the psychological, in view of the fact the Black situation in the United States has been such as often to give rise to suppressed anger. In the United States, so many factors are compounded in this question that it is difficult to tease out a cultural component, but we will examine the related situation in South Africa after we have

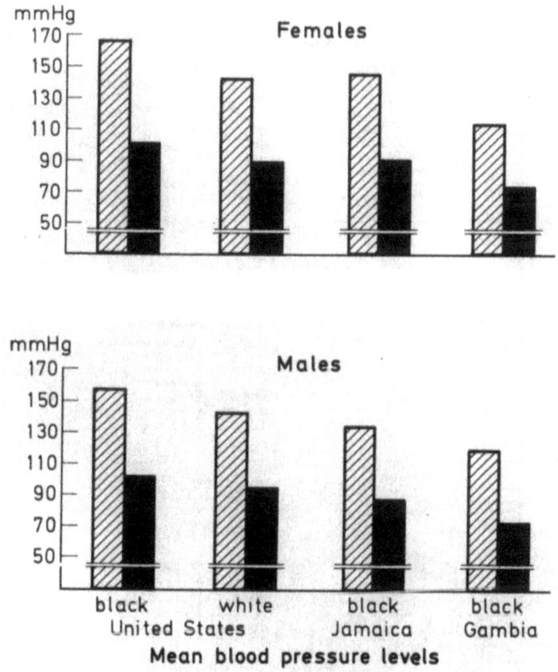

Fig. 9.4. Comparison of mean blood pressure levels, for persons aged 45–54, by sex, in United States, Caribbean, and West African Blacks, all of supposedly the same racial stock, as compared with levels in United States Whites [24, 396]. ▨, Systolic; ■, Diastolic

looked at the more basic question of the relationship of hypertension to culture change.

The effect of culture change is clearly illustrated by Fig. 9.5, taken from a paper by Cassel [94]. It depicts the mean blood pressure levels in three pairs of societies, each pair sharing the same cultural background but representing a different race. The chains of white dots give the mean readings for the societies which are living in the traditional style – what Cassel calls "remote" – and those of black dots for societies which have been more affected by contact with an industrial culture. It is clear in this figure that, almost regardless of age and sex, the "remote" groups have lower blood pressures (both systolic and diastolic) than the others. Also, whereas the systolic rates of the culture-contact groups tend to rise with age as one expects in Western societies, those of the "remote" groups generally do not. This finding of an increase in blood pressure as a people becomes more "modernized" is by no means universal – rural agricultural workers and fishers in Japan have higher mean levels than the urban population [250], and in the New Hebrides the people near the capital, Port Vila, do not have higher levels than those in one of the remoter islands [465]. Also, a higher mean blood pressure level in the population does not inevitably signify a higher percentage of persons suffering from hypertension. Nevertheless, the finding is sufficiently common that we should ask what it means, and in particular what significance, if any, it has for psychosomatic theories of hypertension.

When asking such a question it is wise, as noted previously, first to assess what somatic factors might be operating. The shift to a more urban setting usually results in an increase in weight and in salt consumption, both of which are known to be related to blood pressure. If the shift is to an urban slum, there may be an increase

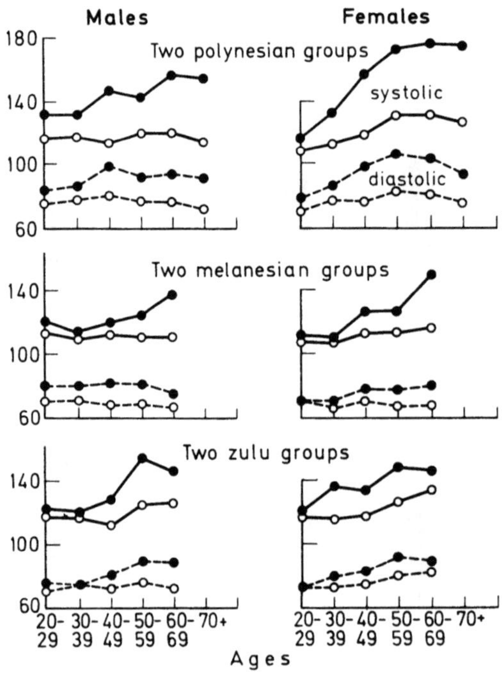

Fig. 9.5. Differences between the mean blood pressure levels of population samples considerably affected by recent contact with Western civilization ("culture contact") and samples of the same racial origin that were little affected by such contact. From Cassel [94], ●—●, Culture contact; ○—○, Remote

in kidney infection and hence the risk of hypertension secondary to this. If occupations have become more sedentary, with less physical activity, this could be relevant, and if the diet has become more starchy there may be an increase in hyperglycemia. In some instances where such matters have been investigated, the somatic factor has been thought sufficient to account for the whole difference. Thus, differences in body weight were thought to account for the whole blood pressure difference when Cape Verde migrants to the United States were compared with nonmigrants [196]. Mostly, however, as in the matter of salt consumption in the Cook Islanders [502], identified somatic factors have not been thought sufficient, and there may be two or more factors working in opposing directions. For instance, although the urban Zulu consumes more salt than the rural one, he tends to expend more physical labor. Also, most urban groups have better access to medical care than the "remote" ones. Therefore the researcher who wants to investigate the effect of culture change or urbanization on blood pressure must remember that he has many such factors to take into consideration before he can confidently link any difference in levels to a psychosocial one.

In the face of so many potentially etiological factors of a somatic type, the most convincing epidemiological evidence of psychosocial factors affecting blood pressure relates to the Tokelauans, a Polynesian people who have been migrating quite actively from their small islands to New Zealand and have been made the subject of a prospective study by Ian Prior and his colleagues in Wellington. The mean level of blood pressure in the original island population was low and showed only a doubtful rise with age, whereas that of their migrants to New Zealand was significantly higher and is showing a marked rise with age. This difference could have been due to a tendency for the more aggressive to migrate while the more peaceful stayed at home (a possiblity which most discussants of blood pressure in migrants appear to forget); or it could have been due to differences in diet and in resultant body weight or salt intake. To assess how far involvement in New Zealand society was linked to the rise in blood pressure, a 12-item social interaction index was developed on the basis of semistructured interviews carried out by anthropologists in the Tokelauan language [38]. It was found that the third of the sample that had the most interaction with wider New Zealand society had significantly higher systolic blood pressure levels than the third that had the least involvement with that society, allowance being made for age and sex. Moreover, after the weight/height ratio and the duration of stay in New Zealand were allowed for, the correlation between the social interaction score and blood pressure was significant for both systolic and diastolic rates, and in both sexes, although more marked in the males.

These findings make a strong case for a psychosocial factor having an etiological role, but they do not give much indication of what that factor is. Although the sheer amount of new stimuli impinging on the members of the group appears to be the most obvious variable, the data do not exclude the possibility of it being the character of these stimuli rather than their amount which is crucial, and neither do they exclude the possibility of self-selection determining simultaneously (a) the blood pressure level; (b) the degree to which new contacts with New Zealand society are sought; and (c) the way in which these new contacts are perceived. Regarding whether it is mainly the amount or the character of the new stimuli which is more relevan, it is not possible at the time of writing to draw much more from the Pacific Islands data although we will find some clues to that problem when we turn to the African data. Regarding the questions of self-selection and the ways in which social experiences are perceived, however, there is a cross-cultural comparison from another part of the Pacific which is instructive.

In the Micronesian island of Saipan there are two main peoples, the Chamorro and the Carolinians. They were the subject of a psychiatric and psychological comparison in the late 1940s [285] and have recently been included in a hypertension survey [488]. They are of the same racial group, but the Chamorro had an unfortunate colonial history from the seventeenth century onwards which had turned them into a comparatively distrustful, inhibited people while the Carolinians, whose original communities were on neighboring islands although they have been for some generations in Saipan, escaped the heavier colonial persecutions. When Joseph and Murray undertook their mental health study, they found the Carolinians both more mentally healthy and more outgoing, and when I visited the island in 1978 I got the same impression. For instance, it became clear that the Chamorro were afraid to take steps to seek aid for an abused or a mentally ill member of their extended family if they had not been requested to do so by an immediate relative, lest that "interference" result in retaliation, whereas the Carolinians, like most other Micronesian and Polynesian peoples, would take such steps as a matter of course.

The blood pressure survey on Saipan showed the Chamorro to have only slightly higher mean blood pressure readings than the Carolinians when weight was disregarded. However, obesity, which is an admired characteristic in this population, is a major factor in producing hypertension there and only 60% of the Chamorro aged 30

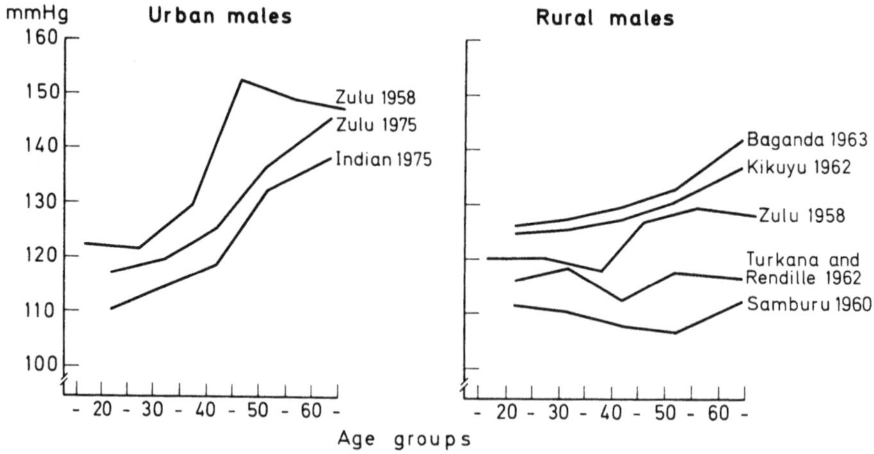

Fig. 9.6. Age curves for the mean systolic pressures in male samples from various South and East African peoples [547, 548, 549, 562, 563, 660]

and over are overweight by international standards as compared to 72% of Carolinians. When only persons not more than 16% above their "ideal weight" in relation to height are considered, 20.4% of the Chamorro sample aged 30+ had hypertension as compared to 8.5% of Carolinians [488], a difference significant at the 0.005 level. Accordingly, we have here an instance where migrational self-selection has not played a part and where the two groups have been exposed to about the same degree of "modernization" during the present generation, but where a culturally promoted tendency towards mistrust is associated with a much higher rate of hypertension (after weight has been allowed for) than a culturally promoted tendency towards openness and trust. It may be true that the Chamorro have greater reason for being distrustful than the Carolinians do, but the burden of the evidence is in favor of it being the attitude towards others that is associated with hypertension, rather than the behavior of others.

Reference to how the behavior of others may affect hypertension brings us back to the situation of the Black under various degrees of freedom and subordination, and although data from the Americas or from West Africa such as those sampled in Fig. 9.4 might be used to explore this, I prefer to use material from South and East Africa, since it enables us to examine certain features which are not as clear elsewhere. Figure 9.6 presents male mean systolic pressure curves for a number of samples from South Africa, Uganda, and Kenya, the corresponding female curves not always having been available, either because the women could not be as representatively studied or because their abundance of metal armlets, etc., interfered with the sphygmomanometer. The curves are divided into urban and rural, and the data fit very well the theory that blood pressure is related to the degree of exposure to socio-cultural change. On the urban side, the Zulu of 1975 were more familiar with urban conditions than those in 1958 had been, a greater proportion of them having been born in the city, and the Indians were even more adapted to urban life although also treated as *Untermenschen*. On the rural side, the Baganda sample was obtained from within 10 miles of Kampala and hence had been affected by city life, while a number of the Zulu had also worked in the city or the mines. The Kikuyu sample had virtually no urban experience, but they had been disturbed by enforced concentration in new villages during the 1950s, so that culture change had been imposed on them, while the Samburu, Turkana, and Rendille samples were drawn from pastoral tribes relatively undisturbed by modern change. Studies have been carried out regarding the relationship of body weight and diet in a number of these samples but they have been found to correlate poorly with the blood pressure measurements, and hence the probable importance of the psychological factors is increased.

Among these hypothesized psychological factors, the volume of new social stimuli appears to carry relatively little weight, at least if one considers the short-term effect on blood pressure. Samburu recruits into the Kenyan Army maintain surprisingly low blood pressure levels for their first year or more [564], despite the fact that it is in this period that they must make the most adjustments. (In America also, migrants to Chicago from the southern United States maintain blood pressure levels below those of the locally born for many years after arrival [585].) Perception of many of the new stimuli as threatening seems more pertinent, certainly for the urban Zulu. There is no doubt that for the latter, the urban environment carries many threats against which their upbringing has not provided adequate defences, threats arising from the discriminatory government regulations on the one hand and from the criminal subculture on the other. Moreover, these threats engender a permanent sense of mistrust, something well illustrated in responses such as the following which De Ridder obtained to a modified T.A.T. card in Johannesburg about the same time as Scotch was measuring blood pressure in Durban.

> The evening lights of a White suburb are reflected on this man ...
>
> The poor fellow has been overworked, exploited and underpaid. He fears going to the buses or the taxis, lest he be reluctantly compelled to expose his earnings to some unreliable eyes. It won't be long anyway walking home in the safety of these lights and quiet atomosphere. But the poor fellow fears even his shadow when he comes to think that at the end of this suburb will be the beginning of the stench, noise and unsafety of his township – lurking with darkness and unseen shadows. But providence saves him when a policeman flashes a torch upon his face and demands his pass. He tells a lie that he has none so that he can spend the night in a cell .... [145, p83]

Neither Scotch nor Seedat, from whom the urban data in Fig. 9.6 are derived, attempted to assess whether there was any association between such fears or mistrust and the blood pressure level, but Scotch did show that the latter was higher in urban females who admitted to believing themselves to have been victims of sorcery than in those who did not admit this [547], something which points in the same direction.

Most tribal Africans, however, have relatively low blood pressure levels despite the fact that so many feel threatened by supernatural forces (as was noted in Chap. 5). Also, the life of the Samburu pastoralists possesses many more real dangers, thanks to predators, famine,and tribal raids, than that of the ordinary Western urbanite with so much higher blood pressure. In addition to the question of perceived threats, therefore, we have to consider firstly the degree to which the individual feels that they can be coped with, and secondly whether the response which they arouse can be acted on immediately or has to be suppressed. If one compares the pastoralists with the Baganda and the Kikuyu, one difference is certainly that traditional social structures and the confidence accorded them persist in the first tribe, whereas these have been seriously shaken in the other two. Hence, insofar as the East Africans look to others to act on their behalf, an attitude which may be pertinent among the Japanese, as we will see, they must be less sure of this among the Kikuyu than among the Samburu, and must have almost completely abandoned such a belief among the urban Zulu. However, the second point, namely whether feelings of anger and frustration are customarily suppressed or able to be acted out, is probably the more important. In South African cities the Black cannot risk reacting directly against the police, bosses, and delinquents most likely to anger him, and so such feelings probably came out all the more in response to the innocuous T.A.T. cards. In rural East Africa, on the other hand, we are told by Edgerton that anger is relatively little suppressed.

In his study of eight cultural subgroups in Tanzania, Kenya, and Uganda, Edgerton found plenty of conflict between individuals, but he remarks regarding the modified Rorschach test material which he got there that "in all tribes there was a remarkable lack of hostile responses, and there were still fewer overtly aggressive ones. Even such characteristic non-Western responses as two animals fighting over something were quite uncommon, while actual conflict between humans was mentioned *only twice* out of several thousands of responses that were given" [163, pp203-204]. Although Edgerton interprets this as indicating that the Rorschach was not tapping unconscious sources in these peoples, other test results which he reports suggest that it was, and a more orthodox view would be that because aggressive feelings could be given relatively direct expression, they did not need to be expressed through the very indirect outlet which the Rorschach provides. Furthermore, in the Samburu, who have lower systolic pressures than any of the other East African peoples surveyed in this fashion (Fig. 9.6) although they are renowned warriors, there is evidence to suggest that that culture has prompted a special method – a culture-bound syndrome, we might call it – for relieving suppressed irritation.

Shaper, who drew attention to the Samburu's low blood pressure, tells us that they are pastoral nomads, and he explores without success the significance of their unusual diet to their blood pressure [563]. (They consume much milk, and blood tapped from the neck veins of their cattle.) He might have been better to have drawn our attention to the fact that they represent one of the most highly organized gerontocracies in the world. Not merely political decisions, but a majority of wives and of cattle, are in the hands of the older men, thanks in part to tradition and in part to their supposed power to cause harm by cursing [579]. Men under the age of 30 are forbidden to get married, each male starts what we would call adult life in a quite subordinate position, and through a strict system of age grades each is assured of a wife, cattle, and usually respect as he grows older, without having really to compete for these. In such a social structure, shared to a lesser extent by the Turkana and Rendille whose blood pressure curves are only slightly higher than that of the Samburu, it is easy to see that threatening and anger-provoking experiences are likely to decline as age progresses in these males. This could very well be one reason why the pressure curves do not rise with age in this society, and a similar argument would apply in other stable gerontocracies, societies in which one also tends to find relatively low blood pressure curves. However, by the same token one would expect a significant rise of blood pressure among the younger males, kept under the orders of elders who take most of the women for themselves and against whom the young dare not rebel for fear of being cursed.

That such higher blood pressure does not appear in the young Samburu males may be due to two traditions. One consists of regular dances for the young at which the two sexes and various age bands compete, at which a great deal of energy is expended, and of which Spencer writes that as the dance progresses the behavior becomes more and more juvenile, suggesting a form of regression to the childhood in which the strains of young adult life had been absent. (The analogy with the rites involved in dances frequented by certain groups of urban Western youth invites comparison.) The other tradition is a form of dissociation which starts with a shivering and proceeds to a shaking so severe that the person may have to be held to prevent him from harming himself. The subjects claim to lose consciusness, but they do not claim to be possessed, bewitched, or fearful; rather they regard this as an expression of manliness, and they see an association between the shaking and anger. The shaking can occur in private but often occurs at dances, and Spencer writes: "During the dances of display in particular, where the moran (i.e., the young men) say they are angry, their chorus is a rhythmic growl – almost a suppressed bellow not unlike a bull's – and at each sound they press their heads forward and up so that their throats are considerably constricted; this corresponds fairly closely to their behavior when shaking." "The term for 'to be angry' is *a-goro* which is the inflexive form of the verb 'to strangle'." "Thus there seems to be a definite verbal association between the emotion they associate with this (anger) and the behavior they display when shaking" [579, pp 263–264].

That the Samburu's low blood pressure is related to the dances, the shaking, and the hierarchical structure is an untested hypothesis, but one which receives a little support from the fact the Samburu who join the Kenyan army and are cut off from these traditions experience a considerable rise in blood pressure if they remain more than a year or thwo without returning [564], although they show no rise in pressure during the first, nominally most stressful army year. However, there is another, very different, way in which cultural teachings might reduce the risk of hypertension, one which is pertinent to the question of the relationship between that condition and peptic ulcer.

Almost all the hypotheses concerning a possible psychosocial factor in hypertension which were mentioned at the beginning of this section involved the assumption that blood pressure rises when an individual prepares for "fight or flight" after encountering something which is interpreted as threatening; and most of them further assume that essential hypertension will develop if this readiness for action becomes chronic and unrelieved. However, societies (and individual families) vary considerably in the degree to which they teach children to act for themselves or expect others to act for them, and we might therefore expect the level of preparedness for action in vace of threat ot be greater in some societies than in others. As will be shown in the next chapter (pp 265 et seq.). American children are earlier taught to act for themselves than Japanese ones are, and Japanese adults are more encouraged to act on behalf of others than Americans are. Between American and Chinese culture is a similar but lesser difference. In a laboratory study during the 1940s, American subjects of Asian and Caucasian (White) origin had various physiological measurements taken while they were undergoing a stressful experience, enamely watching a 6-foot hammer drop close to their fingers [596]. The White subjects showed significantly greater changes in pulse rate and hand movement than the Japanese subjects, with the Chinese being intermediate. The Asian subjects, however, showed greater changes in the galvanic skin reflex. Although this is another instance where the research calls for replication, and although transient changes in blood pressure could not at the time be recorded, these results are in line with what has just been said about childrearing. If we infer that blood pressure is more likely to fluctuate in harmony with pulse rate than with GSR, and if we further infer from Cannon's classical studies that emotionally produced changes in the skin are likely to be accompanied by flushing and secretion in the stomach, then we have reason for thinking that Japanese childrearing practices may reduce the risk of hyptertension, but correspondingly increase the risk of ulcer, in comparison with American childrearing practices.

Such a line of thought permits us to understand how the Japanese might have a high rate of peptic ulcer even though their childrearing imposes no oral deprivation and although their mean blood pressure level is comparatively low in relation to their high salt intake [250]. It also, in my opinion, helps us to understand how hypertensive and ulcer mortality might significantly correlate at an international level while showing an inverse correlation at the individual level, as the Czech and Israeli reports indicated. Certain types of stress or pressure may be considerably higher in one country than in another, resulting in differences in national rates of psychosomatic disorder, but in many countries family differences in childrearing practices may result in the stomach being more vulnerable in some individuals and the blood pressure in others. I find it potentially significant that the two countries from which the inverse correlations at the individual level were reported are multicultural, and are also ones whose ulcer mortality has never been high. However, the Japanese and Americans differ markedly respecting another psychosomatic condition, ischemic heart disease, and the question remains whether the evidence regarding that much-studied condition harmonizes of clashes with what has just been said.

6 Ischemic Heart Disease: Finns and Japanese Americans

For the disorders that have been discussed so far in this chapter, the most that it has been possible to offer have usually been hypotheses regarding psychological factors in their etiology, and some demonstration that such hypotheses are able to account for the international, cross-cultural, or historical variations no less well than hypotheses which ignore the psychological dimension. This has been so, in the first place, because research into these disorders has rarely handled more than two presumptive etiological factors at a time, although we have good reason to believe that the etiology is multifactorial, and in the second place because there have been no satisfactorily quantitative methods of assessing the psychological factors which we suspect to have been at work. Coming to ischemic heart disease, neither limitation fully applies and it is thus possible to say something about the degree to which cultural factors appear likely to be playing a role, alongside other factors which we now know to be relevant.

Ischemic and coronary heart diseases only became recognized as major causes of death after World War II, and while it has been argued that this was merely the result of inadequate diagnoses in prior times, there is good reason to think that Western society has suffered a true "epidemic" of such deaths since about the 1930s, an epidemic which is now dying down in like fashion to the epidemic of male peptic ulcer deaths preceding it. When I was at medical school in the 1930s, the emphasis was all on rheumatic (valvular) heart disease, with nonfatal angina pectoris also important but with myocardial infarction and coronary occlusion given little emphasis, the marked increase in mortality from heart disease which had occurred since the beginning of the century (a threefold increase in Massachusetts from 1910 to 1940) being attributed mainly to the rheumatic and syphilitic forms. In addition, as I have pointed out elsewhere [437], there was a marked shift in the sex ratio for angina pectoris between the nineteenth and the twentieth centuries, women contributing less than 10% of cases before 1900 and approximately 40% later. However, there has not been an adequate recounting of these changes, far less an attempt to relate them to dietary, social, and cultural trends, and the matter is too debatable to treat here as I have treated peptic ulcer. (For instance, a comparison of Montreal autopsy data found a lower rate of coronary occlusion in the 1920s than in the 1890s [400].) Instead, we can have recourse to the official mortality statistics for the 1960s and 1970s, by which time a reasonable uniformity of diagnostic criteria had been achieved, and more particularly to the relatively numerous, international and cross-cultural studies of multiple variables in large population samples.

To Ancel Keys must go the credit for recognizing already in the early 1950s the value of carrying out international comparisons of heart disease involving several variables at the same time, comparisons which enable us to tap a much wider range of mean values than we can usually find within single societies. The 10-year follow-up of the over 21 000 subjects in his Seven Countries study [303] has revealed an almost tenfold difference between the incidence of death from coronary heart disease (CHD) in Finland and in Japan, and has also shown the importance of diet in producing this difference. Although the single measures of serum cholesterol taken from each subject at the start of the study predicted individual deaths from CHD quite poorly (most probably due to the intra-individual variability in serum cholesterol levels), the mean levels in each sample predicted the 10-years male mortality rate from CHD quite effectively, 64% of the variance between samples being able to be "accounted for" on this basis. Moreover, when national mean cholesterol levels were estimated on the basis of the production, import, and export of different types of food in 20 countries, 53% of the variance in national rates for male CHD mortality was "accounted for" on the basis of diet [89]. The association between CHD death rates and mean cholesterol levels might have been lower if a different set of countries had been chosen for Keys' study – France and Israel, for instance, instead of Holland and Greece – and in the later 20 countries study [89] a considerably lower percentage of the CHD variance could be accounted for by diet on the female side than on the male – 31% instead of 53%. Nevertheless, these percentages are sufficiently high for psychiatrists and behavioral scientists who aim at identifiying psychological factors in CHD incidence to be looking at factors affecting the cholesterol level as well as factors that are independent of it, as appears to be true respecting what the 'Jenkins Activity Survey' and the 'Type A Behavior Pattern Interview' measure.

The effect of psychological factors on preferences for cholesterol-rich or cholesterol-producing foods is a subject which has received almost no attention, despite the fact that there is in many countries a tendency for the aggressive, competitive individual to choose a high meat diet (the Brahmin's avoidance of meat is based partly on its association with aggressivity), and although comparable factors have been abundantly studied in relation to obesity. There appears to me to be a possible association between the fact that the Franch workman links masculinity to an abundance of wine drinking rather than to an abundance of meat eating, and the fact that the French CHD mortality rate is exceptionally low in relation to the proportion of animal fats in the national diet; but that is mere conjecture, lacking data. A subject on which we do possess data is the degree to which people of different countries yield similar responses to questionnaires or interviews concerning behavior thought to be " coronary-prone"; but these have not been successfully used to account for the differences which remain between national rates of CHD after diet has been allowed for, and it has also not been demonstrated that national answers mean the same thing. Thus, when Swedes and New Yorkers answer that they *"often"* brood about certain problems, or find the emotional climate at their place of work *"not bad,"* as is reported in one study [474], we cannot judge from the available information whether they are using these descriptors similarly or very differently. However, there are a few comparative studies in this field which are succeeding in yielding new and useful data. Let us consider some subcultural differences that have been explored in a people with an unusually high CHD rate, the Finns, and one with an unusually low rate, the Japanese.

The high *Finnish* CHD rate is almost certainly linked to their high consumption of animal fats, and there has also been a suggestion that it is linked to an adverse calcium-magnesium ratio in their drinking water [292]. However, the Lapps who live to the north of them have just as high a percentage of animal fats in their diet and just as high a mean serum cholesterol level [613] without having the same high CHD mortality rate. Also, an excess vulnerability is to be found among Finnish migrants (and their descendants) in Canada [1] and in Norway [613], so that neither the diet nor the magnesium balance are sufficient explanations. A genetic predisposition to the disease invites serious consideration, but against this is the fact that there is a marked difference between the CHD rate of the eastern (Karelian) and the western Finns even though they are thought to be equally Finnish. The stereotype of the Finn is of a person with powerful muscles who enjoys the peace and loneliness of his great forests, who is little communicative, and who acts with great deliberation except when drunk. This is a picture very different from that of the "coronary-prone personality" as described in American literature and it would seem that that personality theory would be unable to contribute to an understanding of this people's high vulnerability to coronary disease. However, when the reputations which the eastern and western Finns possess inside their own country are compared, there are indications that the "coronary-prone personality" concept may not be entirely irrelevant, particularly if one allows for historical change.

In the nineteenth century the eastern Finn (Karelian) was described in a book widely used in Finnish secondary schools as "more open, friendly, lively and enterprising, but also more talkative, bragging, inquisitive and touchy. He likes travel and business, makes long tours in his own country, and sends his goods to Russia" [617]. Between the two World Wars the Karelians, judging from the homicide statistics collected by Verkko [634], seem to have lost their amiability and become quite violent, particularly under the influence of alcohol, their homicide rate being much higher than those in other parts of northern Europe. After World War II, during which many were displaced by the change of boundaries with Russia, what chiefly characterized them seems to have been the diligence and drive with which they established new lives for themselves in other parts of the country, and in the 1970s it is said [505] that they are known as the "must" people, i.e., those with an obsessional need to behave as tradition or as their inner standards demand. By comparison, the western Finns are today seen as more flexible, less persistent and, to hark back to a point which was made in the previous section regarding the Samburu, as passing on to their young men more in the way of games and strenuous competitions which might provide means for the release of aggressive drives [534].

These regional stereotypes need not mean much, but a questionnaire study suggests that they may hold some truth, and the reference to the Samburu is not entirely irrelevant either, since the Karelians, as well as having a much higher CHD mortality rate than the western Finns, have a substantially higher prevalence of hypertension. (Whether the eastern group have also significantly higher serum cholesterol levels than the western seems in some doubt, owing to these levels varying much more with the season of the year in the former than in the latter [304].)

The greater prevalence of hypertension is shown in the upper parts of Table 9.4, and in the lower part are summarized the answers obtained both from CHD patients and from males to a "coronary behaviour profile" questionnaire. In the lower part one sees that the self-reports of the eastern Finns indicate significantly more competitiveness, striving, and time urgency than the self-reports of the western Finns, which is in accordance with both the regional stereotypes noted above and "coronary-prone personality" theory. However, the eastern Finns also indicate themselves to be the more satisfied with their work situation, something which is not contrary to the regional stereotypes but might be contrary to the coronary-proneness theory, depending on which authority one turns to. In a different study involving only myocardial infarct survivors, it was found that Finnish patients expressed significantly more dissatisfaction with their life situations than Swedish and American patients [518] and had judged themselves as having less time urgency than the Swedish and American subjects did; but this does not cast light on the difference between the eastern and western groups.

Neither does it cast much light on the more general question of the high Finnish vulnerability to this disease, since job dissatisfaction is a debatable part of the „coronary-prone personality" theory. The Finnish studies have not yet made any real attempt to combine personality and other factors in the type of multivariate analysis which research into psychosomatic disorders demands; and they have not developed their own model of the local, coronary-prone individual which would correspond to the American "Type A" or to the more psychoanalytic picture which Dutch authors

Table 9.4. Differences between eastern Finns (Karelians) and western Finns with respect to coronary heart disease mortality, hypertension, and responses to a "coronary behavior profile" questionnaire; males only

A. Morbidity		Eastern Finns	Western Finns	
	N	728	806	
Diastolic BP of 100 mmHg [293]		19.9%	6.3%	
B. Mortality	N	728	806	
Dying from CHD within 10 years [303]		6.8%	2.5%	
C. Coronary behavior profile scores [505]	Infarct survivors		Healthy[a] controls	
	Eastern Finns	Western Finns	Eastern Finns	Western Finns
N	40	46	345	479
Overwork	1.02	1.34	1.46	1.44
Striving and competitiveness	2.62	2.39	2.76 – c –	2.34
Time urgency	2.95 – b –	1.95	2.56 – c –	2.04
Work dissatisfaction	0.90 – c –	1.50	0.97 – c –	1.52
Life dissatisfaction	8.18	7.71	7.56	7.39

Percentages in (A) and (B) relate to disease-free males aged 40–59 at entry into study, and are age-standardized

[a]By "healthy" is meant free from cardiovascular disease

[b]Difference significant beyond the 0.05 level

[c]Difference significant beyond the 0.01 level

have provided [312]. There is a need for someone to be asking what there could be in the Finnish psychological background which could lead to them being so much more vulnerable to the disorder, after allowance is made for diet and smoking, than neighbors like the Swedes, Lapps, and Russians. The obvious point from which to start would seem to be the demands made on them by their harsh environment and the psychological defences which are developed, particularly in Karelia, against that environment, when compared with the defences developed by their neighbors; but another starting point might be the way in which their use of alcohol differs from that of their neighbors.

Turning now to the unusual *Japanese* resistance to CHD, and to the disappearance of that resistance as Japanese-origin men become fully americanized, we find that there has been some attempt to explain the facts on the basis of cultural psychology [385] and that multivariate analysis is being employed. Most of the research here has focused on men who developed some form of CHD without dying from it, whereas most Finnish research focused on men dying from it, so that the two sets of studies are not necessarily concerned with the same problem. (Angina pectoris and myocardial infarction do not have the same demographic distribution.) However, a comparison of the findings is instructive.

The main studies of ischemic heart disease in Japanese-Americans consist of a cross-sectional survey of 3809 males aged 30-64 living in California [380], and a longitudinal study of 8006 men aged 45-68 living in Hawaii [678], although there were a number of prior comparisons of Japanese, Japanese-Americans, and American Whites which verified the differences in CHD incidence between these three groups and recorded considerable other differences relating to serum cholesterol, weight/height ratio, blood pressure, etc. In the two main studies of Japanese-Americans, measurements were taken of blood pressure, serum cholesterol, glucosemia, smoking habits, and relative weight; and in each of them information was gathered from which estimates were made of the degree to which subjects were more American in cultural orientation. In the Hawaii study, in addition, 2437 men completed the Jenkins Activity Survey (JAS) at the time of intake [116], and measures of coronary proneness given by that instrument could be compared with the CHD data collected then and subsequently from the same subjects.

Table 9.5 gives a selection of the key findings from these studies. In the first part of it one can see that after allowance has been made separately for serum cholesterol, smoking history, and weight, the subjects who were more Japanese in their cultural orientiation had less coronary heart disease at the time of examination than the subjects who were more American in orientation. Similar differences could have been shown with allowance being made for blood pressure, serum triglycerides, and serum glucose. The second part of the table shows that cultural orientation affects the development of coronary heart disease, fatal and nonfatal, in men who had been found free from such disease of first examination. Neither study, unfortunately, has yet compared the percentage variance "accounted for" by the cultural orientation factor with the percentage "accounted for" by the different physiological factors, but such a calculation can be expected.

These findings confirm what had been inferred from earlier studies, namely that the Japanese have no inherent, genetic, resistance to CHD, and that the closer they come to an American way of life the smaller becomes the difference between their CHD risk and that of other Americans. However, the protection which Japanese cultural tradition gives against coronary disease could operate in a number of ways, not all psychological. There could be key elements in traditional Japanese diet which protect against CHD, elements which operate either in childhood or currently. There could be differences in occupational affiliation between the more Japanese and the more American-oriented groups; and there could also be differences in social experience, such as support by a minority group or rejection by the White majority. However, there could also be persisting differences in types of autonomic arousal, along the lines indicated by the experiment of Stratton and Henry [596] mentioned earlier, or there could be differences in value orientation which affect the attitudes underlying "coronary-prone behavior." The researchers involved in these studies have undertaken many analyses in an attempt to assess which line of association is the more probable, and their results are interesting. Culture of upbringing proves of greater importance than current cultural preference, and probably also than current diet. Subjects who had a predominantly Japanese upbringing but who at time of examination expressed preference for American food exhibited five times *less* CHD than subjects with a predominantly American upbringing who expressed a preference

Table 9.5. Frequency of coronary heart disease in Japanese Americans as related to knowledge of Japanese culture and to certain other variables

A. California: point prevalence [380]		Age 30–44				Age 45–64			
Predominant cultural orientation[a]		Japanese-oriented		American-oriented		Japanese-oriented		American-oriented	
		N	CHD%	N	CHD%	N	CHD%	N	CHD%
Serum cholesterol	220 mg%	294	1.4	483	1.7	335	3.9	355	5.1
	220–259 mg%	144	0.7	308	4.5	261	0.8	304	4.9
	260 mg%	49	2.0	98	9.2	101	4.0	129	8.5
Smoking history	Never smoked	113	0.9	212	1.9	191	2.6	212	1.9
	Ex-smoker	176	2.3	345	4.9	268	3.6	300	7.0
	Current smoker	208	1.0	339	3.8	240	2.1	259	6.2
Weight/height ratio	Low	188	2.7	215	0.9	263	1.1	196	2.6
	Medium	204	0.5	375	4.8	256	2.7	346	4.3
	High	102	1.0	305	4.6	183	5.5	252	9.1

B. Hawaii: 6-year incidence [678]		Age 45–59 at entry				Age 60–68 at entry			
Birthplace		Japan		Elsewhere		Japan		Elsewhere	
Number of years in Japan	10+	93	1.1	548	1.8	26	4.1	108	4.6
	1–9	45	2.2	863	2.2	40	10.0	136	7.3
	0	–	–	4412	3.6	–	–	719	7.5

[a] By "orientation" is meant upbringing rather than current interests; see original paper for the complex approach employed.

for Japanese food with its lower animal fat content. Socioeconomic status, which could have been a complicating variable, proved not to be of real significance, but the cultural orientation of the subjects' milieux was of considerable importance, particularly in the 45-64 age group, since those involved mainly with other Japanese-origin persons had by far the lowest morbidity [380].

Regarding the responses of the Hawaii Japanese-Americans to the JAS, the first point of interest is that only 15% of the total group fell into the "Type A" category, as opposed to 50% of California Whites, but that they scored higher than the White criterion group on Jenkin's "H" scale from the same instrument, a scale labeled "hard driving" and supposed also to indicate coronary proneness. The JAS is a self-report instrument, telling us how the subject sees himself (of perhaps how he would like to be seen), in contrast to the Rosenman and Friedman Type A Behaviour Pattern Interview which relies on the judgement of clinicians observing the subject's behavior. However, the findings are in harmony with what other comparisons of Whites and Japanese-Americans [96] have reported, and if one recognizes that there is a distinction for the Japanese between "hard working" and "hard driving" in the American sense, they would lead us to predict that the Japanese group would have the lower CHD rate. As numerous psychosomatic studies have indicated, the hard work undertaken by the Western, coronary-prone, individual seems to be in part an outlet for aggression and in part either a defence against prohibited feelings of passivity or a need to feel in control of the situation. In Japanese culture, work is seen more as a form of enjoyment. "The Japanese are confident of the inexhaustibility of energy emanating from the inner core of the self or *hara*, the vital center of the body. Many a Japanese finds his satisfaction in work deriving from energy expenditure [and] attaches moral significance to a steady flow of physical or mental energy" [342, p 163]. This image of work and of potency can lead to other psychological difficulties, but it enables the Japanese-educated person to relax without feeling guilty or frustrated, which is what the coronary-prone personality is supposed not to be able to do.

The second point of interest about these data, to date, is that although the JAS standard scales, based on Californian Whites, do not correlate significantly with the distribution of CHD observed among Japanese-Americans, a scale based on the Japanese-American responses alone does do this [116]. Naturally, one will have to wait and see whether that new scale can be validated, and it is in any case probably not going to be as effective as a scale whose items are based on clinical experience with Japanese and Nisei patients. However, the general direction in which this work is pointing is clearly valuable. By comparing across cultures the personality characteristics of CHD-affected individuals with the characteristics of those that escape the disease despite possessing many of the physiological "risk factors," we can hope to come closer to identifying the key psychological mechanisms conducing to the disorder, while getting rid of the false clues which have resulted from culturally based associations between these mechanisms and other psychological attitudes or processes. Moreover the fact that after migration the Japanese vulnerability to cardiac ischemia increases, as was noted earlier [286], makes them particularly suitable for an investigation of this type.

The studies just cited offer the best research model of any which I have made use of in this book, and as such ought to be pursued further. However, they are very costly and the psychiatrist or psychologist who seeks to have future studies of this type include measures of personality or cultural value orientation will have to present a strong case, something which will be difficult to do as long as we are in disagreement about the validity of our own instruments and about what they are measuring. Self-report instruments such as the JAS can probably continue to be used for certain purposes, but in cross-cultural comparisons they can yield deceptive results and it may be better to attempt development of more objective measures of such variables as time urgency, following the lines which Glass [223] has pioneered. Also, once one thinks cross culturally, there are a number of much simpler methods of testing many hypotheses, for instance by replicating and extending the stress experiment [596] that was conducted in the 1940s, or by comparing childrearing patterns among the eastern and western Finns.

7 Conclusions

International and cross-cultural comparisons of the psychosomatic disorders, despite all the difficulties which they involve, hold many lessons for psychiatry and thus deserve to be kept more fully in view than is currently fashionable at psychiatric conferences. One of the lessons which this chapter should have adequately brought home is that national cultures change over time and that the physiological predispositions to disease can change quite markedly as the result of this. I have tried to show the same thing respecting depression, but the evidence on that can be challenged whereas it is difficult to challenge the changes in mortality which this chapter has dealt with. A second lesson is that both at the theoretical and at the methodological level, we need to find better ways of handling pluricausality, i.e., the fact that diseases are often the result of several equally important causes rather than of a single indispensable cause and some auxiliary ones. Western medicine achieved notable advances by assuming the existence of indispensable causes – bacilli, etc. – and attacking these, but at the present time a wide range of the more important diseases affecting the industrial world do not fit this model, and the major mental disorders probably do not fit it either. In this chapter it has at times been a convenient fiction to imagine that a disorder such as hypertension has a number of purely physiological roots and a single psychological one, but most of the evidence points away from there being only one important psychological mechanism or cause involved in each disorder. To defend ourselves from the accusation of being too imprecise, in our talks with our somatic colleagues, it may be desirable in a given situation to argue for only one of the psychological factors which we see as involved; but among ourselves we should recognize their plurality and should also recognize more constructively than we have done in the past the plurality of causes in such purely psychiatric conditions as schizophrenia and obsessional neurosis.

Such a recognition calls for much new thinking, and the examples of hypertension and CHD deserve particular attention since it is with them that we see this new type of thinking most clearly. On the one hand, the recognition means that the absence of a particular causal factor in some patients says nothing about its importance for other patients, and if we believe that we have found some psychological factor operating in one group we need not stop pursuing it simply because it has been shown to be absent in another. The fact that mistrust plays a negligible role in producing hypertension among the Carolinians says nothing about its importance for this disorder among the Chamorro, for instance, and nothing about its importance for our understanding of psychosomatic mechanisms in general. On the other hand, recognition of pluricausality calls for much more cooperative effort than in the past, and also for more effort at distinguishing one psychological (causal) factor from another. The cooperation is needed to ensure that when we are attempting to assess the importance of a favorite factor that we know how to measure, the masking effect of other factors which we do not know how to measure is adequately allowed for. A greater differentiation of one causal factor from another and, more importantly, from inessential concomitants, is necessary because when one is dealing with many factors at the same time, the risk of error is much greater than when one is pursuing a supposedly indispensable factor with all other influences being secondary. Brief reference was made to the confusion which resulted from the assumption that a single serum cholesterol reading would represent an individual's mean level; a similar confusion may have arisen from assuming that the "hard driving" of the coronary-prone personality is necessarily reflected in answers dealing with "working hard."

In the search for better differentiation of psychological mechanisms or factors, international and cross-cultural comparisons are going to be valuable. When such factors are sought within a single society – and in particular when factor analysis is a major statistical tool – it can be extremely difficult to differentiate associations which reflect a common psychological mechanism or attitude from associations which reflect a common cultural indoctrination. When the matter is pursued in a number of different societies, an association depending on cultural indoctrination is much less likely to persist across them all, while an association dependent on a basic psychological mechanism will. Moreover, if one is seeking to assess whether a psychological element is organ specific or is a general stressor, as one might still wish to do more accurately with respect to the achievement motivations which Rudin started exploring, the best way of approaching the matter might be by cross-cultural comparisons. The Japanese drive towards achievement has been shown to be different from the Western type [147], and perhaps less stressful.

Chapter 10 Neuroses and Other Minor Disorders

The ways in which international comparisons can contribute to our understanding of the minor mental disorders differ considerably from those in which they contribute to the major ones. With the latter we have been dealing with fairly distinct syndromes and fairly uniform methods of identifying them in a population, even though these methods do not operate everywhere and though some ambiguity remains. Much could therefore be done in the way of comparing incidence rates or considering cultural variations in the characteristics of those who display the core syndrome, both in historical sequence and across contemporary societies. With the neuroses and other minor disorders there has been no such agreement either past or present. Prior to 1900 the term neurosis carried mainly the neurological connotation given it by its inventor, Cullen, in 1784, so that one found it embracing not just hysteria and the neurasthenias but Parkinsonism and chorea; and even the classic term hysteria was not applied in any uniform fashion, for instance being used for males by some writers but not by others. Today Cullen's organic concept of neurosis persists in some Pavlovian schools, but even if one ignores the latter and considers the term to apply only to conditions in which there is no evidence of a relevant organic disorder, i.e., psychoneuroses, one finds that there are markedly different ways in which it is employed, so that different interpretations need to be applied to reports which, if they had dealt with the psychoses, could probably have been given a uniform interpretation. If this were merely a problem of nosology, i.e., a problem of deciding which clinical pictures to include under each heading, we might be able to circumvent it by focusing on precise syndromes, but it was one of the early discoveries of psychoanalysis that when one syndrome was "cured" – for instance by hypnosis – a different one would appear. Viewing superficially different syndromes as distinct entities thus becomes of doubtful value, and it seems much better that we should attempt to compare whole classes or categories of syndromes, perhaps only between those societies in which a uniform nosology reigns. However, although the latter is sound in principle, one is still liable to find that the criteria whereby this nosology is applied vary considerably both within and between these societies.

What is regarded as a neurosis in Western societies today differs significantly depending on the category of professional involved and the setting in which he is working, the main relevant categories being general physician, private or clinic psychiatrist, psychoanalyst, and sociologist. For the general medical practitioner and internist the term neurosis may merely imply that there has been no success in attributing the patient's complaints to a definite somatic source; and a prevalence survey using general practitioners is liable to bring to the fore the somatizations but not those syndromes whose features are wholly psychic. For the psychoanalyst a conceptually sounder definition is likely to reign, perhaps that given by Fenichel [183, p18], but the social selection that determines which patients reach a psychoanalyst is so biased that we cannot take the patients whom he sees as representative of those in the general population. The psychiatrist may also use a conceptually sound definition of neurosis and he usually sees a broader sample of the public; but it has been shown that some psychiatrists apply the term to anyone seeking psychotherapy for whom a more precise diagnosis is not apparent, and neurotics who do not seek psychotherapy are unlikely to be known to them. Finally, if our sampling of neurotics is through a household mental health survey, something most often guided by sociologists, we will find well-represented, persons who are able to directly verbalize their symptoms in response to the questions which the surveyor poses, but not those whose symptoms fall outside the range enquired into (which is usually restricted) or those who cannot verbalize their problems. Moreover, cultural groups can vary considerably in response style, and household surveys can yield deceptive cross-cultural comparisons, as was found in the Midtown Manhattan Survey [583] whose small Puerto Rican sample, as was noted earlier (p 52), apparently contained no healthy person.

It is thus from quite restricted sources such as an army (see Table 5.1) that we can expect to get reasonable, quantitative, data on the neuroses, and even from such a source there are important categories of disorder that are liable to be missed, for instance the obsessional. Rather than pursue data on incidence, therefore, it is better for Comparative Psychiatry to undertake other types of enquiry regarding the neuroses. One such alternative objective is the study of syndromes which are common in a very few cultures and rare in all others – the so-called culture-bound syndromes. By exploring why these should arise so much more in some societies than in others, we may be able to uncover new clues to the etiology and mechanisms of the neuroses. Another possible objective is the testing of what might be called the social relativity theory of the neuroses, i.e., the idea that neuroses are an internal reflection of external – social – conflicts, varying with the latter and having no essential character of their own. It was probably the Scottish psychiatrist, R.D. Gillespie, best known for his textbook with Henderson [255], who enunciated this theory most clearly when he wrote that "psychoneuroses are in the ultimate analysis social disorders of individuals. They are symptomatic of a disturbance of social relationships mentally 'introjected'." [218, p36]. More recent authors who have written in a similar vein are R.D. Laing [330] and Thomas Scheff [537]. Gillespie did not mean, of course, that predisposing factors were irrelevant – he wrote considerably on constitutional predisposition – or that precipitating events were all merely an aspect of social conflicts. However, he does appear to have meant that the nature and symptomatology of the neuroses depend less on events in infancy or on recent traumata than on the character of the social conflicts around the patient and the conventions which the society employs for controlling such conflicts.

That social relativity theory is one which Comparative Psychiatriy is particularly suited to test. We will therefore examine the stability of the neuroses first in relation to an apparently uniform and powerful precipitating factor, and then in relation to early childhood experiences in different societies, asking to what extent contemporary social conflicts appear to be affecting the symptomatology.

1 Battle Neuroses from One War to Another

Of the two broad categories into which the neuroses are most often divided, i.e., the traumatic neuroses and the psychoneuroses, the epitome of the first is the battle neurosis in which there has been physical trauma and in which there is also a real threat against life which can only be avoided by rebelling against powerful social demands. This is what the armed forces experience during wartime; and when these armed forces are given sufficient medical services, those resulting neuroses which impair military efficiency are quite unlikely to escape attention. We know from World War II studies that after a certain length of time in the frontline virtually no one remains healthy and efficient, and the same applies to combat air sorties, indicating that the presence of predisposing factors is unimportant. According to conventional theory, therefore, neurotic breakdowns under these circumstances should be quite uniform, while with the social relativity theory they might be expected to vary with the social background. The best comparisons would be among frontline soldiers who develop neuroses, but such data are not sufficiently available and we must make do with the neuroses developing in total armies during war. I am calling these "battle" neuroses, which is a slight distortion of the term, to differentiate them from the neuroses of wartime civilians and peacetime soldiers.

The first war in which the medical services were sufficiently developed to supply us with moderately full details of sickness as well as of deaths and injuries was probably the *American Civil War* (1861-1865). When one searches the medical literature regarding it one finds two main disorders of psychiatric interest, the first labeled "nostalgia" and the second "pseudo-rheumatism," but one finds almost no mention of what became called war neuroses 50 years later. For the total Northern Army, not just the units engaged in fighting, cases of nostalgia were admitted to hospital about as frequently as asthma or epilepsy and twice as frequently as melancholia [670], from which it was routinely distinguished. It is described as having been a disorder of young recruits, who developed "great mental dejection, loss of appetite, indifference to external influences, irregular action of the bowels, and slight hectic fever," followed by "hysterical weeping, a dull pain in the head, throbbing of the temporal arteries, anxious expression of the face, watchfulness ... and a general wasting of all the vital powers" [489]. The same writer goes on to state that "The Hospitals of New Orleans and its vicinity, during the past summer, were filled with such cases, complicated with fevers and diarrhoea." The pseudo-rheumatism was recognized by the authorities of the time to be made up of a great variety of conditions, including a form of scurvy, but to include

"a very large group of cases ... in which scientific examination fails to detect any disease whatever. The patients complain as loudly of pain in the back and limbs as in the most decided cases of genuine rheumatism ... but they appear well nourished, have a good appetite, devour their full ration of food, and present none of the grave constitutional symptoms described in connection with the cachectic neuralgias we have considered. Nor are any of the symptoms of chronic rheumatism present." [671, p324]

Neither of these clinical pictures fits what we normally consider to be a war or battle neurosis, the first being too frankly depressive and the second not sufficiently crippling when the patient thinks himself unobserved. Woodward appears to be expressing the opinion of the army medical hierarchy when he labels the men who exhibit the second condition not as neurotics but as malingerers. He states that "malingering of every kind has been exceedingly common" and that "the whole military system of the country during this period favored and encouraged it" since the "enormous bounties which a mistaken patriotism offered for recruits" [671, p325] led to many enlisting merely to get the bounty and then attempting to leave the armed forces again as soon as possible. Psychiatrists are well aware of certain types of army medical officer who regard all mental disorders as forms of malingering, and we must be on guard against this possibility here, but that does not detract from the striking fact that in this war the medical authorities were not seeing typical anxiety or dissociation neuroses in sufficient numbers to comment on, although they were seeing plenty of depressed (nostalgic) reactions.

The next war from which data should be available is the Franco-Prussian war of 1870, but I have been unable to find anything sufficiently specific from that time and it is possible that the fighting was over too quickly for observations to have been made. During the *Boer War* in South Africa (1899-1902), however, it is apparent that many of the types of war neurosis that were to develop in World War I were already quite familiar. A report mentions that "disordered action of the heart is very commonly diagnosed;" that "emotional outbursts, which sometimes take the form of irresistible fits of weeping on the slightest excitement" occurred particularly in officers; and that "functional disorders causing contractures and paralysis occurred in a certain number of wounded patients" [65, pp128-132].

One gets the impression that some of the conditions were iatrogenic – most obviously the "disordered action of the heart," which was a conventional diagnosis at that time, and some neurasthenia – but that most were not. An obvious difference between the Boer War and the American Civil War was that the American troops were in their own country and served in very loosely organized units, so that they could easily run away or hide if that seemed the easiest way of resolving their intrapsychic conflict, whereas the British soldiers in South Africa faced more dangers in running away than in staying with their units; but risk of somatic trauma (concussion) was about the same in each.

From the *Russo-Japanese War* too few details of mental disorders were forthcoming to permit useful conclusions, although one gets the impression that the Japanese had few psychiatric problems apart from those secondary to somatic illness (e.g., typhoid and beriberi) while the Russians had more cases of various sorts, particularly reactive psychoses [20, 408].

World War I, in contrast, produced a flood of psychiatric reports on both sides, one which fortunately becomes manageable for today's researcher thanks to a book of abstracts of the literature from nine countries published in 1918 [75], and to a valuable series of annual reviews of the German literature by Birnbaum in the *Zeitschrift für die gesammte Neurologie und Psychiatrie* from 1916 onwards.

The first thing which strikes one in this World War I literature is the rapidity with which "shell shock" became an important, polymorphic, syndrome on both sides, despite the fact that the respective medical authorities had started off with different approaches to war psychiatry. The second point which strikes one is the slowness with which "disordered action of the heart" was publicly recognized to be a neurosis, and the large number of patients who escaped the frontlines with the aid of this label. The German psychiatric services were the most prepared for the war, but also seem to have been the earliest affected by an upsurge of battle neuroses. Their preparations were based on the expectation that the main problem would be the rapid evacuation and disposal of psychotics [652], and in the very first months this seemed to be borne out, with only 6% of psychiatric casualties being labeled neurotic [408]. However, subsequent papers indicated clearly that the main problem was to be the dissociation or conversion hysterias, and "shell shock" or what was seen as a postconcussional syndrome [473]; and in the first 8 months of the war there were at least 20 papers devoted to these and related matters in the German medical press.

French psychiatric preparations for the war were less clearly planned, perhaps because a War Department consultant, Professor Régis of Bordeaux, had placed emphasis not on the relatively straightforward organic side but on the emotional aspects of battle stress, with the possibility of "terrified and distracted soldiers fleeing automatically, disoriented, unconscious, sometimes hallucinated, no longer knowing what they were about, a prey to these new forms of disease akin to the traumatic and hysterical neuroses of industrial origin" [510]. In the first 8 months of the war, only three papers appear to have been published regarding "shell shock" and other war neuroses in French soldiers as compared with the 20 published regarding German ones, which *may* indicate that these conditions were less frequent on the French side. However, by the spring of 1915 the high command had found it necessary to organize special teams of enquiry on the problem, and by the end of 1915 it was possible for one centre alone to report on 1000 cases of war deafness in which there was neither cranial injury nor auricular lesions [340]. The British entered the war slightly later with a small professional army, and in the first 8 months they also published only three papers on our subject, each referring only to a few cases, and there is one slightly later paper [189] suggesting that war neuroses were surprisingly rare. The British official medical history of the war [367] supports that view, while omitting to mention that the low neurosis rate in 1914-1915 was accompanied by a very high rate of desertions [10, p273]. However, with the Battle of the Somme in July 1916 the problem suddenly assumed alarming proportions.

> "In the first few weeks several thousand soldiers were rapidly passed out of the battle zone on account of nervous disorders, and many of them were evacuated to England. When this great influx of patients arrived in England 'shell shock' had become a generally recognised term, as if it were a new disease ... In fact, misguided public opinion had raised the psycho-neuroses to the dignity of a new war disease, before which doctors seemed well-nigh helpless. This view became rapidly widespread among the soldiers in France. Officers, men, and even in some instances medical officers, imbibed the new doctrine." [367, p 9]

In due course the term "shell shock" was forbidden to be used, but by then it had entered into popular mythology, and for years after the war finished, new cases of alleged "shell shock" or war-caused neurasthenia come forward to claim and receive pensions, for instance 1594 in the year 1921-22 [411].

In all the armies, the main precipitator of the neuroses was being knocked down and perhaps half buried by the blast of a high-explosive shell, but the resultant symptomatology varied. Sixty percent of the British cases were estimated to fit the picture of a vague neurasthenia with "headache, dizziness, failing powers of

Table 10.1. Types of neurosis in the Austrian Army, 1914–1918, by ethnic group [496]

	Germans	"Viennese"	Czech	Northern Slavs	Southern Slavs	Hungarians	Jews
	%	%	%	%	%	%	%
Traumatic neuroses	3.3	6.4	3.3	2.6	7.0	3.7	2.6
Hysterical neuroses	56.7	53.6	59.7	65.3	34.9	57.4	52.1
Reactive depression	7.2	4.0	1.6	6.5	13.9	5.6	6.0
Other neuroses	23.0	23.2	13.1	20.4	20.9	33.3	20.5
(Malingering)	(9.8)	(12.8)	(22.3)	(5.2)	(23.3)	–	(18.8)
	100.0	100.0	100.0	100.0	100.0	100.0	100.0

Same data source as in Table 4.1., but not following the same diagnostic divisions.

concentration, inefficient memory for details, a sense of helplessness when faced with the necessity for making an effort, a constant state of irritability, and an irregularity of sleep associated with nightmares or a riotous mental activity during the night" [367, p21]. This is the classic picture of a traumatic confusional state, and only about 10% showed any form of dissociation hysteria – usually psychogenic deafness or mutism – while the remainder exhibited little more than a simple exhaustion which passed with rest and encouragement. Among the French forces, however, the literature suggests on the one hand that differentiation of malingering from neurosis was a serious problem – over a quarter of 72 French papers sampled deal with the subject as compared with less than 10% of equivalent German and British papers sampled [75] – and on the other hand that dissociation or conversion hysterias comprised a substantially larger proportion than any theory of the traumatic neuroses would predict [138, 523]. In the German and Austrian forces, if one takes Pilcz's analysis of 7500 psychiatric admissions to the military hospital in Vienna [496], it would appear that more than half of the cases assumed the form of a hysteria (Table 10.1), the proportion being highest among the Czechs and lowest among the Southern Slavs whom we have seen (p 99) to have had a high percentage of reactive psychoses.

It must be remembered that Pilcz was reporting from a base hospital, and that the term "hysteria" could be embracing vague somatic as well as the frank dissociation symptoms. Also, it is theoretically possible that this predominance of "hysterias" in the Vienna case load was due to inclusion of functional cardiac disorder, which in France and Britain tended to remain the province of the cardiologist. (Over 40 000 men received some postwar pension or payment in Britain because of "disordered action of the heart" which the war had allegedly induced [411].) However, that is not the impression which one gets from the general German-language literature or from an eye-witness report of Berlin services by a Dutch visitor in 1916 [682]. There were three main schools of treatment for the neuroses in Germany at that time, one which administrered brutal physical treatment with electric shocks and shouting, a second which simply kept the patients hospitalized in the hope that the condition would improve by itself, and a third which sympathized with the soldier's fear and discharged him home as soon as permitted. The cardiac neuroses would be accepted as such by members of the third school, but it seems likely that more dramatic symptoms would have been required to merit inclusion as a war neurosis at the clinics of the other two.

After World War I was over, as has already been noted, new cases of war neuroses continued to appear for many years, some of them perhaps merely seeking the same compensations that their fellow survivors had received, but others afflicted by the reliving of the initial trauma in nightmares, which is a well-known feature of the true traumatic neuroses and which Simmel [185, p32] thought to be a defense against psychosis. Between the two World Wars, however, the British and American medical services, with to a lesser extent the German and French, had realized the great harm that was being done by allowing soldiers to believe that explosive blasts were liable to produce permanent, invisible, damage to the brain, and it was decided to change the psychiatric approach. In the first place, soldiers (and their officers) were to be encouraged to recognize that an emotional disturbance was not unnatural during heavy bombardment or fighting; in the second place treatment was to be started as close to the front line as possible, to avoid the neurotic thought patterns becoming established. At the same time, considerable emphasis was placed on the need for better psychiatric screening at recruitment, and the organic aspects of the war neuroses – all that the French had written regarding the *confusion mentale de guerre* – were largely ignored.

In the *Second World War*, German and French psychiatry which had contributed so much previously to the study of the war neuroses now contributed very little. In the French case this was because of the occupation of the country; in the German case it seems to have arisen in part because it was claimed that the New Reich did not produce neurotics [594], and in part because the main new approach to the war neuroses in that country, that of the psychoanalysts [185], had been virtually exiled. The most that one can get from the German side, therefore, is that the dissociation hysterias had largely been replaced by "organ neuroses," so that whole military companies were formed of individuals sharing the same gastrointestinal, cardiac, or genitourinary complaints [146]. However, the Anglo-Saxon countries produced an abundance of studies which make up for that lack.

Because the Second World War was so much more mobile than the First, without the long months in heavily shelled trenches which made the former so stressful, it might be thought that the incidence of war neuroses would be less. Moreover, the new United States/United Kindom doctrine of providing psychological first-aid close to the frontline should have resulted in fewer of the psychiatrically affected needing hospitalization. Insofar as they can be compared, however, the psychiatric hospitalization rates seem to have been higher in the Second than in the First World War, and discharges from service on psychiatric grounds accounted for a higher percentage of armed forces personnel, both in Britain and the United States, exceeding all other medical categories [10]. Dissociation hysterias came to comprise a very small percentage of the hospitalized – 2,5% during the North African campaign [415] – while simple anxiety or confusion states comprised three-quarters of the cases in most regions and mixed states initially provided most of the remainder. As the war progressed, however, a relatively new syndrome claimed increasing attention, one which had rarely been mentioned previously. This was called the "reactive depression in old soldiers" or "old sergeant syndrome" (although it affected all ranks), and it occurred mainly in men who had had many months of combat, had had good premorbid personalities and who were often the last survivors of their company or platoon [361, 578]. The symptoms were fear and tremulousness, loss of self-confidence, loss of what had previously been a high level of combat effectiveness, and conflictual guilt feelings regarding the latter; but whereas other neurotic patients grasped at any chance to leave the battle zone, these ones resisted being sent back and often had to be forced. There is every reason for calling their condition a war neurosis and they had all been under heavy enough fire to justify a World War I diagnosis of *commotio*, but although their state was produced in part by exhaustion, it was also produced by the loss of all their comrades, a loss of belief in those who were leading them, and a loss of belief in the principles they had thought themselves fighting for.

This "old sergeant syndrome" is in striking contrast to what had been the popular image of the "old soldier" in World War I and in previous wars, i.e., the image of someone who knew how to look out for himself, did not allow himself to become attached to anyone, and believed neither in his superiors nor in their values. It reflects a change in mental climate, one which can be seen by comparing World War I cartoons (in the British weekly *Punch*, for instance) with those of Mauldin in World War II; and it provides just one example of the importance which trust played in preventing or precipitating war neuroses in 1939-1945. In the European Theater of operations where United States troops could regularly be withdrawn to rest conditions approximating those at home, there was a strong positive correlation between the rates of wounded and psychiatric casualties, reflecting the psychological impact of bombardment and fear [415, p363]; but in the same battle the ratio of psychiatric casualties to wounded could be twice as high in one unit as in another, among the fresh as well as among the long-service troops [415, p340]. Among the Americans the key to this appears to have been the degree of satisfaction which the leadership provided, something which adds a psychiatric dimension to the sociological findings of Stouffer et al. [595]; but the British data reproduced in Fig. 10.1 suggest that the cultural composition of the troops is of equal importance.

The general inference to be drawn from Fig. 10.1 regarding the last 2 years of the war is, as expected, that when the fighting was active in a zone the casualty rate was higher than when it was inactive. In all ethnic groups, for instance, the 1945 rates are lower than the 1944 ones in the Mediterranean, but higher in Southeast Asia. However, one also sees that Indian troops had a lower rate of psychiatric admissions than British ones not just in Southeast Asia, where they would feel more at home, but in the Mediterranean where they must have felt less at home than the British or Canadians. Moreover, African troops in Southeast Asia, where they were just as foreign as the British ones, had lower rates of psychiatric casualties than the latter, while in the Mediterranean the Canadian troops, who were given more combat duties than the British, had higher psychiatric rates than the latter. (The strikingly high rate of psychiatric breakdown among the African troops in the Mediterranean theater in 1944 derived less from battle conditions than from the strain of being conquering troops in a European society, within which they were expected to adhere to European standards of conduct.) From psychiatric reports on the Indian troops, particu-

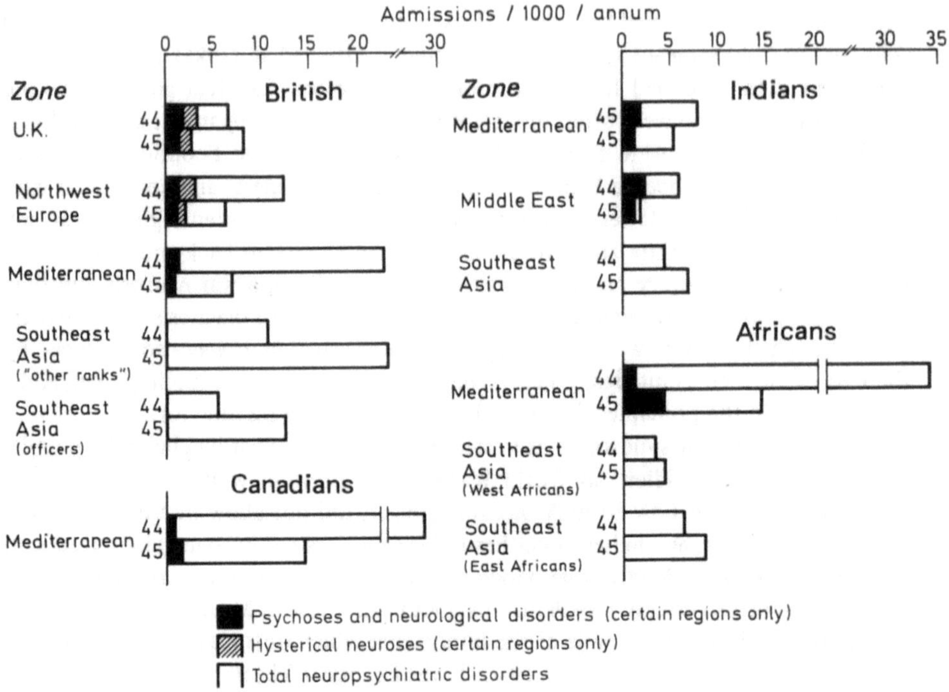

Fig. 10.1. Neuropsychiatric casualties in the British Army and other forces using the same medical services, 1944 and 1945; by origin and zone of combat. [From various tables in official history (405).]

larly that by Williams [659], it is clear that the rates of mental breakdown were lowest among the combatant Punjabi, who accord strong loyalty to their British or Indian leaders (so long as the latter do not betray that loyalty too flagrantly), and were highest among clerical N.C.O.s with a good service record and apparently good premorbid personality, but long service. One can interpret the lower Indian and African rates on the assumption, adopted by some writers, that they had insufficient education and imagination to anticipate fear. However, American Black troops usually had higher psychiatric casualty rates than the White troops under comparable circumstances, although they were likely to have had less education, and in one instance where the Black incidence rate was six times that of the White, this was to a large extent explained by social discrimination, poor leadership, and lack of identification with either the army or the reasons for the war [513].

Psychiatric data from the Korean War are not satisfactory, but they are available for the *1965-1971 war in Vietnam*, and make most enlightening reading. In the first 3 years of that war, the incidence of psychiatric conditions among the troops there was only 9% higher than among those in the United States [458, p46], despite the extremely anxiety-provoking conditions of combat. In a news release in 1967, the authorities – carefully avoiding any reference to Vietnamese civilians – announced that neuropsychiatric illness was affecting only 12 per 1000 per year, compared with 37 per 1000 during the Korean War and between 28 and 101 per 1000 (depending on the theater and year) for the United States troops during World War II [133]. The fact was used to bolster the argument that the war had the support of United States youth, since it was thought that if they had been fighting with troubled consciences they would have had more mental illness, but as we now know a wholly different type of mental disturbance was building up behind the authorities' backs: illegal drug-taking. As was noted in Chap. 8, it has been estimated that 43% of troops in the last years of the war had used heroin at least once, and 29% had used it regularly [515]. This is an important fact, making nonsense of the claim that these forces had good mental health, but it does not necessarily imply that the war neuroses were simply coming forth in a new form. Soldiers who had been under heavy fire do not seem to have been more prone to use drugs than those who had not been, and the "old soldiers" who proved vulnerable to a particular type of war neurosis in World War II used drugs *less* than the rest. Regarding possible, delayed effects such as the repeated nightmares reported by one category of sufferer from a battle neurosis, there has been considerable attention paid to the failure of some Vietnam War veterans to readjust to civilian life, but the evidence suggests that this is due less to combat experiences than to identity problems and to the fact that the homecoming men came to be seen as fools rather than heroes in some quarters. When battle neuroses did develop, they assumed the now familiar form of anxiety, agitation, and confusion.

The wars of the past century can thus be seen to have produced a much wider variety of battle neuroses or combat reactions than could be expected from the variations in the types of physical trauma (concussion from different types of explosive, for instance) or variations in perceived threat to life. The range of these neuroses is not infinite; one does not get, for instance, obsessional neuroses or sexual neuroses particularly associated with the battlefield even though impotence may be an incidental feature. Nevertheless it is much too wide a range for us to be able to say that the symptoms are all attributable to the precipitating somatic and psychic stresses. Even the simple incidence of reported battle neuroses, with symptomatology disregarded, shows too wide a variation to be accounted for on the basis of intensity of battle stresses, since although that incidence tends to increase in proportion to the fierceness of battle when we consider only soldiers of a homogenous cultural background in a particular war, the ratio of psychiatric to nonpsychiatric casualties can vary widely between groups of different cultural backgrounds when they are exposed to the same stresses in the same war, as Table 10.2 shows. There we see that in the Mediterranean theater in World War II the ratio of psychiatric to nonpsychiatric casualties was 25/100 in the British troops and 2.5/100 in the Indian, a tenfold differ-

Table 10.2. Neuropsychiatric casualties and wounds from enemy action in forces under British command, Mediterranean theater of war, 1944 [405]

	British	Canadian	New Zealand	Indian	African
	Rates per 1000 strength				
Injuries from enemy action	91.0	179.2	229.0	308.8	188.2
Psychoneuroses and psychoses	23.2	31.3	22.5	8.0	34.5
Psychiatric cases per 100 wounded	25.5	17.5	9.8	2.6	18.3

ence. Even within people of the same cultural background that ratio can vary markedly with the war. The American ratio in World War II (with a somewhat different definition of "casualty") was 56/100 in the Mediterranean theater, while during the American war in Vietnam it was only 21/100.

Differences in predisposition to mental disorder stemming from childhood or from genetic inheritance do not account for the variations in battle neuroses any better. If we assumed that such predisposition was the key factor, we would likewise have to assume (a) that East Indian genetic predispositions and childrearing patterns were much healthier than British ones in the earlier part of this century; and (b) that American childrearing patterns underwent a marked shift in the 1930s. The first of these assumptions is needed to explain the differences in Fig. 10.1 and is not in itself impossible; but we will see below that Indian males in civil life are very vulnerable to neuroses, and Kakar [288] has argued convincingly that there is so sharp a contrast between the Indian boy's first and second 5 years of life, that, according to psychoanalytic theory, fixation at a pre-oedipal stage becomes considerably more likely then in most Western cultures. The second of these assumptions would be necessary to explain the marked change in American battle neuroses between World War II and the war in Vietnam; and we have no evidence that such a change in childrearing took place. Even if one argues that the character of battle neuroses should be attributed neither to the precipitating stress alone nor to the predisposing factor alone but to the combination of the two, the variations which we have been reviewing do not appear any more explainable.

That leaves the way open for Gillespie's social relativity theory of the neurose, but it does not thereby prove that such a theory is correct. At first glance Gillespie's reference to "a disturbance of social relationships mentally 'introjected' "might seem to refer in the present instance to an introjection of the wars themselves or of the national rivalries, and in that case we do not appear any further advanced. Up to a point one can argue from the data that the more a people feel their own society directly threatened in a war, the more their soldiers tend to be vulnerable to battle anxiety and confusion states. (The American Civil War implied little threat to Northern society; Indian soldiers in the Mediterranean did not see India as threatened; and so on.) But the high rate of anxiety states in American forces during World War II is a major obstacle to such a theory, as is also the relative absence of frank anxiety states among the French forces in World War I. However, Gillespie's "disturbance of social relationships" would normally be taken as referring to something more intimate than national rivalries. Do the data fit that concept any better?

Disregarding for the moment the question of symptomatology, an answer to that question can be sought by asking whether there were any types of disturbed social relationship that were more common in the armed forces with high battle neurosis rates than in those with low rates, allowing for intensity of battle stress. The highest comparative rates appear to have occurred in the British and French forces in the Somme battle of 1916; in certain United States Black units in the Pacific during World War II; and perhaps in the African forces in the Mediterranean in 1944, although their psychiatric casualties may not have been mainly battle neuroses. The lowest rates appear to have occurred in the British Expeditionary Force of 1914-1915; in the Indian forces attached to the British Army in World War II; in the

American forces in Vietnam; and perhaps during the American Civil War if one discounts the nostalgias and pseudo-rheumatisms. When one asks whether the first group suffered from any particular type of social disturbance or conflict to a substantially greater degree than the second group, the only thing that seems at all pertinent is distrust of leadership. This distrust showed itself most clearly in the mutiny of numerous French army units in the months subsequent to the Somme battle and in the reported attitudes of United States Black units in the Pacific, while it can be argued that African forces in the Mediterranean probably had good reason to withhold trust from their (White) officers. Conversely, trust of leadership was a striking feature in most Indian combat units, particularly those from the northwest, and appears to have been high at the regimental level in the British Expeditionary Force (1915), while the American soldiers in Vietnam seem to have trusted their immediate superiors. However, it is clear that many Vietnam soldiers did not trust their political leadership; that British soldiers in 1915 and Northern soldiers in the American Civil War were quite ready to desert; and on the other hand it is doubtful whether the United States Black soldiers had any particular distrust of Roosevelt. Furthermore, even if we recognize that trust at some level or another may be a factor here, it is by no means clear whether this constituted a social disturbance which was then introjected as Gillespie would have conceived. Another, potentially more fruitful way of viewing the factor of trust in the forces with high and with low comparative rates of battle neurosis is to ask what mental state develops when that trust is present and is absent.

The basic difference between someone who trusts his leader and someone who does not is that the former can leave many difficult decisions to the leader while the latter has to take these decisions for himself. The mental activity most susceptible to disturbance by trauma, fatigue, or toxins is, as Kurt Goldstein [227] has taught us, the taking of higher-level decisions. In the commonest type of battle neurosis one finds the patients complaining of (to repeat a description cited earlier) "failing powers of concentration ... a sense of helplessness when faced with the necessity of making an effort ... [and] riotous mental activity during the night" [367, p21]. These are complaints likely to be met from people attempting to take decisions and finding their powers of doing so impaired; or of people attempting to regain self-mastery. Another familiar symptom of the ordinary battle neurosis, namely the reliving of the traumatic event in nightmare or hallucination, can also be interpreted as an effort at regaining self-mastery, according to Simmel [185]. When one looks into the question of which categories of armed forces personnel are most vulnerable to battle neurosis, one finds that it is not those most often called upon to act alone, or those most subordinate to the orders of others, but those who are most often called upon to take decisions for people whom they know personally. In the British forces during World War I from 1916 onwards the officers had proportionately more battle neuroses than their men; in the Indian troops in Southeast Asia the most vulnerable were the administrative sergeants (*havilars*); in the American Army in Europe during World War II, as we have seen, it was the long-service soldiers to whom the others looked for guidance that were particularly affected. Furthermore, the evidence suggests that the incidence of battle neuroses is comparatively low when important decisions have to be made privately but where the alternatives are fairly clear cut, as is the case where it is easy to desert, or when the individual can accord himself a type of "moratorium" (in Erikson's sense [171]) from taking important decisions, as appears to have been the case among the American soldiers in Vietnam who knew that if they followed orders and survived for 12 months, they could then return to determining their own lives again.

These considerations may cast some light on the variations in the incidence of battle neuroses between one army or another, but do they cast any light on the reasons for the variations in *type* of neurosis? Seemingly not, since the dissociation and conversion hysterias of the Boer War and World War I do not easily lend themselves to being interpreted as a struggle to regain decision-taking powers. Yet it is the shift to this form of neurosis from the nostalgias of the American Civil War and the further shift out of the conversion states to the anxiety and confusion states of World War II that calls most for explanation. Are we to treat these shifts as casual and unimportant symptom shifts induced by the attitudes of the army medical services at the different periods, or do the dissociation and conversion states reflect an etiology essentially different from that of the anxiety neuroses of war? This question can be tackled purely in terms of battle neuroses, but it can be argued that it is more logical to see these dissociation and conversion states within the wider context of the hysterias. Although I appear to be making quite a detour, therefore, I propose to consider the international and cross-cultural distribution of these states more generally, and only after that to attempt to answer the question which opened this paragraph.

2 Hysteria and *Latah* – India, Mexico, and Malaysia

The term hysteria has been employed to cover so wide a range of syndromes that some authorities have recommended its complete abandonment [111], and there is little point in attempting to compare incidence rates internationally. However, if one sets aside the so-called hysterical personality, the vague somatic sydromes to which the term has been applied for want of any better, and the transient states of loss of emotional control typified by the Eskimo "piblotoq" [202] and the Latin American "ataque" [129], then there remains a core group of syndromes whose distribution it is interesting to compare at least impressionistically, relying more on clinical reports than on statistics. This core group comprises the dissociation and sensori-motor hysterias, and shares the common characteristic that a limited part of the body or mind which is normally fully coordinated with the rest becomes isolated from that coordination, either functioning independently or being blocked from functioning. The group also shares the characteristic of being reproducible through hypnosis. The best known facts regarding the distribution of these syndromes are that (a) they occur much more in females than in males; (b) among males they occur more in members of the armed forces during war than in other sections of the population; and (c) they are commoner in people with little education than in people with much. For each of these features a different explanation is usually given, resulting in a rather untidy theory, but when one looks at certain other, largely overlooked, features of their distribution there appears a common element which in my opinion points towards a more coherent explanation for the different peculiarities.

One of these distributional features which we have already considered concerns the relative frequency of the dissociation and conversion hysterias in different wars and armies. Because they were less frequent in World War II than in World War I, and because the soldiers in the second war were on average better educated than those in the first, it is generally thought that amount of education is the key here. However, these particular hysterias were almost certainly less frequent among the forces during the American Civil War than among the British forces during the Boer War, although there is no reason to think of the former as better educated, and in World War II there was another difference which cannot easily be attributed to level of education. In the German forces in that war, as was noted above, the hysterical forms of battle neurosis had been largely replaced by organ neuroses (palpitations, enuresis, dyspepsia, etc.) or by simple anxiety states (*Kriegszittern*)[146, 325]. The main report which we possess regarding neuropsychiatric casualties in French soldiers, however, states that 30% comprised conversion hysterias, and the details provided in that report [601] suggest that this is not the result of the diagnosis being applied too loosely. The little else which has been published about neuropsychiatric casualties among the French in that war, plus impressions gathered from colleagues working with the different forces then, persuades me that the battle neuroses were more liable to take this form among the French soldiers than among the German, American, or British. But there is no reason to think that the French were less educated than the Germans, or that their army medical services were so much harsher that their soldiers had to produce particularly dramatic disabilities in order to gain attention.

A second example of a difference in the apparent frequency of hysteria when one might have expected a similarity concerns women in India, Mexico, and Central America. In India, numerous psychiatric reports such as that of Veeraraghavan [632], and anthropological ones such as that from Opler [470], indicate that the classical dissociative and conversion hysterias are relatively common, affecting the higher as well as the lower castes [156]. For Mexico and Central America, a search of the literature and consultations with colleagues who have worked there indicate that these forms of hysteria are little known among the Indian (Amerindian) women, although they can be encountered among the usually better educated women of mixed Spanish origin (ladinas, mestizas). The Amerindian women in that region are quite vulnerable to neuroses, either the *ataque* mentioned earlier or a mixed anxiety and depression state with somatic symptoms which goes under the labels of *susto* [524], *espanto* [619], and a variety of local terms; but these neuroses do not have what characterizes core hysteria, namely that a part of the body or mind is isolated from the rest. Here again, there is no reason to think of the East Indian women as receiving less education than the Amerindian ones. Similarly, to turn to psychoanalytic theory, there is no reason to think of them as having been more subject to sexual stimulation during childhood than Mexican women are.

The third instance of a difference in frequency which I wish to draw attention to here relates not to true hysteria, but to a condition which shares certain of the same clinical characteristics and which may be etiologically related, the "culture-bound" syndrome *latah*. In latah, subjects exhibit brief episodes of loss of self-control during which they either utter remarks which they would never utter normally (coprolalia) or imitate whatever appears to be suggested to them by persons whom they observe (echolalia, echopraxia). Although the disorder has some of the characteristics of an exaggerated startle reaction (the exclamations which people utter when startled by a loud bang) and also some of the characteristics of Gilles de la Tourette's syndrome (the echopraxia) it shares with hysteria the fact that the victim has not consciously willed the behavior, denies responsibility for it, and proves to be highly sensitive to conscious or unconscious suggestion. Latah-like conditions have been recorded in many parts of the world under different names, but one of their features is that they tend to become much more numerous over a limited period of time and then die down again, while another is that although at low-prevalence times they are, like hysteria, found mainly in women, at times of highest prevalence they tend to affect males as much as or more than females. One such condition ("jumping") affected French Canadians in New England during the 1870s-1880s [39]; another (*miryachit*) showed an upsurge among Siberians a few decades later [134]. The best documented instance of the rise and fall of such a condition, however, concerns latah itself in Java and Malaya.

As I have shown elsewhere [427], latah appears to have been virtually unobserved by European residents and travellers in these countries prior to 1860, but during the 1880s and 1890s it was stated from Dutch-ruled Java that "the condition is so common that one can find many women with it any day in the streets" [628], while similar statements were made from British-ruled Malaya. In the latter country it seems to have been met as often in males as in females, and one writer noted that "the latah sufferer is usually intellectually superior and more alert than his fellows" [195]; but it was at that time by no means the trivial condition it became later. One man is reported to have killed his infant daughter and another to have seriously burnt his hands while helplessly imitating someone else's actions [427]. By the 1920s a survey of 600 doctors in the Dutch East Indies showed that the condition had become much less common in areas under Western influence, and occurred predominantly in domestic servants [630], a significant fact in view of the role which patients from that class played in the development of nineteenth century ideas about hysteria and hypnotism [167]. Outside areas under Western influence, we know that it continued in milder form, these milder forms still being found in the villages in the 1970s [568]. Superficially, the decline in the prevalence of the latah-type conditions in different countries appears to be related to improved education, but at the height of the epidemic writers were commenting that the educated were as vulnerable as those without formal education, and that the introduction of Christian mission schools had not reduced its frequency. Moreover, the evidence suggests, as with the "jumping Frenchmen" in New England, that there was an earlier period when the condition was much less prevalent, perhaps even unknown.

The difference in the prevalence of hysteria in Western soldiers, the difference in the prevalence of hysteria in non-Western women, and the latah-type epidemics have been placed together in this section, because I think that they share a concealed etiological feature, one which also has a bearing on the religious possession states which many authorities have in the past treated as hysterias. The feature is most clearly recognized in the Western armies.

In World War I, the French and the German armies had trained their soldiers in very similar fashion, and they had, as far as can be judged, similar rates of battle hysteria, although the German rate may initially have been higher than the French. For World War II, the French used much the same training, one which assumed the war would be between opposing masses. The Maginot Line exemplified that view. The *Wehrmacht*, however, was training for a land war of depth and movement in which not just tanks but small groups of infantrymen and machine gunners would be expected to operate in relative isolation from their officers. The French soldier, therefore, was trained mainly to obey orders promptly and completely without asking himself whether these orders made sense, while the German soldier was trained to interpret his orders in the light of information which he knew his officers might not have. If one now turns back to a comparison of the American Civil War army and the British one in the Boer War, a similar difference appears. The British Army was a small professional one for the most part, trained to a strict obedience of orders and glorying in the absurd legend of the "Thin Red Line." The American Army was made up of recently recruited civilians who had learnt from childhood to take their own decisions rather than obey orders.

Passing to the East Indian (mainly Hindu) and the Amerindian women, one finds that the former had had drilled into them from early childhood the need to conform to a series of rules which could not be rationally deduced from life experience but were dictated by their religion – rules relating to pollution, relations between castes, subservience to the male, etc. Moreover, conformity to these rules was important for achieving greater happiness or freedom from distress in future lives, in comparison with which the trials and benefits of one's present life were unimportant. The Amerindian women of Central America were not less affected by religious and supernatural beliefs, but these beliefs had not given rise to a set of rigid rules of behavior, and the benefits which one might acquire in a future existence were for them considerably less important than those belonging to the present. One could be punished for breaking some taboo or neglecting some Spirit's needs, but these Spirits were arbitrary and it was necessary, therefore, always to be alert to the possible significance of what one was observing, a significance which could not be reacted to on the basis of a few rules learnt by rote. There are other factors contributing to the development of neuroses in both groups, but this question of whether one learns blindly and by rote or learns by trial and error appears the most pertinent to the fact that neuroses assume a predominantly hysterical character in the one group and not in the other.

In the first of the above illustrations, hysteria was proportionately higher in the group that had been encouraged to submit blindly to the orders of officers, than in the group that had been encouraged to make their own interpretations of their situation, even though, as we saw in the previous section of this chapter, the latter teaching was liable to induce a greater susceptibility to other forms of battle neurosis. In the second illustration, a higher frequency of hysteria occurred in the group that had been taught to follow blindly a set of religiously prescribed rules affecting all aspects of life, than in the group which did not believe that sticking to rules could enable one to avoid the malice of the gods. Coming to the Malays and Javanese, the first point to note is that the conversion to Islam some centuries earlier had resulted in the gradual dissemination of schools in which learning by rote rather than by understanding was the rule, and was tied to a better life in the hereafter, just as with the Hindus. However, a point which has more pertinence to the upsurge of latah at the end of the last century is that it was at this time that the major peoples of the region became reconciled to the presence of Europeans among them, and sought to copy these Europeans as a way of acquiring a better material life, this copying being easier done through automatic imitation and obedience than through attempting to understandand the reasons for the Europeans' orders and way of life. A third point of relevance is that the culture of the region has a long, probably pre-Islamic, tradition of puppet play and of handling children as puppets [36], i.e., of encouraging children to submit their bodies entirely to the manipulation of an adult, this tradition being probably linked to another which states that one's behavior should always conform to the situation, no matter how differently one might feel. It is my opinion that when we meet a sudden upsurge of latah-type behavior, as in Siberia and Maine as well as in Malaya and Java, this is when a less powerful or wealthy people comes in contact with a more powerful or wealthy one and seeks to acquire the latter's advantages through imitating them or carrying out their orders without initially attempting to understand these [430]. Later, when it is realized that automatic obedience or imitation earns fewer rewards than seeking to learn the principles underlying the model, the form of learning changes as the incidence of latah-like behavior decreases, although the condition does not necessarily disappear. Isolated instances of latah-like behavior can be found in most societies, but usually only when there is some slight secondary gain similar to that obtained from clowning [568], and most such cases barely merit being called pathological.

With these points clarified it is now convenient to return to the questions left unanswered many paragraphs earlier, namely whether the dissociated and conversion battle neuroses can be interpreted on the same basis as the anxiety and confusional ones, and whether the changes in form of neurosis from one war to another support Gillespie's social relativity theory of the neuroses. Taking the second point first, the evidence suggests that Gillespie's theory is in part correct and in part wrong. The character of battle neuroses varies with the social setting and seems determined in part by the internalization of elements in that setting, but it is not the internalization of social disturbances which appears important. Rather it is the internalization of teachings regarding how best to respond to disturbances and other types of problem. Regarding the other question, it seems clear that the soldier with a dissociation neurosis is not attempting to work out his own decisions, but he could be said, like the other neurotic soldiers, to be attempting to master his situation by applying to the fullest the method he has been taught, in this case opening his mind to orders or suggestions which, in the event, come more strongly from his own unconscious than from his superiors. The excessive stresses of battle lead to excessive efforts at mastering the personal situation, and these efforts turn pathological. The lowest levels of neurosis for a given battle stress should presumably occur when soldiers are encouraged to share decisions, neither trying to do too much on their own nor leaving too much to their superiors.

The demanding of automatic obedience from soldiers explains how they, particularly in battle, have in the past exhibited much more dissociation and conversion hysteria than other males. The fact that most educational systems teach mastery by understanding in place of mastery by automatic learning explains why persons with higher education exhibit less hysteria than persons with little education. But why, in the light of the foregiong theory, should women exhibit so much more hysteria than men in civil life? The Hindu women referred to earlier were not more fully indoctrinated in religious conformity than their men, and Javanese boys received more training in rote (automatic) learning than their sisters. Kretchmer [324] assumed that women had a "constitutional " predisposition to hysteria, and psychoanalytic texts generally attribute the sex difference in this matter to the fact that female sexuality, even in infancy, being for anatomical reasons more passive than male. Should we take it that there is a sex-linked factor in hysteria which is present from infancy or is the difference based on the roles to which men and women are customarily assigned?

In searching for cross-cultural material which might contribute to answering this question, I have thought it most pertinent (as with depression) to ask whether there are any societies in which men have as much as or more hysteria than women, without more neurotigenic stress. I have not been able to find any such example involving frank and socially handicapping psychopathology, and this fact is important. However, when one extends the concept of hysteria to cover other types of dissociation, the result is different, and it therefore appears worthwhile examining briefly this wider picture.

3 Trance and Possession States: Bandari and Abelam

The great majority of cases of trance and possession which are to be found in non-Western societies ought not to be labeled pathological. They are much more comparable to the trances which a Western hypnotist induces either as a form of treatment or for the entertainment of an audience, even though the "hypnotist" may be the cult group rather than a single individual, the ceremony may have a religious significance, and the "entertainment" may occur more frequently than we are used to. A substantial minority of persons entering trances learn the practice after suffering from a neurotic – some would say psychotic [338] – illness, but few dissociate without some type of instruction. In most societies where male participation in trance and possession equals or exceeds female, the dissociation symbolizes power. The subject's initial episode may have the character of a personal malady, but there will be a well-established local tradition regarding how one should convert this apparent malady into an asset, and it tends to be males rather than females who follow that path, for instance by becoming shamans, although there are important cults, particularly in Africa, through which women acquire power or prestige by such means.

There are a few instances, however, in which males predominate among the tranced or possessed, but do not usually use it as a channel to power. These instances appear to me to fall into two broad types which may have relevance for the problem of the sex difference in pathological hysteria. The first of these types of situation is exemplified by the Bandari living on islands in the south of Iran and belonging to the Zar cult. Zar is a possession and healing cult which is widespread in the Horn of Africa, Egypt, Arabia, and parts of Iran. In almost all its branches one finds women rather than men belonging to it, and they join it seeking help for some illness or other misfortune which becomes attributed to spirit possession [301]. Among the Bandari the same basic beliefs exist, but is men rather than women who seek the cult's aid, men with depression, hysterical blindness, and a variety of somatic complaints, not particularly young but all of very low socioeconomic status [212]. When one enquires what distinguishes the Bandari from other peoples among whom Zar beliefs are found, one learns that they are not merely poor, as is true of most of these others, but are a small group treated as semi-outcasts by the Arab and Iranian majorities around them. In other instances known to me where older males feature prominently as clients in healing cults a similar situation exists, i.e., the cultural group to which they belong is markedly disadvantaged when compared with their neighbors.

The second type of situation is when the dissociation or trance states occur mainly or exclusively among young males, something exemplified by the Samburu who were referred to in the previous chapter [579], and by the Abelam of New Guinea [353]. In these instances there is usually no concept of spirit possession involved, and the abnormal behavior consists of shaking violently, having pseudo-epileptic seizures, or running about wildly. In other peoples of New Guinea in which such "shaking sickness" occurs, women seem to be affected more than men although the male episodes are more dramatic [270, 507], but in the Abelam where it is predominantly young men who are affected we are told that it is associated with sexual deprivation, the same state as applied to the Samburu, and probably also dictated by a gerontocracy. In both the Abelam and the Samburu, it seems clear that the dissociation is permitting the venting of anger or aggressive feelings, and that these feelings are linked to a sense of sexual deprivation.

There is a suggestion here, therefore, that dissociation is particularly likely to arise in people who feel themselves disadvantaged in comparison with the others around them, who are prevented from taking direct steps to correct that disadvantage because the powers which enforce it are too great, and who have learnt that they are more likely to attain their modest desires if they submit to these powers than if they rebel against them. The instances just cited have referred to males who feel this way, but there is a large literature, particularly from Africa [126], indicating that the high participation of women in healing cults which use trance or possession arises from the same factors. Such cults "may provide a channel for social mobility, allow the 'voice of women' to be heard in a male-dominated society, and occasionally enable participants to enjoy benefits to which their status would not normally entitle them" [126, p 204].

If this is the case with the less pathological forms of dissociation, one must ask whether it might not also be the case with the more pathological, i.e., with true hysteria, even though one is dealing not with organized cults but with isolated individuals. The cross-cultural evidence is too weak to build a sound argument on, but there is a suggestion here that the reason women have more hysteria than men relates not to some "constitutional" factor, as Kretchmer assumed, and not to experiences in childhood as Freud proposed, but to certain disadvantages which traditional society almost everywhere has imposed on them. These disadvantages are in part sexual, since women are expected almost everywhere to wait for the male to initiate sexual contact rather than take the initiative, and in part related to the fact that men hold the greater power (outside of matrifocal societies such as the Minangkabau). Women thus usually learn that they can achieve more by accomodating themselves to male ideas and by making themselves desirable to the power holders than by taking their own independent decisions, and what has been presented above indicates that this subordinating attitude is associated with a heightened risk of hysteria. It is true that as respects heterosexual gratification, the female is at a biological disadvantage in all mammalian species, insofar as she is unlikely to achieve satisfactory intercourse with a disinterested male, while a sexually aroused male can obtain his own gratification from a disinterested female or even a subordinate male. This has contributed to the submissive posture which sexually aroused females in most species assume, and which might be said to be a biological characteristic conducing to greater submissiveness in general [52]. However, among humans it is the social rather than the biological restrictions on sexual and other forms of gratification from which women mainly suffer, and one must ask whether the roots of the female predominance in hysteria do not lie here rather than in biology or in childhood. A partial answer might be obtained by studying the prevalence of the disorder in matrifocal societies, but this has not yet been done.

4 Phobias –– British, Japanese, and Eskimos

By the study of individual patients, psychoanalysis (and psychiatry generally) has been led to accord a major role in the development of different forms of neurosis to childhood experiences, and to the degree to which current stressors strike a chord which resonates among the memories of these experiences. From the evidence presented so far in this chapter, a strong impression has arisen that the distribution of certain types of neurosis is determined less by childhood experiences and their links to current stressors than by other forces in the patient's contemporary social setting. That evidence, of course, does not exclude childhood experiences from having participated in the development of the neurosis, and there are plenty examples of patients with battle neuroses or (somewhat less plentifully) with addiction to trance or possession states, in whom a relationship between the current condition and some childhood trauma can be demonstrated. Nevertheless, the international variations which we have so far considered appear to have been more strongly linked to differences in social forces affecting the adult than to differences in the social (familial) forces affecting the child, and this is surprising. Cultures differ greatly in the traumatic experiences to which children are exposed, and one might have expected that these differences would have had a marked influence on the vulnerability of particular cultural groups to specific neuroses. However, I know of no evidence to suggest that British males are exposed to more traumatic experiences in childhood – either in general or of a particular type – than East Indian males, despite the differences in their vulnerability to battle neuroses; and neither do I know of any evidence to suggest that East Indian females are more exposed to sexual arousal in childhood than the Amerindian children of Mexico and Central America.

One possible explanation for this lack of evidence is that within-culture variation in such matters is greater than between-culture variation, but most anthropologists would not agree with that proposition and a more probable explanation is that we have not been looking at the appropriate types of neurosis. Psychoanalytic thinking is much more developed respecting phobias, obsessional neuroses, and sexual disorders than respecting the traumatic and hysterical neuroses. I therefore propose now to see to what extent some international differences in the distribution of particular phobias can be linked to childhood variables, and follow that with a brief reference to the sexual neuroses and the Oedipus complex.

In delimiting what to regard as true *phobias* for the purposes of international comparison, it is not enough to exclude cases with irrational fears which do not interfere with social life, and cases in which phobic symptoms are subsidiary to a more widespread disorder. One must also exclude instances in which fears which strike ourselves as irrational are viewed as relatively justifiable by the patient's society. When such fears exist, for instance of ghosts, foreigners, and venereal infection from a toilet seat (depending on the society), it is still possible that some persons are truly phobic in these respects while the majority of their neighbors treat the matter more casually [244], but at the national or cultural level it is best to regard the whole class of such fears as nonpathological and when one does this historically, a curious point arises. European history offers many isolated examples of persons notorious for some phobia, as Robert Burton [81] showed, but if one excludes fear of witches and other supernatural agents, then one finds that it is only around 1870 that what we would call phobias today seem to have become sufficiently common to merit serious medical attention. More specifically, this is when agoraphobia first entered medical literature, [651], that phobia which has since become the most familiar to European psychiatrists. In the 1960s, a British radio program on agoraphobia resulted in such intense public interest that a society of agoraphobics called the Open Door sprang up with about 1500 members. We need not think of all these as truly handicapped, but a sampling of 80% of them revealed that 67% had consulted a psychiatrist because of the problem, 56% were avoiding crossing streets and open spaces, and 23% were virtually housebound because of the condition [379].

Other studies of phobias among Anglo-Saxons indicate, as has been stated, that this fear of open spaces is more frequent, and usually more refractory, than other phobias such as of animals, heights, and knives. However, in other societies the predominant phobias may be quite different. For instance, in Iran a survey of phobic symptoms in over 600 mental patients with different diagnoses revealed that fear of open spaces comprised only 1% of these symptoms, while fear of darkness comprised 24%, of corpses 16%, and of animals 16% [139]. Among the North American Apache there is reported to be a widespread, irrational fear of dogs, even small puppies, and of an unaggressive bird called the whippoorwill (L.B. Boyer, personal communication). In Japan, fear of looking someone in the face and fear of having an offensive odor are reported to be remarkably common and sometimes quite handicapping, 19% of neurotic Kyoto University students seeking psychiatric aid having been found to suffer from a more general "phobia of interpersonal relations" (*taijin kyofu*) to which these symptoms belong [294]. It is not being suggested that so high a percentage of neurotics in Japan are suffering from a true phobia in the sense given earlier, but it is clear that many do. Because Japanese childhood experiences have been compared with Western ones, and because *taijin kyofu* has been discussed in a number of accessible papers, it is convenient to compare the latter with agoraphobia in Anglo-Saxon societies and explore how far the differences in symptomatology can be linked to differences in childrearing.

Despite their common nature as phobias, agoraphobia and *taijin kyofu* show considerable differences in matters other than the presenting symptom. Taking the writings of Marks [378], Kasahara [294], and Kimura [308] as guides, it can be said that the former affects mainly women while the latter affects both sexes equally; that the former neurosis has its onset most often in the mid-20s and runs into the 40s and later, while the latter starts soon after puberty and is rare after the age of 40. *Taijin kyofu* appears to have been increasing in Japan after World War II, at least until the late 1960s, and to affect first-born more than later-born, while agoraphobia has probably not been increasing and is not linked to birth rank. Agoraphobia is associated with panic attacks, fear of fainting, and problems of will; *taijin kyofu* is associated with feelings of shame, fear of harming others, and what may happen accidentally rather than by will. Unsatisfactory sexual life is reported by a substantial proportion of agoraphobics, despite the fact that they are usually married, and psychoanalysts such as Edoardo Weiss [648] attribute most cases to sexual conflict while making virtually no reference to dependency conflict. *Taijin kyofu* patients do not appear to be troubled by sexual dissatisfactions, and psychoanalytically trained Japanese authorities such as Takeo Doi [153] see dependency conflicts as crucial to that disorder. If childhood experiences are major factors in the phobias, therefore, there should be considerable and pertinent differences between Japanese and Western childrearing; and we need to consider in some detail what these are.

The main comparisons of Japanese and Western childhood and mother-child relations are to be found in the series of studies directed by William Caudill, and continued by his colleagues after his death. In the first months of life there is already a clear difference between the two cultures respecting the infant's vocalizations [95], and by the age of two-and-a-half similar differences can be observed in various other aspects of the child's relations with its environment [98], differences which have been shown to arise from the mother's behavior and not to be genetic [97]. In the early months, American mothers talk much more to their babies but have less physical contact with them than Japanese mothers of equivalent social class do, providing less in the way of spontaneous care but responding more to the infant's attempts at signaling for care. As a result, although Japanese and American infants spend about the same proportion of time in unhappy vocalizing, American ones spend much more time in happy and exploratory vocalizing [95]. As time passes, the American child finds itself increasingly left alone to amuse itself, increasingly encouraged to play at adult roles, and increasingly reprimanded when it does something which the parent does not like, while the Japanese child is less often verbally reprimanded and is given greater encouragement to indulge itself and seek care from the parent, a behavior to which the Japanese apply the term *amae* [153]. By the age of six, the American child is much more accustomed to adults attempting to coerce him into action and to resisting that coercion or attempting coercion on his own behalf, than the Japanese child is, and he experiences more in the way of positive interaction, physical as well as verbal.

These studies make no reference to sexuality in childhood, but from others [147, 339] it can be inferred, firstly, that family members are more likely to sleep in the same room, even a widow and her grown-up son and daughter, and to bathe naked together in Japan than in America or Europe, so that adult genitalia are more familiar to the Japanese than to the Western child. Secondly, parental sexual intercourse is very discreet in Japan, for instance with the husband entering his wife from the rear while they are both lying on their sides under the covers. There is thus less likelihood than in the West of a child being excessively aroused by the sight, or interpreting such intercourse as an attack on the mother, or of being shouted at because it has intruded at an embarrassing moment, experiences which Western psychiatrists identify as traumatic. Thirdly, there appears to be little difference between the cultures in their treatment of sexual play, touching of genitals, or masturbation in children (allowance being made for social class), apart from the more general difference in the character of warnings if these be used, the Japanese being more likely to refer to people not liking the child and Westerners being more likely to refer to abstract naughtiness or bodily harm. I can find no information on the relative probability of a child being sexually molested or seduced. Incest is known in Japan just as in the West but varies very much with social milieu.

Western psychoanalysts have tended to see the phobias of all types as rooted not merely in early childhood but in the sexual experience at that age. Japanese psychoanalysts, while agreeing on the importance of childhood, have tended to see the phobias as rooted in dependency conflicts rather than sexual ones. From the above summary of childhood differences, it is easy to see that the middle-class Western child might be more liable to view his nascent sexual feelings as dangerous, forbidden, or conflictual than the middle-class Japanese child, so that emotionally loaded sexual memories would be more liable to surface in the Western psychoanalytic patient than in the Japanese one. However, that should not, in principle, affect etiology. Some Western authorities would say that although the sexual element in Japanese phobias is less apparent, it is no less important and must have been missed. Asian authorities such as Doi [153] and Neki [461], on the other hand, have frankly remarked on what they consider to be their Western colleagues' insensitivity to, or fear of, dependency feelings; so that one might equally infer that it is dependency conflict rather than sexual conflict which underlies Western phobias. From one angle the Japanese child might be expected to grow up not with more but with fewer dependency problems than the Western child, thanks to his mother's more ready acceptance and gratification of his dependency needs in infancy. However, it was noted above that although the Japanese mother may give more care, the Western infant expresses greater happiness, so that this judgment regarding dependency needs may be premature. These are points which we must come back to, but first it is desirable to examine whether there are other differences between the two cultural traditions which might explain the difference in phobias, without involving the early childhood experiences that the psychoanalysts see as the key.

Regarding *taijin kyofu* there is one feature in Japanese cultural history which I feel to have an obvious bearing on the symptomatology. It is not mentioned in any of the psychiatric papers on the subject which I have read, and I can only assume that it is so familiar a part of Japanese history lessons that their psychiatrists take it for granted. This is the fact that for centuries, upper-class Japanese women were expected to conceal their faces and all other parts of their bodies from the view of men other than those in their immediate families, and men might likewise conceal their features from women under certain conditions. Thus, although extramarital sexual relations were common, it appears to have been not unusual for lovers to have slept several times together without ever having seen each others' faces clearly, and in that same tradition personal scents assumed great importance as means of identifying people, both fabricated scents whose recipes were closely guarded secrets, and natural body odor. Moreover, the tradition gave rise to phobias not so different from *taijin kyofu*. In the fifth book of Lady Murasaki Shikibu's magnificant psychological novel, *Genji Monotagari*, written around 1000 A.D., is the following passage: "She was a very unusual girl, shy beyond all reason. It was only by the greatest effort that she could bring herself to let even her mother really see her, and in general she carried the dislike of being looked at to the verge of insanity. Yet she had no defect either of person or intelligence which could have prompted her to behave in this fashion." [416, p759]. Later it is mentioned that the girl's stepfather, who had been married to her mother for many years, had never seen her, but had only spoken with her behind a screen. *Taijin kyofu* affects males today quite as much as females, but it would still seem not unreasonable to think that this courtly tradition has contributed both to the avoidance of face-to-face contact and to the over-sensitivity to body odor which are its most prominent symptoms.

The availability of a tradition on which patients can model their symptoms, however, does not mean that that tradition is etiological in the true sense, and I know no comparable British tradition which could help explain agoraphobia. One thus still needs to ask if there are specific features of modern Japanese childhood or adult life which would lead to this particular model being seized on. On this subject Doi has drawn attention to a minor aspect of Japanese mothering which may be relevant and which has acquired greater significance thanks to research that has appeared since his book [153] was written. His point is simply that *taijin kyofu* can be viewed as an exaggerated expression of *hitomishiri*, which loosely translates as shyness or bashfulness but implies fear of strangers or of the unfamiliar, rather than the adherence to proper decorum and the fear of performing in front of others which the English terms can imply. *Hitomishiri* is used by a Japanese mother to refer to the negative responses which infants exhibit around the age of 8 months towards stangers, and Doi implies that she tends to use the term approvingly, as indicating both an attained stage in mental development and a proper attachment to her and the family. Now, this aversion to strangers is normally seen as the earliest sign of social anxiety, and in its mildest form is shown by the infant averting its gaze [643], the same behavior as typifies *taijin kyofu*. Not all babies exhibit aversion to strangers, and the same baby may do so under some circumstances but not others. Among the theories which have been offered to explain these variations, a plausible one is to the effect that less anxiety is provoked if the infant has some feeling of being able to modify the adult's acts through its own behavior than when it has no such feeling [64]. For instance, while aversion tends to occur when the stranger moves toward the baby, no such aversion occurs if the stranger stays still and the infant's movements take it in the stranger's direction. The research of Caudill's team, noted above, indicated that Japanese mothers were more prone than American ones to act on the infant's behalf whether the infant had signaled a need or not, and were less apt than American mothers to respond to the infant's attempts at signaling, the most probable reason being that "In Japan the mother views her baby much more as an extension of herself, and psychologically the boundaries between the two of them are blurred. The mother feels that she knows what is best for the baby, and there is no particular need for him to tell her what he wants because, after all, they are virtually one" [95, p43].

Because the Japanese infant is given less training in manipulation of adults' actions through its own behavior, it could very well be that anxiety toward strangers is more intense than it would be for the average Western infant. If the Japanese mother then encourages the anxiety, up to a point, in place of helping to master it, psychoanalytic theory would predict fixation at this stage. In later years, both Japanese and Chinese children are taught much more strongly than is the case in the West to avoid involvement with strangers (I have met some of the symptoms of *taijin kyofu* in Chinese patients) and the Japanese children are additionally encouraged to indulge themselves within their family setting (*amaeru*), so that that fixation could be reinforced, this encouragement being greatest for the first-born who, as was noted above, is more prone to *taijin kyofu* than the others. Doi has suggested that the reported increase in *taijin kyofu* since World War II, which might appear paradoxical if one thinks of the disorder as linked to cultural traditions, may be due to the normal gratification of certain aspects of dependency having declined, so that individuals needing such gratification become more disturbed.

Between *taijin kyofu* in Japan and agoraphobia in Europe there is more of a similarity than simply that they are both phobias, since each is often found to be linked to a desire to remain within the shelter of the familiar home. However, agoraphobia attacks women some years after they have left the parental home rather than at the time when they are leaving it; it does not affect the firstborn more than the laterborn; it is more chronic than *taijin kyofu* or most other phobias; it showed a sudden upsurge at the beginning of this century which invites explanation; and although a minority of agoraphobics fear being close to strangers, the majority are affected not so much by the presence of people as by their absence. One should no less be able to explain these features of agoraphobia on the basis of Anglo-Saxon (or European) culture than explain the *taijin kyofu* features on the basis of Japanese culture.

That the agoraphobic is often disturbed by the absence of people rather than by their presence is a difficult feature to explain if one assumes that the condition is based on sexual conflict, and this difficulty is increased by the fact that many agoraphobics are more comfortable in darkness than in daylight. If thoughts of rape or sexual temptations were a dominant factor, as they seem to be in some other forms of phobia in women, an open space in daylight should be reassuring and a dark doorway threatening. Yet it is in the open space that agoraphobics are most likely to develop a panic, and they can often obtain relief by reaching the side of the square and sheltering in some doorway. Some clinicians have attempted to explain the fear of open spaces as a fear of being seen by everyone (implying sexual exposure) but the panic can be still greater if the patients think there might be no one there to see them. It thus seems to be the emptiness of the space and the patients' feeling of isolation there rather than the presence of others which is stressful, an unusual feature but one which is shared by another neurosis, *kayak-angst*, which affects the Eskimos of the eastern Arctic. So let us consider this similarity briefly.

Kayak-angst is an acute panic state which can develop in someone sitting fishing alone in his kayak with the water smooth, the sun shining and land within sight. It is unlike other culture-bound anxiety states such as Australian Aborigine's *malgri,* insofar as it is unassociated with beliefs in witchcraft, supernatural spirits, or water monsters, and for that reason it has been attributed to sensory deprivation [238]. However, to be exposed to the quiet sound of the waves, the touch of the wind, and the glint of reflected sunshine is not what is usually considered to be sensory deprivation, and the intense fear which the subject feels differentiates the condition from the state called "highway hypnosis" or "horizon hypnosis" which can occur in people whose sensory inputs become too monotonous. A more likely explanation is that the subject has suddenly become aware of the extreme loneliness of his present situation at a time when he is not preoccupied with any particular task, has allowed his mind to wander, and hence has left a relatively open channel between the unconscious and the exterior. With both *kayak-angst* and agoraphobia the anxiety tends to be relieved when the subject is reached by others and helped to a place where there are others around him, but *kayak-angst* is not a chronic disorder with the subject fearing to go out to sea lest an attack occur, whereas agoraphobia is among the most chronic of phobias and anticipation plays a major role in it.

At first consideration there is virtually no similarity between the backgrounds of Arctic Eskimos and urban Anglo-Saxons, so that the similarity between *kayak-angst* and agoraphobia might seem coincidental. Eskimos are thinly scattered in small groups across an empty land almost untouched by man, while urban Anglo-Saxons are crowded into man-made environments. Eskimo infants are kept close to the mother's body and treated as an extension of that body, as among the Japanese, with considerable initial indulgence, while the Anglo-Saxon infant has relatively little body contact and is from very early on treated as a separate individual. Yet psychological testing shows Eskimos and Anglo-Saxons to share one mental trait which distinguishes them from most Central European groups on the one hand and most Amerindian groups on the other, namely the degree of "field independence" which they show [666], a trait associated with individualism, and social studies suggest that this derives from a shared emphasis on the development of self-reliance during childhood. This is well known for the Anglo-Saxons, being illustrated in the "Four Families" film referred to in the previous chapter [397], as well as in many other studies. Among the Eskimos the training does not start as early, but childrearing is by no means as casual and permissive as is sometimes thought. A review of the literature concludes that "the mother exerts subtle but powerful demands for control over certain behaviors. While generally permissive in form, socialization includes frightening, teasing and some forms of external emotional cruelty. The child learns that ... the real power in living with people lies in dissimulation when needed and bullying when possible." [261, p109]. Even in the kindest families, training in self-reliance and responsibility begins early, perhaps at the age of three or four, when the child may be left alone for considerable periods, for the simple reason that in the harsh environment with which the Eskimo must cope, irresponsible behavior may threaten the survival not just of the individual but of whole families. Projective testing suggests that suppressed feelings of helplessness and passivity, as well as hostility, can underlie the Eskimos' apparent competence and cordiality [261].

One experience which Eskimos and Anglo-Saxons have in common and which could be related to the panic attacks which empty spaces can provoke, therefore, is that of being left alone in early childhood and of being expected to be self-sufficient when alone. That the Eskimo disorder is so much less chronic than the Anglo-Saxon one (agoraphobia is probably the most chronic of the phobias in Western society) can be explained on the one hand by the Eskimo's first experience of being left alone occurring at a later age than among the Anglo-Saxons, and on the other hand by the Eskimos becoming so much more familiar with being alone in empty spaces as they grow up. This could also explain why *kayak-angst* is an unanticipated panic state rather than a phobia of anticipation, and why it virtually never occurs when the person is fully occupied with what he is doing, regardless of the surrounding emptiness. If we take the child's panic at being left alone as a crucial factor in both conditions, however, how does this help explain the other features of agoraphobia noted above?

The fact that agoraphobia affects women so much more than men can be explained along similar lines to those we have just followed, namely that although boys are probably left just as much alone in Anglo-Saxon cultures as girls, the former are given ample encouragement and experience in exercising their powers of self-reliance in subsequent years, while parental attitudes towards the development of independence and self-reliance in girls has traditionally been ambivalent. Boys are taught to admire the idea of being a lone pioneer; girls are taught that being alone is unpleasant. The fact that agoraphobia was so little known prior to the 1870s and has shown such a (relative) upsurge since the beginning of the present century fits well with what was noted in the previous chapter regarding the changes in childrearing practices in Britain and the United States (p 216). As may be remembered, a marked switch took place around that time from teaching mothers to be indulging and comforting to teaching them to be strict and "scientific." The latter doctrine emphasized leaving babies alone and not picking them up when they cried, so as to develop greater self-reliance [43]. It was hypothesized in Chap. 9 that this shift in childrearing contributed to the development of peptic ulcer in males but not in females, since males were expected to resist dependency feelings in adult life while females were encouraged to indulge these. What is now being hypothesized is that although women were not under pressure to resist dependency feelings and could usually have their dependency needs gratified in one sense, they remained vulnerable to feelings of loneliness when the marriage within which they sought protection became insufficiently supportive (80% of the "Open Door" sample of agoraphobics were married, and an unusually small percentage were employed outside their homes [379]). The development of phobias rather than peptic ulcers can then be explained by the fact that no independence conflict is involved. Such a hypothesis is in harmony with the fact that agoraphobia tends to develop later in life than *taijin kyofu* or some other phobias, the shift from the protection of the parental to that of the conjugal home having been done at the person's own rate, and usually being initially felt as gratifying.

What we have learnt from comparing agoraphobia and *taijin kyofu*, therefore, supports the psychoanalytic theory that childhood experiences contribute importantly to the development of the neuroses, even though the data we considered on the other types of neurosis did not support that theory. There is little in the life situations, cultural expectations, and cultural models presented to adults in the two societies we have been comparing – apart from the earlier customs followed by Japanese court ladies – which would lead one to expect agoraphobia in the one setting and *taijin kyofu* in the other, whereas there are definite differences in experiences during childhood which would lead one to expect these particular phobias. Furthermore, the comparisons we have been making do not suggest that the differences between the two phobias are superficial and inessential aspects of a single disorder. Both syndromes appear linked to the small child's anxieties resulting from the disappearance of the familiar and the proximity of the unfamiliar, but the picture is not such that if, for example, the symptoms of *taijin kyofu* were removed by hypnosis, one would expect symptoms of agoraphobia to take their place. What this comparison of phobias has not supported, however, is the psychoanalytic belief that childhood sexuality is of direct relevance. Agoraphobics do quite often exhibit evidence of sexual conflicts – frigidity, for instance – but they do so less often than European patients with some other phobias, and such conflicts seem unimportant in *taijin kyofu*. The final question to be tackled in this chapter, therefore, will be whether Comparative Psychiatry can cast any light on this other important element in psychoanalytic theory. Is the European psychoanalyst's inclination to find the roots of neuroses in early sexual experiences merely a product of his own and his patients' background, or is it a sensitivity to an etiological principle which is important everywhere?

5 Sexual Neuroses and the Oedipus Complex Theory: India, Laos, and the Celebes

During the 1920s, a debate between Bronislaw Malinowski and Ernest Jones on the universality of the Oedipus complex provided one of the earliest examples of an attempt at employing cross-cultural data for the testing of psychiatric theory. Although involving other matters such as the sister-brother incest taboo, the main question was whether it was the father's sexual relations with the mother which the small boy resented, or his power. Jones argued that it must be the sexual aspect of the father's position; Malinowski, on the basis of observations in the Trobriands where the biological father was merely the mother's husband and it was the mother's brother who acted as male head of the family, argued that it was paternal power that was the key, tension being greater between young men and their maternal uncles than between them and their mothers' husbands. Because Jones and others of the orthodox school saw Malinowski's ideas as a threat to the doctrine of the importance of infantile sexuality and a return to Adler's belief that sexual drives were secondary to a power drive, they did not open their minds sufficiently to the significance of Malinowski's observations, and the Oedipus complex theory hardened around Jones' position. (The debate is well summarized in Anne Parson's paper on the subject [486].) Malinowski's field observations have been replaced by others in matrifocal societies, for instance the study by Corin in Zaire [125], and the universality of the Oedipus complex theory as it refers to personality development or metapsychology has been explored in various cross-cultural analyses [592, 655], with ambiguous results.

Insofar as the Oedipus complex theory is concerned with normal personality development, it is of only marginal relevance in this book. Insofar as it relates to psychopathology, however, it is something which Comparative Psychiatry can appropriately examine and if possible test. Even as late as the 1930s, Freud regarded most other forms of anxiety as stemming from castration anxiety [205], and saw most neuroses as having their roots there, so that even though the topic is receiving relatively little attention today, judging from publications, psychoanalytic trainees are taught to assume its universality. In the comparisons employed so far in this chapter, there has been little evidence to suggest that factors likely to affect early castration anxiety are associated with the variance of the neuroses across populations, but this could be because that evidence has been too thoroughly masked. Can we find examples of unmasked castration anxiety or related sexual neuroses and link them to childhood experiences?

The major sexual neuroses – those marked by impotence, frigidity, and the more extreme sexual deviations – are not brought for medical attention with sufficient consistency to make cross-cultural or international comparisons of incidence possible, and the subject is still too embarrassing in most societies to be included (with likelihood of honest answers) in community mental health surveys. Moreover, cultural differences in the encouragement which girls receive in the attaining of orgasm [382] make frigidity a doubtful indicator of neurosis. However, there are two categories of sexual neurosis in males which are almost "culture-bound" and which have so clear a character that they are unlikely to be prevalent in other societies without us knowing about them. These are the *koro* group and the *jiryan* group, the one rare but dramatic so that cases are unlikely to go unheeded, the other exceedingly common in its harboring society but regarded as a disorder needing treatment. It would seem profitable to see whether the distribution of these conditions coincides with the distribution of certain practices affecting childhood sexuality and castration anxiety, or is associated with quite different factors.

The commoner set of syndromes, under such labels as *jiryan* and *dhat* in India, *prameha* in Sri Lanka, *shen k'uei* in China, and *naeng* in Korea, has as a common theme the fears that the strength which is embodied in the semen (or what some local cultures regard as the female equivalent of semen) is being lost or disturbed, that general health is consequently being affected, and (again in some cultures only) that death may result. The anxiety appears most strongly in a zone stretching across the Indian subcontinent from Karachi to Dacca; but in modified form it can be found in Sri Lanka, China, and Korea as the afore-mentioned terms indicate, being linked to the doctrine of humors and bodily essences which underlies most Asian medical systems. The further from northern India one gets, the more the belief has been modified, so that in China the fear may focus on the male's kidney rather than on his semen [648a], while in Korea [566a] and in Sri Lanka [465a] it may be less males than females (with leukorrhea) who comprise the majority of patients, and swelling of the joints may feature prominently in the diagnosis. The last point leads one to think of gonorrhea, which used to result in arthritis in about 5% of cases before the days of penicillin. But in northern India this type of neurosis affects almost only males and does not seem linked to gonorrhea.

There are numerous illustrations of its high frequency in the most affected Indian areas. Thus, 25 out of the 36 male Hindu informants and six out of the nine Moslem ones employed by Morris Carstairs in his study of a high-caste community [92] during the 1950s either thought themselves to be suffering from *jiryan* or had taken special measures against it. In Chandigarh in the 1970s, 48% of lower-class males considered nocturnal emissions to be abnormal, perhaps due to physical illness, and about 35% thought that such emissions called for medical treatment [371]. In a survey of male 1st-year students in Karachi, 20% reported having consulted doctors, hakims, or "sexologists" about sexual problems of which *jiryan* was the most common [247]. As one gets further away from that part of India, however, the frequency gets much less. Reports which I have regarding student health in Sri Lanka make no mention of such a condition, although we know it to occur in the less literate sections of the population; and although Wen and Wang were able to collect 23 cases of the *shen k'uei* syndroms at a urology clinic in Taipei [648a] this does not appear to occur in nearly as high a frequency as its equivalent in India.

Throughout the societies in which these syndromes are found there is a general belief that semen represents a distillate of blood and blood a distillate of food, so that the loss of a single drop of semen is the equivalent to the loss of much food or energy. From that derived a widespread but esoteric and rarely practiced teaching for effecting sexual intercourse without emitting semen. However, in China and Sri Lanka the common belief is usually that it is only the man who practices too frequent or prolonged sexual intercourse, or who masturbates too often, who is in danger, whereas in northern India anxiety is often aroused by nothing more than occasional nocturnal emissions or even by the thick sticky drops of secretion which can precede or follow micturation. Why should the northern Indian male be so much more anxious on the subject?

One contributing factor is probably the Shaivite religious tradition which has been part of Hinduism for as long as the latter can be said to have existed, which has affected popular thinking in Pakistan, and in which sexuality and asceticism are simultaneously opposed and equated. Siva (or Shiva) is the god on whom Hindu ascetic behavior is modeled, but he is also the god whom the scriptures depict as most actively and explicitly sexual. In his semen was stored much of his power, and ordinary men were thought to follow him in this, but that stored power was much greater when the semen was activated by sexual temptation, and it was therefore Siva's task, and that of ascetics modeling themselves on him, not to shun that temptation but to embrace and master it. In the present century the Shaivite tradition is still operative, as illustrated by Gandhi's decision to have a young girl sleep near him so that he could assure himself that he had conquered his sexual desires [610]. Carstairs' Hindu informants all "referred wistfully to the ideal of unbroken celibacy; or failing that, of sleeping with one's wife only once in a lifetime," but they recognized that most people could not attain that ideal and that "The best they can hope for is to order their lives so that their acts of piety suffice to compensate for the inevitable wastage of soul-stuff and semen" [92, p87].

But although Shaivism is known throughout the subcontinent, its base was not in the north where *jiryan* is most common but in the south where it is much less so. Also, although these living religious beliefs must greatly affect Hindus who aspire to true asceticism, there seems no reason for them to engender so much anxiety in the general population. Shaivism does not appear to offer an adequate explanation in itself, therefore, and in psychoanalytic eyes *jiryan* would seem definitely to be a condition wherein manifest anxiety and religious belief are masking castration anxiety. In many Indian families the father is a distant, forbidding figure not just toward his children but toward his wife sometimes, and Carstairs was expressing what would be an orthodox psychiatric opinion when he wrote that an "extreme emphasis upon the Oedipal situation pervades many aspects of Hindu social life" [91, p131]. Moreover, Indian family structure is different in the north from what it is in the south, in the sense that in the north the head of the family tends to be the single autocrat toward whom all others look up, whereas in the southern (Dravidian) family tradition there is a multiplicity of statuses within each extended family; and that would lead us to expect fear of the father to be greater in the north than in the south. Nevertheless, there are obstacles to the application of the classical castration anxiety theory here. For one thing, the anxiety is focused not on hetereosexual intercourse or on relations with mothering figures but on the loss of a few drops of semen, with no idea of sexual competition involved. Secondly, there are many other societies where the father can be equally as strict and forbidding but where the *jiryan*-type syndrome is unrecorded. It is always possible to argue, as some psychoanalysts do with remarkable ease, that the anxiety has been displaced onto a different symptom or even syndrome, but before one so easily imposes a European-based explanation on the picture and assumes that this is a clear instance where a non-European neurosis must be grounded in childhood castration anxieties, it seems better to take a closer look at the evidence.

The average younger Indian adult is given good reason to suffer from a sexual neurosis, but this reason lies in the attitudes of the elders when he marries rather than in direct or masked castration threats during childhood. A majority of newly married Indian couples in the past (and maybe even today) remained in the boy's parental home, were forbidden to exhibit signs of mutual affection while in the presence of others, had scarcely known each other prior to the marriage, and in other ways were discouraged from becoming too attached to each other, since such attachment might weaken the boy's loyalty to his parental family. There was no honeymoon, and it has always been surprising to me that the young couple were able to function sexually at all, in such families. The mother's desire to retain her adult son for herself is a major factor in this situation, but there is also something more, something archetypically existing in the Siva legends themselves. In one such legend, found in several texts, the senior Aryan gods (Siva was not a member of the original Aryan pantheon) ask Siva to produce a son by his wife so that the son might kill a demon who was challenging them. However, when Siva and his wife were enjoying intercourse and the son was about to be conceived, the earth shook so much that the older gods were disturbed and realized that a son born to a couple embodying so much power would be a threat to themselves just as much as to the demon. They therefore sent one of their members to interrupt the intercourse (for which they were duly cursed) and to ask Siva to produce a son in another fashion, something which he did by letting his seed fall on the ground, i.e., by something analogous to what is complained of in *jiryan*. Similar references to powerful figures being induced to give up the power which would have enabled them to overturn the older or more dominant generation are found in other parts of the Hindu scriptures. Ascetics who have acquired too much power by their austerities have temptresses sent them by the now fearful gods, to induce them to have intercourse or to lose semen in some other way. One thus finds that in this tradition, and to a lesser extent in the Buddhist traditions which passed from India to the east and south, semen symbolizes not so much sexual rivalry as power rivalry. Carstairs' picture of his *jiryan*-plagued informants indicates clearly that fathers are feared and resented not just because of a hypothesized sexual rivalry in childhood but because they exercise power over their adult sons' daily lives, while descriptions of family relationships in the south of India point more toward sibling rivalry as a problem. These observations suggest that *jiryan* could very well arise from suppressed hostility toward the father, but that it is the power of the latter which is important, as Malinowski argued, and not his sexual rights.

The *koro* group of disorders are mainly found in south China, Indochina, and the Celebes, although isolated cases have been reported from many other locations. In essence, the neurosis consists of a fear that the penis (or less commonly other external genitala) will shrink into the abdomen or disappear, and that death will result. Attacks tend to be acute, perhaps repeated, but rarely prolonged. Earliest European references to the disorder were from the Dutch East Indies in the nineteenth century but it is thought that the concept reached there from China, even though Tseng apparently did not find a mention of it in his search [621] of old Chinese medical texts. Among the Chinese and among the Makassarese of Celebes (Sulawesi) it is sufficiently well known for traditional healers and some lay families to possess a special instrument whereby the penis can be gripped and prevented from shrinking into the abdomen. The syndrome is met in its purest form among the Makassarese, where it can affect the labia and nipples of the women as well as the male penis, and where cases appear formerly to have been neither rare nor occurring particularly in epidemics [631].

The Makassarese are a people with a strict social hierarchy in which the separation of sex-linked roles and the establishment of sexual identity has gone to unusual extremes, males and females very rarely undertaking the same tasks [102]. Males follow a very aggressive model (their ancestors were notorious pirates) in which sexual prowess is important, and there is great sensitivity to insult, at least within the upper strata. Females are taught to submit completely to their elders, to avoid drawing men's attention to themselves, and to be ashamed of any sexual desires. Both sexes have considerable suspicion of marriage (the men perhaps because it calls for gentleness rather than aggressivity) and Chabot [102] states that even after marriage there may be difficulty in persuading the couple to have sexual intercourse. Relations between father and son, and mother and daughter, are stated to be poor, and there is an institutionalized form of male homosexuality for boys who choose not to conform to the dominant male model. They would appear to be a very likely people in which to find childhood-based castration anxieties of such an extreme degree that they break through the customary disguises and appear in open form. When they do break through as *koro*, it seems most often to be because a man has found it too difficult to maintain an adequate male self-image – that of someone who will not let pass the slightest lapse in the respect which others must accord him on the basis of his hereditary status – so that he fears loss of identity, an identity symbolized by the genitals. No female cases have been described in sufficient detail to reveal the dynamics in that sex, but it may be that a threatened loss of female identity is the precipitant among them as well.

Among the Chinese, the corresponding syndrome goes by a name variously spelled *shook-yang, suk-yeong*, and *suo-yang*, the variants deriving partly from anglicization and partly from dialect. In southern China, including Hongkong and Taiwan, it appears to be a rare disorder, since it took Yap 15 years to collect 19 cases [679], and the affected males were usually neurotic in other ways as well. They appear to have had weak fathers rather than strong ones, a number of these fathers died early, and there is no evidence of a real challenge to the patient's maleness from other males either in childhood or in adult life. The average background is thus very different from that reported in Celebes, and one gets the impression that the genitals are merely sharing in the somatization with other organs, the specific fear of them shrinking into the body deriving from folk beliefs. In Singapore in 1967, however, there was an epidemic of *shook-yang* which affected over 500 persons during a 2-week period, including a small percentage of women and of non-Chinese men [239, 464]. The epidemic was occasioned by a rumor regarding pork alleged to have come from pigs suffering from swine fever; the majority of patients showed no neurotic symptoms apart from the fear of shrinking genitals; only a quarter of them admitted to having heard about *shook-yang* previously; the English-educated were as much affected as the rest; and most patients recovered with reassurance only. What happened was obviously an outbreak of epidemic hysteria affecting relatively healthy persons, as such epidemics usually do, but as with all such epidemics it still remains to be explained what had generated the free-floating anxiety that crystallized so easily around this symptom, and why it was this particular symptom that was the focus. Because the imagined result is so similar to that of castration, one explanation for the choice of symptom might be that Chinese family relationships (in Singapore, at least) must be particularly prone to generate castration anxiety. However, quite apart from failing to explain the timing of the outbreak (and the Singapore physicians had offered no explanation for this) this hypothesis does not harmonize well with the findings from the next *koro* epidemic that occurred.

That further epidemic occurred in northeastern Thailand in 1976, in a district to which many Vietnamese had fled in the 1950s, and which had recently received an additional influx of Laotian refugees. The latter brought with them the story that the new Communist rulers were attempting to control male potency and fertility through diet and native herbs and were also encouraging sexual freedom [603]. Soon after this, rumors began to spread that the Vietnamese refugees were poisoning food, riots occurred during which Vietnamese shops were stoned, and an epidemic of *koro* broke out, estimated to affect perhaps 2000 persons. It affected the same low percentage of females as the Singapore epidemic did, and spread to children through the emotional reactions of their teachers, but what is significant for present purposes is that although ethnic Chinese comprise about 10% of the local population, not one is stated to have developed the condition. The symptoms were much like those of *koro*-type disorders elsewhere, except that the sensation of penile shrinkage was preceded briefly by vertigo or abdominal discomfort. I have not been able to ascertain whether local folk-medicine traditions include the description of something like *shook-yang* derived from the Chinese, but the point is not of great relevance. In 1979 there was a small outbreak of similar cases in Lagos, Nigeria, men believing that their genitals had magically disappeared after they had been spoken to and touched by a stranger in the street(O. Morakinyo, personal communication), and there is no reason to think that Chinese beliefs had extended there.

The Singapore, Lagos, and northeastern Thailand outbreaks all have the characteristics of an epidemic hysteria, and it is well known that the symptoms displayed by the index cases in such epidemics are of considerably greater importance in determining the symptoms complained about by the other victims than the latters' personal predispositions. However, these were outbreaks occurring in general populations in which a wide variety of possible models were available, not outbreaks in schools or factories where only the index case was likely to offer a recent model, and so the question remains: why did the *koro* model catch the public's imagination at this particular time? Guided by other studies of epidemic hysteria [570], we can say that there must have been either (a) a strong pointer towards the genitals being vulnerable to the supposedly noxious agent; (b) strong but unconscious anxieties focused on the genitals; or (c) the genitals comprising the most suitable symbol onto which could be displaced other anxieties which were too threatening to be openly faced. There is no evidence for (a). The Oedipus complex theory points to (b), but castration anxiety from this source is usually disguised and attains direct expression only when prior displacement has failed, as in psychosis. Displacement theory points to (c), but requires that the repressed fear be greater than fear of castration, something which psychoanalytic writing does not appear to contemplate. The literature on the Singapore Chinese and my own private sources (I did research on the childhood of the affected generation, in the 1950s) do not indicate either that castration threats in childhood were extreme or that psychotics exhibited castration fears in other years, so that (b) is difficult to support. On the other hand there is some evidence that the northeastern Thai and the Singaporeans could have had repressed fears regarding their very survival as peoples, at the time their *shook-yang* epidemics broke out, something which fits alternative (c).

The picture is clearer for the Thai. The risk of military invasion by the Vietnamese was an admitted fact in the mid-1970s, but what was not openly discussed, although indicated in a number of ways, was the economic threat posed by the Vietnamese refugees who had arrived in the 1950s. These had come to dominate some sections of the economy and penetrate others to such an extent that the local Thai might find themselves forced to abandon some of the traits which characterized them as a people, in order to compete. Elsewhere in the world, the term "genocide" is regularly being used today to describe situations in which one people is being given the chance of better material reward through adopting the life-style and values of another, but where its survival as a distinct people is thereby made doubtful. The use of so strong a word to describe that type of situation indicates how deeply the anxieties aroused by such a possibility lie. The Thai outbreak of *shook-yang* was blamed on the Vietnamese, who were concurrently attacked, and it died out when food from Thai as well as from Vietnamese farmers began to be boycotted in other districts. In the Singapore Chinese it is possible that similar, repressed, fears regarding survival as a separate people might have existed. Singapore was a small nation with large Malay populations bordering it. In 1965 it had been ejected from Malaysia; in 1966 there had been race riots (Malay/Chinese) in Singapore; at the beginning of 1967 it was announced that the British armed forces, which had provided Singapore with its defences and with much income, were to be withdrawn; and in the summer of 1967 there were Malay/Chinese race riots in Malaysia. There was little open admission that its political or economic survival might be seriously threatened, but Singapore's Premier found it necessary to point out that Pakistan and India were unlikely to attack it, and an article in the *Far East Economic Review* which discusses the situation is entitled "Underlying angst" [21]. In the context of the Chinese/Malay tension it is possibly relevant that the rumored source of the *shook-yang*, pigs, are a forbidden food for the Malays on religious grounds, but a popular one for the Chinese.

Among the Singapore Chinese and the Thai, therefore, it is unlikely that the adult castration anxieties represented by the *koro*-type outbreaks derived mainly from childhood castration anxieties at the time of the passing of the Oedipus complex, although such a derivation does appear quite possible in the case of the Makassarese. What we seem to have with the Singaporeans and the Thai is a displacement of anxiety not from castration to something felt as less threatening, but a displacement *to* castration from something felt as more threatening. Loss of cultural identity and loss of the means of making a livelihood are more serious matters in Asia, where millions die of famine, than loss of genitals. In India, similarly, the father's autocratic power both over the child and over his adult sons constitutes a greater threat and source of anxiety than his real or imagined sexual rivalry. In Europe it may be true that the average boy – or at least the boy of middle-class parents – can imagine no greater threat than loss of genitals after he reaches the Oedipal stage, but for other children there can appear greater threats to their existence, such as the rivalry of their peers. In the otherwise admirable book *Oedipe Africain* [476], doctrinal loyalty leads the authors to attribute most of the neuroses which their Senegalese patients exhibited to rivalry with the father or his substitute, whereas their clinical descriptions make a good case for it being sibling rivalry that is the most stressful and pathogenic.

6 Conclusions

At the beginning of this chapter the question was raised whether we should consider neurosis as a single disease embracing many interchangeable syndromes, or as a family of diseases whose internal divisions are still to be established. It cannot be said that the material marshalled here has answered that problem, since only a few of the many syndromes suggested by the chapter's title have been touched on. Nevertheless, it is possible that our international and historical comparisons have thrown a little more light on the subject.

The evidence which we have reviewed suggests that the characteristics of any neurotic syndrome derive from three main sources. What we may call the *content* is to a large extent determined by the symbolic traditions which the patient has learnt from his culture, purely private symbols being characteristic of psychoses rather than of neuroses. In India, power is symbolized by semen and anxieties respecting power are symbolized by or displaced onto the fear of semen loss. In Japan, the distinction between strangers and familiars was for a long time symbolized in certain strata by the presence or absence of a screen preventing nonintimates from coming face to face, and anxiety about strangers is symbolized by an anxiety about face-to-face contact. What we may call the *structure* of a neurotic syndrome, i.e., the behavioral mode that is involved, is to a large extent determined by the coping styles which the patient has learnt from his society (or a section of it) to employ with general problems. If patients have learnt to rely on ritual or appeal to supernatural powers, then one tends to meet obsessive syndromes, as has often been described. If patients have been taught to allow important decisions to be taken by those whom they regard as their superiors, then dissociative or hysterical syndromes are likely. Finally, what we may call the *purpose* of the syndrome, i.e., the avoiding of certain types of pain or (less often) the obtaining of certain types of reward, is going to depend mainly to the pains and rewards to which the patient's society exposes him, but also on the ways in which he has been taught to perceive them. Chronic exposure to the risk of death and injury in the frontline while others outside the battle zone are escaping that risk will induce a syndrome of a type likely to result in departure from the battle zone rather than one increasing risk of injury, but the probability of such a syndrome developing is greater when life is viewed as enjoyable and death as termination than when life is viewed as punishment and death as merely a transition from one life to the next. In Anglo-Saxon societies where mothers are taught to leave their children alone from very young, finding oneself alone in unfamiliar conditions is liable to reawaken memories of the anxieties caused by the initial aloneness, and to provoke defences against this reawakening.

Stated in that fashion, with the content, structure, and purpose of neurotic syndromes all being in large part reflections of what the individual learns from his society and with there being an almost infinite variety of societies, it would seem that comparative studies tell us that there cannot be distinct neuroses but only a vast variety of ways of malfunctioning, i.e., social relativity. That need not be so. Common experiences sufficiently painful to arouse neurotic defences may fall into a limited number of categories, and the choice of coping styles sufficiently effective to become part of cultural tradition is almost certainly quite limited. The range of symbolic substitutions which man can employ is probably infinite, particularly since symbolization of something by its opposite is not merely possible but frequent (calling a tall man "Shorty," for instance); but a typology of the neuroses is possible without considering content. There is thus no need for the neuroses to be viewed only in terms of cultural relativism, once the definition and boundaries of the concept are agreed to. But what we ought to learn from comparisons such as those offered in this chapter is to avoid assuming that because some men think in a particular way, therefore other men must. When we recognize that a pathogenic process met with in one patient is to be met with in others, we are greatly tempted to generalize from that experience and say that it can be expected in all patients exhibiting certain signs. In somatic medicine such generalization has frequently paid off because the biological differences between one man and another are limited. The psychological differences between individuals and between societies are much greater, and dogmatism becomes correspondingly less warranted.

One subject which has not been dealt with here but which the reader might have expected to be touched on is treatment. The main reason why it has been avoided is that there is almost no agreement on the goals of psychotherapy in the neuroses, or how to assess therapeutic success. Another reason is that while two therapists may claim to use the same method, their actual practices may be very different. However, it can in general be said that a form of psychotherapy which has been developed within the patient's own society is going to be more effective than one developed elsewhere, since it is more likely to make use of symbols and coping strategies familiar to the patient and thus put less of a strain on him to learn new ones.

Chapter 11 Mental Health in Global Perspective

In the foregoing chapters, a variety of mental and psychosomatic disorders have been compared across nations or cultures, and an attempt has been made to show how, for each disorder, this type of comparison could lead us to a better understanding than studies undertaken only within single societies. Insofar as most of these disorders are thought to have distinct etiologies, and insofar as even those with supposedly related etiologies, such as depression and suicide, prove to vary relatively independently at the international level, there would seem to be little point in attempting to generalize about them, except perhaps with respect to research methodology. However, one of the hopes implicit in the pursuit of Comparative Psychiatry is that it might contribute to preventive action, and when one looks at preventive psychiatry one finds that it has addressed itself less to reducing specific disorders than to promoting general mental health. In the previous chapters I have for the most part avoided referring to mental health, since the term carries two quite different meanings, both rather vague. Nevertheless, there are two good reasons why a book on Comparative Psychiatry should include some reference to possible differences in society-wide mental health or ill-health. One of these reasons is that there are certain nations or cultures that appear to suffer more, or to suffer less, from a wide spectrum of psychopathological disturbances than might be expected from the chance association of factors affecting different diseases. The other reason is the increasing demand at both a national and an international level for what are called "quality of life" measures, i.e., ways of assessing societal effectiveness which tap more refined aspects than merely the economic; and much of what comes under that heading overlaps what is usually meant by mental health, as was recognized by the (U.S.) National Commission on Mental Illness and Health when it sponsored the first large-scale survey of "quality of life" [237].

There are no adequate ways of comparing mental health at a national or international level at the present time; but this is not to say that such ways cannot be developed. Whether psychiatry should take the lead in this matter is debatable, but certainly it should participate in whatever attempts are made. For this reason I propose in this final chapter to explore the various ways in which comparisons of mental health might be undertaken, both in its customary sense of total psychopathology and in the more positive sense. I shall ask:

(a) Is it feasible and logical to cover all forms of mental disorder in a single measure of psychopathology applicable to different cultures; or alternatively are there specific and measurable aspects of psychopathology which recur in most mental disorders and which we might take as representing the more general concept?

(b) Failing that, is it feasible and acceptable to combine indicators of different aspects of the psychopathological spectrum so as to yield an operationally useful scale for the purpose of comparing national societies?

(c) Does the impression that some peoples are unusually vulnerable, or alternatively resistant, to mental ill-health in general stand up to closer scrutiny?

(d) If so, are there general factors which might explain this?

(e) How far can measures of mental ill-health be taken, by inversion, to reflect positive mental health?

1 A Scientific Measure of General Mental Ill-Health?

The most obvious and logical way of comparing the level of psychopathology in two or more societies is to combine the rates for all categories of disorder which fall under that rubric. To do this, however, implies (1) that we have rational or agreed standards whereby each category can be assessed as present or absent; (2) that we are agreed which categories to include; and (3) that we are also agreed on the relative weight to assign to each category. The first of these demands is one we have already encountered – what constitutes schizophrenia; what constitutes an anxiety state, etc. – but it is also one which can be answered, disorder by disorder. We can decide that someone will only be counted as schizophrenic for the purpose of the comparison if he shows specified signs, just as we can decide that someone will only be counted as hypertensive if he has a certain diastolic pressure under predetermined conditions of measurement. The second demand can similarly be met, to a reasonable degree of logic and consensus, some types of disorder being excluded as being of too little importance for the intended goal. (A survey of physical health, for instance, will not usually classify a person as sick because he has a single acne spot on his cheek.) Assigning weights to the different disorders, however, is something which is virtually impossible to achieve either scientifically or by consensus, since value judgments now enter much more into play. If one assigns all types of disorder the same weight, then the more serious and uncommon get obscured by the common but less serious, and the latter tend to vary too easily under the influence of unimportant and temporary factors. If one seeks to assign different weights to each disorder, however, the problem then becomes what principle to apply. Does a traumatic neurosis producing frightful nightmares get weighted more or less than a hallucinatory psychosis that comforts the economically functioning patient with the idea that his favorite saint is talking to him daily?

The two main principles on which various mental disorders might be weighted (or alternatively merged) are those relating to distress and to behavioral dysfunction. We can say that, regardless of diagnosis, one patient is suffering more distress than another, or we can say that the one is suffering more dysfunction. Each of these approaches is going to result in the neglect of limited types of mental disorder which some persons will consider important, and there is no fundamentally sound way of combining the two; yet if measures of both were obtainable this could still be quite valuable, assuming that these measures were reliable. Is it likely that they would be?

Comparing populations on the basis of the proportions of their populations experiencing more than a predetermined degree of distress of psychiatric origin has appealed to many researchers, and it is what most symptom checklist scales seem capable of achieving. The advantages of the approach are that it can be easily applied to general population samples, both treated and untreated, and that it yields a range of cutoff points for different levels of comparison. The disadvantages are threefold. Firstly, distress can arise by reason of factors other than mental disorder and that distress of nonpsychiatric origin needs to be excluded. Secondly, distress is a purely subjective experience and we have, strictly speaking, no means of comparing one person's subjective experience with that of another: all that we can compare is what they communicate reagrding that experience. Thirdly, one of the defences against distress is to deny it. Each of these disadvantages is capable of seriously distorting the results not just at the individual level, something which could average out over a whole sample, but at the societal level as well.

Regarding the first of these disadvantages, distress due to somatic illness is reasonably easy to distinguish from that of purely mental origin in medically advanced societies, but can be very difficult in somewhere like a Nigerian village where many individuals suffer from chronic infections and infestations, as was pointed out when the first reports of the Nigeria-Nova Scotia comparison surveys [344] came out. Distress associated with unemployment or divorce may be the result of such a state (i.e., be nonpsychiatric) or may derive from a prior mental disturbance which led to that state, so that very much more than the information on current symptoms and demographic characteristics may be needed to permit classification. Regarding the other disadvantages, cultural groups may have very different styles of communicating distress – something which was noted respecting the Manhattan Puerto Ricans in Chap. 3 (p 52) – and they may differ also in the degree to which they attempt to conceal certain types of distress from themselves, becoming involved in additional mental disorder in the process. (In most societies males tend to deny certain types of distress more than females do, and tend more to use alcohol as an aid to that denial, leading them to alcohol dependence.) For all these reasons, it is impossible to say that similar standards have been assured when two or more societies are compared by means of symptom checklists, and hence it is impossible to defend the claim that one society is less mentally healthy than another when only this type of comparison is made.

With measures of behavioral dysfunction we are apparently on more solid ground, since it is in principle possible to have the same external assessors use standard criteria to judge the behavior of the subjects being compared, and it would also seem to be relatively easy under such circumstances for these external assessors to apply uniform criteria to the question of whether an observed dysfunction is mainly of psychic, somatic, or social origin. In practice, however, that has almost never been done, since it would be extremely costly (given the fact that one would theoretically have to observe the subjects undertaking various types of function), and it could also be considered an invasion of privacy. What normally happens is either that one relies, as with the distress measure, on self-reports of impairment, or one makes use of social "filters" whereby only individuals overstepping a certain culturally determined threshold of dysfunction are submitted to this uniform assessment.

Relying on self-reports of impairment is not a method sufficiently developed at the present time for me to be able to say whether it can be used cross-culturally without much additional information. Obviously, for a subject to say that his illness forces him to be absent from work does not signify the same thing for a farmer that it does for an air controller, and it may not mean the same thing in a society where workers' rights are strong as it does in one where those rights are weak. Relying on other members of the society to identify individuals who exhibit apparent behavioral dysfunctions requiring assessment also needs more investigation before one can say whether it can be reliably used for comparing nations and cultures; and at the present time it has been employed in uniform fashion in too few societies to yield immediate comparisons. However, it can be argued that, in most societies, individuals exhibiting more than a certain level of psychiatric dysfunction all get referred to mental hospital or at least for psychiatric assessment, and data on hospital admissions are easy to obtain. While it must be said that we have no proven way of comparing a whole range of psychiatric dysfunctions across societies at the present time, therefore, international comparisons of severe psychiatric dysfunction might be possible to some extent by using hospitalization data only. The weaknesses in such data were discussed in Chap. 2, but a brief reexamination of the question seems appropriate at this point.

The most obvious weakness in using mental hospitalization data as a means of estimating the level of severe psychiatric dysfunction in a society is that societies tend to have established mental hospital beds in relation to what they thought they could afford as well as in relation to what appeared to be demanded. This was what invalidated many nineteenth century attempts at comparative mental health assessment. However, it could in principle be relatively easy to allow for that economic factor, either through a regression equation derived from data such as those shown in Fig. 2.1 or by considering only rich nations as in Fig. 2.2, provided that the degree of dysfunction was the sole or main factor determining which patients get admitted. Unfortunately, this is not generally the case. In most societies the patient without any local family is more likely to get hospitalized than the patient with local family, even though both exhibit the same degree of dysfunction; and societies differ considerably in the extent to which their members remain close to their families. Moreover, the degree to which family and neighbors tolerate a given level of dysfunction can be much greater in one society than in another, regardless of psychiatric bed availability, and national psychiatric services can vary considerably in the degree to which they make the hospital the center of their care-giving system. These factors greatly limit the degree to which hospitalization rates can be taken as reflecting a particular level of psychiatric dysfunctioning in the society, but it could still be possible, particularly as respects the middle third of this century, to use them in this fashion for certain societies, if the degree of severe dysfunction indicated in this way bore a stable relationship to the total psychiatric dysfunctioning in each society. Unfortunately that is not the case. When the prevalence of depression increases markedly in the community as the result of some communal misfortune, and brings obvious disturbances of behavior in its train, the rate of mental hospitalizations may be unchanged, as I have seen [418], since the severely depressed person becomes less deviant than before. Two cultural minorities in the same society may exhibit roughly the same level of psychiatrically based disturbance and yet have very different hospitalization rates, if the disturbed behavior exhibited by the one group takes a form which the social majority regard as illness and that exhibited by the other takes a form which the majority regards only as social deviance.

It is my opinion, therefore, that we have at the present time no single meassure of societal mental ill-health which is sufficiently embracing, conceptually coherent, and reliable to be used for international comparisons. Eventually it may be possible to develop a scale of psychiatric dysfunctioning that would fit that purpose, but for many years to come we will either have to do without such comparisons or we will have to make do with empirically derived scales illuminating limited facets of the mental ill-health concept without claiming to embrace it or reach its heart. This is a type of situation familiar to the social and behavioral sciences which deal so much more with ideal typical constructs, but we have to realize what it means, I have before me a comparison of 27 instruments for measuring anxiety [141], and none of these 27 can be judged as "essentially" better than any other, since we do not know what the "essence" of anxiety is. There would be considerable advantages if we could say that we knew what the essence of psychiatric dysfunction was, and then set out to measure it, but we cannot, and the alternative is to see what we can do with scales composed of a hotchpotch of partial indicators.

2 Aggregated Morbidity Scales: United States and Europe

The question of what one should put into an empirical scale for comparing the level of psychopathology across societies will depend partly on what one seeks to do with the scale, partly on the emphasis to be put on different parts of the mental ill-health spectrum, and partly on what is available. If one seeks to rank many closely related societies on an equal basis, then it is almost inevitable that the items should derive from already-availabe sources, usually governmental, and that the confidence which one can place in the quantification of each item will be of greater importance than the closeness of the items to the abstract construct "mental ill-health." This is because, with such comparisons, a challenge to the reliability of the rankings will usually be more detrimental than doubts regarding whether "mental ill-health" is the best label for what the scale is measuring. For a comparison of only two or three societies, on the other hand, it may be possible to dispense with official and other published sources, and collect one's own data directly from the populations under study, using more precise and appropriate ways of measuring the key variables than most already-available sources can provide. Finally, if one is seeking to test the hypothesis that factor X has an influence on the vulnerability of nations or cultures to psychopathology, then it may be possible to use measures whose separate reliability is less trustworthy, or which are not available for all the chosen societies, but which embrace one's psychopathology construct more closely. (The last is particularly the case when it is only the high and low scorers on the scale that are going to be compared, with the intermediate societies disregarded.)

Techniques for comparing two or three cultural groups on a range of mental disorders or mental ill-health indicators have been referred to in a number of previous chapters, although usually without discussion of whether the results can be considered to reflect total psychopathology. Examples were the comparison of Taiwanese Chinese and Aborigines [354, 512]; Yoruba and Nova Scotians [344]; Chinese, Iban and Malaysians in Sarawak [616]; and Canadians of British, French, German, and Polish origin [441]. They all need field work, which is costly, and hence they are not suitable for comparing many societies. If one wished to compare a limited number of societies, as in Keys' CHD comparison, these methods could be quite suitable but the choice would depend on what one sought to find.

Techniques for ranking many national or cultural groups on a common range of indicators have been developed by social and behavioral scientists rather than medical ones, and statistical manipulation is sometimes claimed to have taken care of the problem of assigning weights. An example of one such approach was given in Chap. 8, with a number of ratable behaviors being assembled for the purpose of comparing levels of drunkenness with levels of anxiety across up to 50 primitive cultures, all data being relatively „soft." For comparisons of more developed societies using harder data we may take as illustration one study assessing the states of the United States on a host of "social well-being" indicators that included a "mental health" factor, and an international study of indicators supposed to reflect anxiety and related concepts.

Comparing the cities or states of the United States with respect to various "social indicators" goes back to the 1930s, but the study including the most items referring to psychopathology is a relatively recent one. In Table 11.1 are listed 47 measures which the geographer David Smith [574, 575] was able to calculate for each of the 48 contiguous states on the basis of data available in the 1960s. One sees that his collection contains quite a number of items of psychiatric or mental health relevance, and that most of them fell conveniently into a single factor when principal component analysis was applied, a factor which accounts for 12% of the total variance. Since the items in factor III are such as can be found from the official statistics of many countries besides the United States, this seems a satisfactory lead towards international comparisons – until one looks at the factor loadings. Three of the four items with the highest loadings carry the negative sign, and tell us that the states scoring highest on this factor have the fewest patients coming into mental hospital and the lowest ratio of general hospital beds to population, so that the scale seems to be measuring absence of (psycho)pathology. The remaining items in the scale – including suicide, divorce, accidental death, and one form of crime – are positively loaded, however, indicating that the states scoring highest on this factor III have the highest levels of these indicators of psychopathology. The scale thus seems to be contradicting itself!

There are a number of ways in which this contradiction might be resolved. One can seek to improve the indicators by, for instance, standardizing for age; one can revise the mental hospitalization data to include some measure of outpatient or sheltered care outside the hospitals; one can combine certain items before the interstate comparisons are started, on the grounds that these items represent alternatives. (An epidemiological comparison of Chicago districts came to the tentative conclusion that suicide might be "an alternative to mental hospital or nursing home utilization" [350, p59].) Finally, one might in this particular case conclude that what factor III is reflecting is not psychopathology at all, but a political or economic variable which happens to express itself through these indicators. Since this study does not deal with

Table 11.1. Principal component clusters of 47 "social well-being" indicators across 48 states of the United States [574]

Factor I		Factor III	
(General socioeconomic well-being)		(Mental health)	
Family income below $ 3000	-.940	Patient days in mental hospitals	-.817
Poor housing	-.908	General hospital expenses/patient	.800
Monthly postretirement benefit	.895	Year-end residents in mental hospital	-.798
Per capita income	.885	General Hospital beds per 100 000 population	-.780
Dentists per 10 000 population	.865	Divorces per 1000 marriages	.632
Dependent family payments	.856	Suicides	.558
Unemployment benefit per capita	.809	Mental hospital expenses/patient	.483
Property value (housing)	.803	Traffic accident deaths	.470
% Households with poor diets	-.799	(Crimes against property	.460)
Infant deaths per 10 000 births	-.799	(Median school years completed	.459)
Public school expenditures	.787	Persons attending college	.455
% Draftees failing mental test	-.783		
Eligible voters voting	.778		
White collar employees (% total)	.775		
Physicians per 10 000 population	.761		
(Median school years completed	.759)		
Factor II		Other items with low loading on main factors	
(Social pathology)		Bank deposits per capita	
		Public assistance recipients (% of population)	
Crimes of violence per 100 000	.838	Union membership (% of labor force)	
Syphilis cases reported	.724	Monthly aid to disabled	
Gonorrhoea cases reported	.672	Monthly old age assistance	
Narcotics addicts	.653	Hospital insurance (% population)	
School segregation	.642	Pupils per teacher	
Registered voters per adult population	-.632	Treated alcoholics per 10 000 adults	
(Crimes against property	.604)	Husband-wife households (% total)	
Illiteracy	.552	Jail inmates not convicted (% total)	
Tuberculosis death rate	.541	Blacks in schools at least 95% Black	
Index of home equipment	-.533	Population per lawyer	

international or cross-cultural comparisons, the interpretation of its data falls outside the scope of this book. However, the type of problem which we see here is one which could easily arise if a similar technique were used for making international comparisons, and one sees that factor analysis does not free one from the need to decide how closely each item in a scale theoretically lies to the abstract concept one is trying to measure. Where factor analysis is helpful with such an approach is in forcing one to reconsider one's assumptions and realize that one's indicators may be more affected by some other influence than by what one assumed to be mainly determining them.

The main international comparisons which have been undertaken respecting abstract concepts related to psychopathology are those of Richard Lynn, who compared 18 countries first with respect to his own concept of anxiety [362] and then to Eysenck's concepts of neuroticism and extraversion [363]. Table 11.2 lists the indicators which he used and the degree to which they correlated with each other across

Table 11.2. Correlation matrix of hypothesized indicators for a comparison of 18 countries respecting "anxiety," "neuroticism," and "extraversion," [362, 363]

Indicators	A Extra-version	B Neuroti-cism	C Anxiety	2	3	4	5	6	7	8	9	10	11	12	13	14	15	16
1. Mental hospitalizations		–	–	*0.72*	*0.57*	*0.58*	*0.50*	*0.49*	0.46	00	0.06	-0.29	0.21	*0.47*	-0.23	0.07	-0.06	-0.32
2. CHD mortality	+	–	–		*0.64*	*0.61*	0.30	*0.49*	*0.47*	-0.10	00	0.02	-0.07	*0.56*	0.01	0.37	0.33	-0.13
3. Vehicle deaths			+			*0.79*	0.44	0.14	0.20	*0.51*	0.08	0.31	-0.02					
4. Calorie intake		–	–				0.26	0.17	0.26	0.30	0.20	0.05	-0.03	*0.55*	-0.26	0.03	0.10	-0.06
5. Suicide mortality	–	+	+					0.37	0.18	0.34	0.14	-0.15	0.19	-0.18	0.43	0.25	*0.51*	*0.61*
6. Cirrhosis mortality		+	+						0.21	-0.20	0.19	0.01	0.12	*-0.61*	0.22	0.18	0.35	*0.64*
7. Cigarette consumption	+		–							-0.26	*-0.54*	0.22	0.15	0.11	0.32	0.29	-0.15	-0.02
8. Peptic ulcer mortality			+								0.02	0.13	-0.23					
9. Homicide			+									-0.36	0.12	-0.12	*0.73*	0.57	00	0.26
10. Celibacy (age 15–49)			+										0.08					
11. Hypertensive mortality			–															
12. Coffee and tea consumption		–													-0.26	0.17	0.10	-0.30
13. Persons in prison	+	+														0.25	0.25	*0.57*
14. Divorce	+																0.41	0.16
15. Illegitimate birth	+	+																*0.55*
16. Total accident mortality	+	+																

Coefficients are taken from the two sources, which do not completely overlap. Columns A, B, and C give the hypothesized relationships of the indicators to the three constructs, i.e., whether the indicator is seen to be related positively (+), negatively (–), or not at all. For definitions and sources of data see original papers. Coefficients italicized are significant at the 0.05 level the 18 countries surveyed. For each of his chosen indicators he cites at least one piece of research which supports (although sometimes rather weakly) his reason for its inclusion, and in this respect he offers a model well worth copying. Moreover, thanks to his having published the correlation matrices from his analyses, it would seem possible from his work to construct one's own mental ill-health rating scale on which to rank the societies which he surveyed, even though he himself might not think this useful. However, although his basic design was sound, its application leaves much to be desired. Although the chosen countries were supposed to be a comprehensive sampling of relatively wealthy, advanced Western societies, Japan was included but Israel not; Ireland included but Iceland not; Austria included but Czechoslovakia not; even though the second fit his basic criteria as well as or better than the first. Substitution of Israel for Japan would probably have altered many of his coefficients quite substantially. Secondly, cirrhosis mortality was taken as reflecting alcohol-associated anxiety; unverified national claims regarding food production, import, and export were taken as indicating the per capita calorie consumption, with some laughable results; and no allowance was usually made for age structure despite what we know about the importance of this for such variables as the crude CHD mortality or the illegitimate birth rate.

For these reasons, Lynn's study offers a model of how one might go about ranking countries on a compound measure of mental ill-health, rather than data from which such a ranking might now be attempted. With better allowance for demographic, economic, and service factors, this approach appears valid and well worth repeating. When it is effected, however, one will still have the question whether (for instance) coronary heart disease mortality should be accorded the same weight as divorce in calculating the national rankings.

3 National Groups with Exceptional Vulnerability or Resistance

While awaiting the achievement of some sort of consensus on the matter just referred to, there might be a different way of making use of international data to assess which sociocultural forces, if any, appear to be having an adverse or protective influence on mental ill-health in general, over and above influences on specific disorders. This is to identify nations or cultures that appear excessively vulnerable to a number of theoretically distinct disorders, without having compensatory good protection against other important forms of mental disorder, and to compare these with ones which have unusually low rates for a similar number of disorders. For this it is still necessary to have some rough idea regarding which indicators of psychopathology should have priority, and the effect of abnormal demographic and service distributions still needs to be kept in mind, but the differences are likely to so great that they can be taken at face value without minute assessment.

My own preference for such a comparison is to put the emphasis on impairment of function rather than on distress, and to give greater weight to duration of impairment throughout life than to the production of complete impairment through death as occurs in suicide and coronary disease. However, since we are now looking for factors affecting many aspects of mental ill-health rather than particular diseases, excessive impairment related almost exclusively to one or two diseases has to be given less weight than impairment arising through several diagnostic categories, and greater weight should be given to disorders which are regarded as wholly psychiatric than to those in which psychological factors contribute only partly to the pathology, as is the case with the psychosomatic disorders, drug dependency, and those forms of delinquency which might be regarded as expressions of mental ill-health. Finally, distress levels as reflected in community surveys must not be forgotten, since they represent an aspect which official sources may not pick up, and I think that greater weight should be given to instances where an unusually high (or low) rate is reported respecting the same people from a number of settings or administrations rather than when it is reported from only one.

In practice, these preferences usually mean putting primary emphasis on the chronic psychoses, which in turn usually means on mental hospitalization rates. We have already considered the weakness of these indicators when taken alone but that does not prevent them from being used, with caution, in conjunction with other indicators. Fig. 2.2 (p26) provides a comparison of two hospitalization measures in territories spending relatively generously on hospital care, and if we set aside the Panama Canal Zone and Caribbean territories as catering too much to transients then we find that the countries with the highest rates on the double measure are the Irish Republic, Finland, Sweden, and Iceland. The lowest rates, conversely, are for Japan, Czechoslovakia, the Netherlands and Italy. The first four countries have admission rates five times those of the second four; they have over three times the psychiatric bed-occupancy rate of the second four; and Canadians stemming from those four countries rank among the five highest subcultural groups with respects to mental hospitalizations (see Table 2.1), while Canadians stemming from Czechoslovakia, Holland, and Italy rank lowest on the hospitalization scale. There are societies not featured in Fig. 2.2 which may have higher levels of psychosis, but for a start I am going to take these two sets of four peoples as representing the extremes of national susceptibility to that type of disorder and I now propose, taking each country in turn, to examine whether the tendency with respect to psychosis is repeated or is inverted in other mental ill-health indicators.

The high *Irish* hospitalization rate derives mainly from their vulnerability to schizophrenia, but we have seen in Chap. 6 and 8 that they exhibit an excess of manic-depressive psychosis and alcohol-associated disorders as well, both in the homeland and abroad. Table 9.2 showed them to be third out of nineteen countries respecting peptic ulcer mortality in 1954-1955; the Twenty Countries Study [89] shows them to rank fifth in age-standardized rates of CHD mortality (seventh when allowance is made for serum cholesterol levels); and WHO tables sampled from the 1960s and 1970s show them to have above-average rates for hypertensive (ICD Nos. 83, 84) and cerebrovascular mortality, age-standardized. According to Lynn [362], Irish students are about average with respect to test responses regarding anxiety, and other reports, including a cross-national comparison [297], by no means give the impression that they are unusually free of neuroses. Where the Irish do have rates substantially below the average is respecting suicide, both in the homeland and overseas (see Fig. 1.1); homicide (if one ignores the killings in Northern Ireland); and vehicle accident death. However, the low suicide rate does not seem to extend to parasuicide, since an Australian study [84] found Irish immigrants to have the highest rates from among 12 immigrant subgroups studied, and the vehicle accident death rate rises from low to average when one calculates it per vehicle-kilometers run. On balance, therefore, the Irish appear to be unusually susceptible to the psychoses, to alcohol-associated mental disorder, and perhaps to parasuicide; above average in susceptibility to psychomatic disease; average with respect to neurotic symptomatology; and below average only with respect to suicide. The last feature does not, to my mind, counterbalance their unhappy susceptibility to the other disorders and I think that we can say that this people suffers from an unusually high vulnerability to mental ill-health in general.

Regarding the *Finns*, it was shown in Chap.7 that they had the highest suicide rate of 30 countries in the 1960s, particularly in comparison with the level expected on the basis of their economic expansion (Fig.7.2), although that high rate has apparently developed only since World War II. In Chap.9 it was shown that they have an exceptionally high rate of coronary heart disease (in the whole population as well as among the Karelians) after allowance was made for serum cholesterol levels; and they also have relatively high mortality and morbidity rates for hypertension and CVA at each age, although below-average rates for peptic ulcer mortality. Alcohol-associated disorders proved to comprise 23.4% of psychiatric first admissions within the age range 25-44 in Helsinki in 1960 [588], as compared with 14.5% for a corresponding group in the Irish Republic; they are disproportionately present in the first admissions of Finnish Canadians; and they have aroused much concern in Finland in the past [634]. Homicide, which is linked to alcohol, runs at almost twice the rate reported for any of the other seven peoples we are comparing, and in the age group 15-44 the death rate from all forms of violence (ICD Nos. AE 138-150) is relatively high. Where the Finns may have below-average rates is for the affective disorders. The levels recorded for these at the national mental health survey in the 1930s [287], and in the 1960 Helsinki one [588] appear low, even allowing for variations in diagnostic practice; the 1969 household survey of 991 individuals [627] found not a single case; and in the WHO-sponsored comparison of general medical practice utilization in seven countries [315] the Finnish sample scored lower than any of the 11 other community samples on a ten item symptom checklist dealing with depression and anxiety. However, judging from the 1969 household survey, the low level of symptom checklist responses is not accompanied by a low level of neurosis. That household survey, which was modeled on the Stirling County and Midtown Manhattan ones, found some degree of neurosis in 56.6% of subjects, and the author considered that the equivalent figure from the Stirling County and Yoruba samples combined was 51.9% [627]. To counterbalance the high vulnerability on other aspects of mental ill-health, therefore, there are only the low rates on affective disorders and peptic ulcer, and there thus seems good reason for thinking that this people suffer from mental ill-health substantially more than average.

With the *Swedes* the picture becomes considerably less consistent, since although they have high rates of mental hospitalization and of suicide both in the homeland and abroad, they do not have rates much above average for any of the psychosomatic disorders; they have below-average rates for homicide or other forms of violent death; and when Leighton and Hagnell attempted to apply to the latter's Lundby population criteria similar to those used in the Stirling County study, they found the Swedes to have a lower level of total mental disorder (mainly neurotic) than the Canadians [346]. There are reasons for thinking that the neuroses in other parts of Sweden may be more frequent than in Lundby, and the question of the Swedes' psychological susceptibility to alcohol and other drugs is difficult to assess because of the strictness of legal controls in the past. On balance, however, the evidence does not indicate the Swedes to have a susceptibility to psychopathology in general which is comparable to that of the Irish and the Finns.

With the *Icelanders*, more care has to be taken regarding what data to use, since official rates vary more from one year to another than is the case with the other peoples, due to Iceland's smaller population. When an 8-year period from the 1960s and 1970s is taken, they prove to have below-average mortality rates for the psychosomatic disorders, a very variable rate of suicide, an above-average rate of homicide; while they may have a moderately higher-than-average rate for alcohol-associated disorders. Helgason's large cohort study (see p 50) yielded a substantially higher rate of neurosis than most other Scandinavian surveys, but he states [253, p174] that when he applies to his material criteria similar to those employed by Fremming in Denmark, most of this difference disappears. When working with Professor Helgason on the possibility of making a comparison between mental disorder in Iceland and Mauritius, I got the impression that public and professional criteria for assessing someone as mentally ill were stricter than in, say, Britain or Canada, and if this were the case the Icelanders should probably be classed as having excess vulnerability to mental ill-health; but until the picture is clearer the matter must remain in doubt.

Turning now to the four peoples with low mental hospitalization rates, those who have read the previous chapters will probably challenge the suggestion that the *Japanese* are unusually free of mental and psychosomatic disorder. We have noted them to have unusually low rates of CHD, but unusually high rates of peptic ulcer, CVA, and at certain periods of their history (see Fig. 1.2 of suicide. Reports on Japanese students such as those in the book *Youth, Socialization and Mental Health* [341] indicate them to have quite high levels of both neurosis and disorders of personality, and mention has also been made of a transient epidemic of drug abuse in Japan (p181). There thus seems little reason to accept them as an example of a people with an unusually low level of mental disorder, even though, judging from Hawaii mental hospitalizations [543], they may have a genuinely low rate of psychosis.

With the *Czechs* the story is somewhat similar, although this is not something which can be verified through my previous chapters. They have a low age-standardized mortality rate for CHD and an average one for peptic ulcer, but their mortality rates for suicide, CVA, and hypertensive disease are high. The fact that their mental hospitalizations in the homeland are low could be attributed to them having a network of psychiatric outpatient services which was reported to be 60% more abundant than in the United States in the early 1960s [503]; and in Australia the mental health of Czech migrants has not been good [326]. There therefore seems little reason for regarding this people as having a broad resistance to psychopathology.

For the remaining two peoples the picture becomes more uniform. In their homeland the *Dutch*, in addition to having low rates of mental hospitalization, have low age-standardized mortality rates from suicide, homicide, CHD, CVA, and hypertensive disease. A community survey identified only 13% of persons aged 15+ as having any mental disorder [214], and their migrants appear to have below-average rates of mental disorder in Canada, the United States, and Australia, the one exception to this rule which I know of relating to what was called "tropical neurosis" among their colonials in Java in the 1920s and 1930s. On the whole, they seem definitely to have a below-average vulnerability to mental ill-health.

The *Italians* are closer to the average, but still on the favorable side. They have low rates of suicide, parasuicide (in Australia), and CHD. Overseas they have comparatively low rates of mental hospitalization and suicide in the United States, Canada, and Australia. Their rate of alcoholic cirrhosis is high (see Fig. 8.2) but there appears to be little mental disturbance associated with this and I am not prepared to accept cirrhosis mortality as a psychiatric indicator. They have an above-average mortality rate for hypertensive disease, but this could be due to local diagnostic preferences since Italian Americans are below-average in frequency of hypertension [521]. They have a relatively high death rate from traffic accidents, something shared by the Dutch, but in both peoples this drops below average when the rate is calculated in terms of million kilometers covered by the country's vehicles per annum, and drops still further when allowance is made for the density of vehicles per kilometer of roadway. There appears reason, therefore, to consider the Italians as above average in resistance to psychopathological conditions.

There are two main conclusions to be drawn from this examination of national groups with above-average and below-average rates of mental hospitalization. The first is that the hospitalization data alone are not adequate indicators of general mental ill-health. The second is that when other indicators are taken into consideration, it does seem possible to identify from official statistics peoples that suffer unduly, and peoples who enjoy unusual freedom, from such mental ill-health. It is now appropriate to ask what might be causing this difference between these peoples, but before we turn to this question we might as well consider whether there are other groups that should be joined with the Irish and Finns on the one hand and the Dutch and Italians on the other, for this comparison.

Of the other peoples cited as having unusually high or low rates for specific disorders in previous chapters, the southwest Croatians appear the most likely to be unduly vulnerable to psychopathology in general. A community survey found them to have high rates for affective and other psychoses as well as for schizophrenia, and hospitalization statistics showed them to have significantly higher rates than the control population with respect to coronary disease, hypertension, asthma, cerebral thrombosis, and some other disorders [302]. However, although that comparison with the control population remains valid after correction for age structure and ratio of hospital beds to population, we cannot really be sure whether the prevalence of the latter disorder is high or low by international standards. A second people whose high rates have been referred to more than once in previous chapters are the Singapore Indians. They have high rates by international standards for suicide, schizophrenia, other psychoses, hypertension, adult asthma, and juvenile delinquency; and probably above-average rates for neuroses. However, other East Indian populations overseas – for instance, in Fiji, Mauritius, and Trinidad – do not appear to share the same vulnerability, and it is doubtful, therefore, whether the Singapore group would have as much psychopathology if they had majority instead of minority status. Regarding peoples that have been cited previously because of their low rates on specific disorders, the Hutterites (p 41) have not proved to be as mentally healthy as first thought, since their low rate of schizophrenia in the 1950s was balanced by an above-average rate of affective disorder, and since in the 1970s they have been showing increasing signs of neurosis [440]. The Malays, who were shown in Chap. 5 and 6 to have low levels of affective and reactive psychosis, plus suicide, have low hospitalization rates for most psychosomatic diseases and would seem to merit inclusion now as a people enjoying an unusually low level of psychopathology. However, it is my impression that they retain this advantage only as long as they avoid economic competition, and that when they must face that competition their rates increase. On the other hand the Tongans (p 72) maintain relatively low levels of mental hospitalization when they go overseas, and they have low rates of suicide, CHD, affective psychosis, and treated neurosis as well as schizophrenia [445], so that they do seem to fit here. They suffer excessively from diabetes due to the fact that obesity is highly admired in their culture, and there is some question whether their favorite drink, the mildly hallucinogenic *kava*, is associated with some form of psychopathology since it makes its users lazy. Nevertheless, the overall picture is one of relative freedom from disorders having a psychological basis.

Regarding other peoples about whom it has been reported that an unusually high or unusually low level of psychopathology exists, nearly all known to me have proved to be less exceptional on review, or are in exceptional circumstances. The Okinawans, for instance, were in the 1950s described as enjoying unusually good mental health, but in Hawaii they proved to have higher mental hospitalization rates than other minorities. A number of Amerindian tribes have in the past been described as suffering from unusually much mental disturbance, but the picture has been changing since they have acquired wealth from mining or oil royalties and have been left freer to determine their own affairs. John Cawte and his colleagues have demonstrated the abundance of psychopathology in certain groups of Australian Aborigines, but they have equally well demonstrated this psychopathology to be linked either to extreme isolation and deprivation, as in the case of the Mornington Islanders [100], or to mishandling by the Australian White majority. By conventional standards the behavior of the Ik of East Africa, as described by Turnbull [623], would appear to be the most pathological in the present-day world; but he has argued that this behavior is relatively functional in the situation of extreme deprivation in which they have been placed. Norfolk Island, an administratively separate territory to the southeast of Australia, made an unusually good impression when I enquired into its mental health in 1977 [436]; but this was probably due to selective migration and would not have extended to Norfolk Islanders resettled in Australia.

4 Features Distinguishing Vulnerable and Resistant Peoples

Although the last remarks indicate that we do not have solid evidence of unusual vulnerability to or resistance against psychopathology in peoples whose data are not conventionally reported, other than ones whose current situation is unusually stressful or favorable, what was presented earlier in the previous section makes it highly probable that the prevalence of psychopathology in different nations varies to a greater extent than would be accounted for on the basis of present difficulties or than might be expected by chance. That means that it is potentially profitable to pursue the methods discussed earlier for ranking nations in terms of psychopathology; but the more immediate question which it raises is whether the differences so far identified can be linked to particular cultural attitudes or traditions.

In Chap. 4, it was observed that the Irish and southwestern Croatians, with high schizophrenia rates, had greater population pressure, poorer soil, more massive emigration, a longer history of foreign domination or interference with their life-style, and much less of a tradition of having important decisions taken communally or by trusted leaders, than the Hutterites and Tongans with low schizophrenia rates. It was suggested that these features must lead to schizophrenia-prone persons in the first two societies being confronted by more difficult decisions or choices than schizophrenia-prone persons in the second two, and to them receiving less communal help with their decisions, so that they would be more likely to respond pathologically. It is relatively easy to envisage these differentiating features affecting mental disorders other than schizophrenia, since it is a fairly common rule in medicine that pathology is more likely to develop in an organ or system that is being taxed than in one which has little demanded of it. Hence if these same features differentiated societies with much general psychopathology from those with little, this would not be difficult for psychiatric theory to handle.

Unfortunately, the features just cited do not differentiate the peoples with much and with little mental ill-health nearly as well as they differentiate those high and low on schizophrenia; and identifying new differentiating features is not easy. Holland faced overcrowding and the need to find land for its surplus population earlier than Ireland did. Southern Italy's barren mountains have been no less inhospitable than western Croatia's, and have inspired a more massive emigration. Although Finland's climate is harsh, it has still resources that are incompletely exploited, as the resettlement of the Karelians demonstrated, and although it suffered foreign domination and interference, like Croatia and Ireland, the same was true of Holland earlier. The impoverished villagers of the south of Italy have been described [33] as no less incapable of cooperative action than those of the west of Ireland.

Nevertheless, there are certain impressions which rise to the surface of the mind when one asks oneself how Finland, Ireland, southwestern Croatia, and perhaps Iceland compare with Holland, Italy, Tonga, and perhaps the Malay homelands. Nature has been considerably less kind to man in the first group than in the second, and has in consequence provoked a much more combative tradition in the first, an attitude of defeat-or-be-defeated which may carry over into human relationships. Another impression is that the mother is seen as considerably more benign in the second group than in the first, regardless of whether families are matricentric or not. In southern Italy, with its Madonna cult, a mother is probably as important for her grown offspring as in Ireland, but in the one society she is envisaged as someone who will always accept and forgive [487] whereas in the other she is more likely to be felt as exigent and provocative [539], a difference which extends to the Croatians and Malays. A third potential difference concerns the degree to which satisfaction can be found in modest accomplishments. Whether among the rich Dutch or the materially impoverished Malays, there is a satisfaction with the pleasures obtainable within the family and the statuses achievable within small circles of acquaintances which does not seem as full among the Finns, Irish, or Icelanders. Banfield remarks regarding the inhabitants of the poor southern Italian village which he studied that what they seemed most to feel the lack of was "... opportunity for those particular kinds of recreation – having coffee in the bar in the public square, for example – which are *civile* (mannerly) and which would therefore identify them as persons entitled to respect and admiration" [33, p66]. By implication they experience contentment when they achieve this modest goal, and I have myself remarked that the Italian Canadian appears to owe some of his relative freedom from psychopathology to "... the readiness of the group to accept work which other Canadians tend to reject but which is well paid ..." [435]. I do not get the impression that there is the same contentment with modest achievements in the other group of cultures.

It would need a much more thorough investigation of national and cultural characteristics than I have undertaken here to assess how far the foregoing impressions are valid and how far they appear to apply to the cultural differences between other societies which have relatively much or little psychopathology. As far as they go, however, they are congruent with the rule suggested earlier, namely that disorders are more likely to develop when an organ or system is taxed than when little is demanded of it. In the societies with much psychopathology that we have just been considering, mothers appear to demand more of their children than in the societies with little psychopathology, individuals appear to strive more for mastery than for harmony (and to be more affected by not achieving it), and there appears to be less satisfaction with modest rewards. It is very possible that other cultural differences operating at a more intrapsychic level, and hence not so apparent on first approach, may be as strong or stronger than those noted. For instance, psychiatric theory would lead one to expect that patterns of upbringing which result in intrapsychic conflicts would be of greater importance than the promotion of different types of striving and ways of valuing rewards. However, this is as fas as I can take the subject at present, and it seems sufficient to offer guidelines toward future research.

5 Psychopathology and Positive Mental Health

In customary usage, we would say that if one society has less psychopathology than another, then it has better mental health; but if the impressions just offered are correct, then employing the latter phrase in this instance poses a paradox. The best known definition of mental health is that given by Marie Jahoda in the monograph [277] commissioned by the (U.S.) Joint Commission on Mental Illness and Health in the late 1950s. Bringing together the opinions of many earlier writers, she concludes that the concept has six main aspects, including self-actualization, autonomy, and environmental mastery. Self-actualization implies being motivated to exploit one's capacities to the utmost; autonomy implies the taking of personal choices and being relatively independent of the social environment; while environmental mastery, in Jahoda's formulation, implies identifying problems, confronting them, and making an effort at solving them. This is not all that the term mental health usually implies, but at face value the elements just cited appear to bear quite a strong similarity to the cultural characteristics of the societies with the most psychopathology, not those with the least. Environmental mastery sounds very similar to conquest of nature. The self-actualizing person is more likely to be the one who is always striving for more than the one who is satisfied with modest rewards. Autonomy means taking decisions for oneself rather than relying on others, and although there is no direct relationship with total psychopathology, such an attitude does appear, judging from the arguments offered in Chap. 4, to be linked to a greater risk of schizophrenia.

It can be argued that the paradox which I see here is a false one, due to the equating of terms which have basically different meanings – "environmental mastery" and "conquest of nature," for instance. It can be argued that although the terms have been employed correctly, my national examples are wrong since, for instance, Holland has conquered nature much more thoroughly than Ireland or Finland has. It can be argued that if I looked further I would find cultures which promoted the mental health ideals just cited and which have low levels of psychopathology. However, it is also possible that the paradox is genuine, in the sense that if we could measure positive mental health this would be found to vary independently of psychopathology or perhaps even increase as signs of psychopathology increase. The mind is not a homeostatic organ; it is best described as an evolutionary one. Abraham Maslow [384] pointed out that as men achieve satisfaction of past needs, they discover or create new needs. Awareness of these new needs creates discontent – symptoms, as I have shown elsewhere [433] – and in exploring new ways of finding satisfaction for these new needs the mind takes risks, just as an athlete takes risks of damaging heart, muscles, or joints when striving for some way to surpass a standard which previously he had merely sought to attain. Positive mental health in the sense of being wholly free from symptoms and dysfunctions may in the absolute sense be not merely impossible but undesirable, and a certain amount of mental disorder may be an inevitable byproduct of mental effort.

I have suggested above that the societies which suffer the most psychopathology put greater emphasis on their members striving for something better, than the societies which suffer the least psychopathology; but that is not the same as saying that the formers' members achieve more with their striving. We have seen in Chap. 7 that a close relationship exists between measures of economic advancement and suicide rates; but this relationship does not extend to other indicators of psychopathology. In the studies of Smith, Lynn, and the Chicago district comparisons referred to above, suicide rates correlated inversely with those for mental hospitalization. It cannot be said that the Dutch or Italian individual achieves less than the individual Finn or Irishman. What seems more likely to be happening is that Dutch and Italian traditions encourage the more ambitious individuals to strive while at the same time encouraging the less ambitious to be content with modest rewards, whereas the Irish and Finns make it more difficult for the less capable and the less active to rest content with what they have. Returning to the athletics analogy, it may be that the societies with the least psychopathology are those which offer the widest range of programs and also have trainers restraining parents from demanding too much of those children without special capabilities, while the societies with much psychopathology have too limited a range of programs and too few trainers guiding the athletes and their parents on what to be satisfied with. However, the difference in attitude does not apply only to striving; it also applies to rewards. I get the impression that societies with more general psychopathology are also more likely to suffer from a type of Nietzschian "*ressentiment*," something which might be interpreted as reflecting not the parent's unsatisfied demands on the child, but the child's unsatisfied demands on the parent.

This chapter began with a reference to international interest in "quality of life" indicators and to the question whether, because the "quality of life" concept overlaps the "mental health" one, Comparative Psychiatry should be attempting to give a lead here. It is now possible to offer an answer to this question. We have seen that it should become possible to rank nations in terms of their levels of psychopathology, and in the more distant future probably to offer advice regarding how national levels of psychopathology could be reduced. We have also seen, however, that characteristics usually associated with superior mental health are more prominent in the societies which we found to have much psychopathology than in societies which we found to have little. What Comparative Psychiatry would propose as suitable models for nations seeking to reduce psychopathology, therefore, might not represent a superior level of "quality of life" or of "mental health" when judged from other angles. Moreover, any attempt by psychiatry to promote particular models of superior mental health could easily lead to an accusation of cultural bias, since what constitutes superior mental health is a value judgment, nor a scientific reality. Brewster Smith has pointed out that this need not trouble us. "Nor need we be embarrassed by the intrusion of values in our focus on various specified aspects of desirable and undesirable psychological functioning. What is to be avoided is the *surrepetitious* advocacy of values disguised under presumptive scientific auspices" [576, p190]. However, it means that psychiatry has no claim to special status here.

Psychiatry has the duty to bring to the attention of society in general the needs of those suffering from mental illness or who are liable to develop such illness. Comparative Psychiatry can and should bring forth evidence to show in what ways different national traditions and policies are affecting these needs, and more particularly affecting the risk of becoming mentally ill. It is up to society at large, however, to decide what weight to give to this evidence in comparison with evidence relating to other aspects of human existence, including what may be called positive mental health. There is no conflict here, but some people seem to perceive one and to discourage the examination of national traditions and policies in terms of their psychiatric effects. That position must be fought since this type of examination can be very fruitful, as this book has attempted to show.

References

The index also serves as an author index. Italic numbers refer to pages on which the paper is cited.

1. Abu-Zeid HAH, Maini KK, Choi NW (1978) Ethnic differences in mortality from ischemic heart disease: a study of migrant and native populations. J Chronic Dis 31:137–146 *(234)*
2. Abuzzahab GS, Anderson FO (1976) Gilles de la Tourette's syndrome: International registry. Mason, St. Paul *(42)*
3. Acheson RM (1960) Mortality from cerebrovascular accidents and hypertension in the Republic of Ireland. Br J Prev Soc Med 14:139–147 *(223)*
4. Acheson RM (ed) (1964) Comparability in international epidemiology. Milbank Memorial Fund, New York *(35)*
5. Achté K (1961) Der Verlauf der Schizophrenien und der schizophreniformen Psychosen. Acta Psychiatr Neurol Scand [Suppl] 155 *(82)*
6. Ackermann L (1905) Trauma and chronic compression of the epigastricum as etiological factor in gastric ulcer. Med News 86:50–56 *(212)*
7. Adelstein AM, Downham DY, Stein Z, Susser MW (1968) The epidemiology of mental illness in an English city. Soc Psychiatry 3:47–59 *(46)*
8. Adler R (1971) Experimentally induced gastric lesions; results and implications of studies in animals. Adv Psychosom Med 6:1–39 *(213)*
9. Adler R, MacRitchie K, Engel GL (1971) Psychologic processes and ischemic stroke (occlusive cerebrovascular disease). Psychosom Med 33:1–29 *(222)*
10. Ahrenfeldt RH (1958) Psychiatry in the British army in the second world war. Routledge & Kegan Paul, London *(246; 248)*
11. Aitken RCB, Buglass D, Kreitman N (1969) The changing pattern of attempted suicide in Edinburgh, 1962–1967. Br J Prev Soc Med 23:111–115 *(174)*
12. Alexander F (1950) Psychosomatic medicine. Norton, New York *(215; 217)*
13. Alexander F, French TM, Pollock GH (1968) Psychosomatic specificity. University of Chicago Press, Chicago *(208; 219)*
14. Amdur MJ, Harrow K (1972) Conscience and depressive disorders. Br J Psychiatry 120: 259–264 *(134)*
15. Amiel R, Lebigre F (1970) Un nouveau test rapide pour l'appréciation de la santé mentale. Ann Méd Psychol (Paris) 1:565–580 *(54)*
16. Amiel R, Mace-Kradjian G (1972) Quelques données épidémiologiques sur la psycho-sociologie et la psycho-pathologie du monde enseignant. Ann Méd Psychol (Paris) 2:321–353 *(54)*
17. Ammar S (1972) Aperçu épidémiologique des troubles mentaux en Tunisie. Inf Psychiatr 48:677–720 *(94)*
18. Andersen T (1975) Physical and mental illness in a Lapp and a Norwegian population. In: Andersen T, Astrup C, Forsdahl A (eds) Social, somatic and psychiatric studies of geographically defined populations. Acta Psychiatr Scand [Suppl] 263:47–53 *(63)*
19. Angrosino MV (1974) Outside is death. Alcoholism, ideology and community organization among the East Indians of Trinidad. Wake Forest University, Winston-Salem, North Carolina *(205)*
20. Anonymous (1908) The Russo-Japanese war; Medical and sanitary reports from officers attached to the Japanese and Russian forces in the field, HMSO, London *(245)*
21. Anonymous (1967) Underlying angst. Far East Econ Rev 57 (July 20th):147 *(276)*
22. Ariès P (1962) Centuries of childhood; A social history of family life. Knopf, New York (Translated from French by Baldick R) *(119)*

23. Arnold T (1782) Observations on the nature, kinds, causes and prevention of insanity, lunacy or madness. Robinson & Cadell, Leicester (Cited in Hunter R, Macalpine I (1963) p 499) *(119; 143)*
24. Ashcroft MT (1977) Prevalence of hypertension and associated electrocardiographic abnormalities in Jamaica and West Africa. West Indian Med J 26:24–32 *(225)*
25. Astrup C, Noreik K (1966) Functional psychoses; Diagnostic and prognostic methods. Thomas, Springfield *(94)*
26. Aviram U, Syme SL, Cohen JB (1976) The effect of policies and programs on the reduction of mental hospitalization. Soc Sci Med 10:571–577 *(25)*
27. Ayuso JL, Martin IM, Fuentenebro-de-Diego F (1979) Analisis etiopatogenico de las depresiones en la tercera edad. Acta Psiquiat Psicol Am Lat 25:187–193 *(135)*
28. Babigian HM (1972) The role of psychiatric case registers in the longitudinal study of psychopathology. In: Roff M, Robins L, Pollack M (eds) Life history research in psychopathology. University of Minneapolis Press, Minneapolis *(44)*
29. Bacon MK, Barry H, Child IL (1965) A cross-cultural study of drinking. Q J Stud Alcohol [Suppl] 3 (whole issue) *(184; 185)*
30. Bagley C, Binitie A (1970) Alcoholism and schizophrenia in Irishmen in London. Br J Addict 65:3–7 *(32; 73; 199)*
31. Bales RF (1962) Attitudes towards drinking in Irish culture. In: Pittman DJ, Snyder CR (eds) Society, culture and drinking patterns. Wiley, New York *(200)*
32. Ball JC, Lau MP (1970) The Chinese opiate addict in the United States. In: Ball JC, Chambers CD (eds) The epidemiology of opiate addiction in the United States. Thomas, Springfield *(181)*
33. Banfield EC (1958) The moral basis of a backward society. Free Press Glencoe, IL *(293; 294)*
34. Barrett GV, Franke RH (1970) "Psychogenic" death; a reappraisal. Science 167:304–306 *(219)*
35. Barry H (1976) Cross-cultural evidence that dependency conflict motivates drunkenness. In: Everett MW, Waddell JO, Heath DB (eds) Cross-cultural approaches to the study of alcohol. Mouton, The Hague *(185; 200)*
36. Bateson G, Mead M (1942) Balinese character; a photo analysis. New York Acad Sci, New York *(111; 258)*
37. Baxter RA (1673) A Christian directory. In: Orme W (ed) Collected works, vol 3 (1830). Duncan, London *(116)*
38. Beaglehole R, Salmond CE, Hooper A, Huntsman J, Stanhope JM, Cassel JC, Prior IAM (1977) Blood pressure and social interaction in Tokelauan migrants to New Zealand. J Chronic Dis 30:803–812 *(227)*
39. Beard GW (1880) Experiments with the "jumpers" or "jumping Frenchmen" of Maine. J Nerv Ment Dis 7:487–490 *(256)*
40. Beaubrun M (1967) Treatment of alcoholism in Trinidad and Tobago, 1956–1965. Br J Psychiatry 113:643–658 *(181)*
41. Becker R (1932) Die Geisteserkrankungen bei den Juden in Polen. Allg Z Psychiatr 96: 47–66 *(121)*
42. Becker R (1932) Bibliographische Übersicht der Literatur aus dem Gebiete: "Geisteserkrankungen bei den Juden". Allg Z Psychiatr 98:241–276 *(120)*
43. Beekman D (1977) The mechanical baby; a popular history of the theory and practice of child raising. Lawrence Hill, Westport *(216; 268)*
44. Beiser M (1977) Ethics in cross-cultural research. In: Foulks EF, Wintrob RM, Westermeyer J, Favazza AR (eds) Current perspectives in cultural psychiatry. Spectrum, New York *(53)*
45. Beiser M, Benfari RCB, Collomb H, Ravel JL (1976) Measuring psychoneurotic behavior in cross-cultural surveys. J Nerv Ment Dis 163:10–23 *(53; 129)*
46. Belgrave TB (1867) The asylums for the insane in St. Petersburg and Copenhagen. J Ment Sci 13:7–19 *(120)*
47. Bell RM (1974) The transformation of a rural village; Istria, 1870–1972. J Soc Hist 7: 243–270 *(70)*

48. Benabud A (1957) Psychopathological aspects of the cannabis situation in Morocco. Bull Narc 9 (4):1–16 *(180)*
49. Benedict R (1946) The chrysanthemum and the sword; Patterns of Japanese culture. Houghton Mifflin, New York *(223)*
50. Bensmail B, Bencharif AK, Bentorki H (1975) Considération sur l'assistance et la morbidité psychiatriques dans l'Est Algérien. Tunis Med 6:393–408 *(94)*
51. Berne E (1964) Games people play. Grove Press, New York *(204)*
52. Bernstein IS (1978) Sex differences in the behavior of nonhuman primates. Soc Sci Med 12B:151–154 *(261)*
53. Berry J (1969) On cross-cultural comparability. Int J Psychol 4:119–128 *(15)*
54. Bickerton YJ (1976) Ethnic group differences at the clientele of a state detoxification unit. In: Seixas FA (ed) Currents in alcoholism, vol 2. Grune & Stratton, New York, pp 357–365 *(190)*
55. Birnbaum K (1906) Über degenerative Verschrobene. Zentralbl Nervenheilk 29:650–658 *(93)*
56. Blackmore R (1725) A treatise of the spleen and vapours ... . Pemberton, London *(116)*
57. Block J, Christiansen B (1966) A test of Hendin's hypotheses relating suicide in Scandinavia to childrearing orientations. Scand J Psychol 7:267–288 *(159)*
58. Bohannan P (ed) (1960) African homicide and suicide. Princeton University Press, Princeton *(154; 162)*
59. Bolander AM (1972) Nordic suicide statistics. In: Waldenström J, Larsson T, Ljungstedt N (eds) Suicide and attempted suicide. Nordiska, Stockholm, pp 57–88 *(156)*
60. Bolton R (1976) Andean coca chewing: a metabolic perspective. Am Anthropol 78:630–634 *(183)*
61. Böök JA (1953) A genetic and neuropsychiatric investigation of a North-Swedish population. Acta genet stat med 4:1–100 *(50; 63)*
62. Bourdin CE (1845) Du suicide considéré comme maladie. De Hennuyer, Paris *(148)*
63. Boussat M, Gueye M, Hanck C, Saibou A (1977) Les psychoses puerpérales; rappel clinique. Méd Afr Noire 24:240–249 *(106)*
64. Bower TGR (1977) A primer of infant development. Freeman, San Francisco *(265)*
65. Bowlby AS, Tooth HH, Wallace C, Calverley JE, Kilkelly C (1901) A civilian war hospital, Murray, London *(245)*
66. Boyer LB, Boyer RM (1972) Effects of acculturation on the vicissitudes of the aggressive drive among Apaches of the Mescalero Indian reservation. Psychoanal Stud Soc 5:40–82 *(201; 202)*
67. Brekke TH, Øgar B (1977) Patients in Norwegian general practice (in Norwegian). Tidsskr Nor laegeforen 97:491–503 *(45)*
68. Bremer J (1951) A social psychiatric investigation of a small community in northern Norway. Acta Psychiatr Neurol [Suppl] 62 *(44)*
69. Briggs J (1970) Never in anger: Portrait of an Eskimo family. Harvard University Press, Cambridge, Massachusetts *(174)*
70. Brill H, Hirose T (1969) The rise and fall of a methyl-amphetamine epidemic: Japan 1945–1955. Semin Psychiatr 1:179–194 *(181)*
71. Britannica Book of the Year (1965, 1966, 1967, etc), Encyclopaedia Britannica, Chicago *(24)*
72. Brody H (1971) Indians on Skid Row. Information Canada, Ottawa *(201)*
73. Brody H (1974) Inishkillane; Change and decline in the west of Ireland. Schocken, New York *(69; 125; 142; 200; 201)*
74. Brown GW, Harris T (1978) Social origins of depression; a study of psychiatric disorder in women. Tavistock, London *(143)*
75. Brown MW, Williams FE (1918) Neuropsychiatry and the war; a bibliography with abstracts. National Committee for Mental Hygiene, New York *(245; 247)*
76. Brugger C (1931) Versuch einer Geisteskrankenzählung in Thüringen. Z Gesamte Neurol Psychiatr 133:352–390 *(59)*
77. Bruun K (1969) The actual and registered frequency of drunkenness in Helsinki. Br J Addict 64:3–8 *(187)*

78. Buikhuisen W (1965) Background to the behavior of young troublemakers (in Dutch). PhD Thesis, University of Assen *(175)*
79. Buonafede A alias Cromanziano A (1761) Istoria critica e filosofica del suicido. Riccomini, Lucca *(147)*
80. Burkitt DP (1969) Related disease – related cause? Lancet 2:1229–1232 *(209)*
81. Burton R (1955) The anatomy of melancholy. Tudor Press, New York (one volume edition of 1621 original) *(116; 262)*
82. Burton-Bradley BG (1977) Longlong. Transcultural Psychiatry in Papua New Guinea (2nd edn). Public Health Department, Port Moresby *(110)*
83. Burvill PW, McCall MG, Stenhouse N, Reid TA (1973) Deaths from suicide, motor vehicle accidents and all forms of violent death among migrants in Australia, 1962–66. Acta Psychiatr Scand 49:28–50 *(12)*
84. Burvill PW, Hobbs MST, Armstrong B (1980) Attempted suicides in immigrants in Perth, Western Australia, 1969–1976. (Typescript 19 pp). Univ. of W. Australia, Perth. *(288)*
85. Buss AR, Lang PJ (1965) Psychological deficit in schizophrenia. I: Affect, reinforcement and concept attainment. J Abnorm Psychol 70:2–24 *(70)*
86. Busse S, Mulloy CT, Weise CE (1978) Disulfiram in the treatment of alcoholism; an annotated bibliography. Addiction Research Foundation, Toronto *(204)*
87. Bustamante JA (1969) Bouffée délirante à Cuba. Evol Psychiatr 34:399–412 *(104)*
88. Bustamante S, Miniet ED (No date) Factores socioculturales en la reaccion psicotica aguda, Instituto de investigaciones fundamentale de cerebro. Loma y 37, Alturas del Vedado, Havana, Cuba (Typescript 13 pp) *(104)*
89. Byington R, Dyer AR, Garside D, Lin K, Moss D, Stamler J, Tsong Y (1979) Recent trends in major coronary risk factors and CHD mortality in the United States and other industrialized countries. In: Havlik RJ, Feinleb M (eds) Proceedings of the conference on the decline in coronary disease mortality. NIH Publication No 79–1610, Washington DC *(288)*
90. Carstairs GM (1954) Daru and bhang: cultural factors in the choice of an intoxicant. Q J Stud Alcohol 12:220–237 *(180)*
91. Carstairs GM (1956) Hinjra and jiryan: two derivatives of Hindu attitudes to sexuality. Br J Med Psychol 29:128–138 *(272)*
92. Carstairs GM (1957) The twice-born; a study of a community of high-caste Hindus. Hogarth, London *(271)*
93. Carstairs GM, Kapur RL (1976) The great universe of Kota. Hogarth, London *(49; 51; 53; 71)*
94. Cassel JC (1974) Studies of hypertension in migrants. In: Paul O (ed) Epidemiology and control of hypertension. Stratton, New York, pp 41–62 *(225)*
95. Caudill W (1972) Tiny dramas; vocal communication between mother and infant in Japanese and American families. In: Lebra WP (ed) Transcultural research in mental health. University Press of Hawaii, Honolulu, pp 25–48 *(263; 266)*
96. Caudill W, De Vos G (1956) Achievement, culture and personality; the case of Japanese Americans. Am Anthropol 58:1102–1126 *(239)*
97. Caudill W, Frost L (1973) A comparison of maternal care and infant behavior in Japanese, American and Japanese-American families. In: Lebra WP (ed) Youth, socialization and mental health. University Press of Hawaii, Honolulu, pp 3–15 *(263)*
98. Caudill W, Schooler C (1973) Child behavior and childrearing in Japan and the United States; in interim report. J Nerv Ment Dis 157:323–338 *(263)*
99. Caudill W, Weinstein H (1969) Maternal care and infant behavior in Japan and America. Psychiatry 32:12–43 *(223)*
100. Cawte J (1972) Cruel, poor and brutal nations. University Press of Hawaii, Honolulu *(292)*
101. Centre National de la Recherche Scientifique (CNRS) (1973) La notion de personne en Afrique noir. Editions du CNRS, Paris *(136)*
102. Chabot HT (1950) Kinship, social status and sex in South Celebes (Thesis) Wolters, Groningen (English translation in Human Relations Area Files, Code No OG6) *(111; 273)*
103. Chance NA, Rin H, Chu HM (1966) Modernization, value identification and mental health; a cross-cultural study. Anthropologica 8:197–216 *(56)*

104. Cheyne G (1733) The English malady: or a treatise of nervous diseases of all kinds ... . Strahan, London *(116)*
105. Chiu TL, Tong JE, Schmidt KE (1972) A clinical survey of latah in Sarawak, Malaysia, Psychol Med 2:155–165 *(50)*
106. Chkili T, El Khamlichi A (1975) Les psychoses puerpérales en milieu marocain. Tunis Med 6:375–392 *(106)*
107. Chopra RN, Chopra GS (1959) The present position of hemp-drug addiction in India. Indian Medical Research Memoir No. 31, Delhi *(180)*
108. Chowdhury N, Hicks RC, Kreitman N (1973) Evaluation of an aftercare service for parasuicide patients. Soc Psychiat 8:67–81 *(175)*
109. Citronblatt A (1912) Zur Klinik und Pathologie des perforierten Magen und Duodenal Geschwürs. Deutsch Zeitschr Chirurg 117:120–124 *(210)*
110. Clark WC (1973) Temporary madness as theatre; wild-man behaviour in New Guinea. Oceania 43:198–214 *(109; 111)*
111. Cleghorn RA (1969) Hysteria – multiple manifestations of semantic confusion. Can Psychiat Assn J 14:539–551 *(254)*
112. Cochrane R (1977) Mental illness in immigrants to England and Wales; an analysis of mental hospital admissions, 1971. Soc Psychiatry 12:25–35 *(17; 124)*
113. Cochrane R (1979) Psychological and behavioural disturbance in West Indians, Indians and Pakistanis in Britain; a comparison of rates among children and adults. Br J Psychiatry 134:201–210 *(124; 129)*
114. Cochrane R, Stopes-Roe M (1977) Psychological and social adjustment of Asian immigrants to Britain. Soc Psychiatry 12:157–164 *(124; 162)*
115. Cochrane R, Hashmi F, Stopes-Roe M (1977) Measuring psychological disturbance in Asian immigrants to Britain. Soc Sci Med 11:157–164 *(17)*
116. Cohen JB (1978) The influence of culture on coronary-prone behavior. In: Dembroski TM (ed) Proceedings of the forum on coronary-prone behavior. DHEW Publication No (NIH) 78–1451, Washington *(237; 239)*
117. Collomb H (1965) Assistance psychiatrique en Afrique (expérience sénégalaise). Psychopathol Afr 1:11–84 *(91)*
118. Collomb H (1965) Bouffées délirantes en milieu africain. Psychopathol Afr 1:167–239 *(102; 104)*
119. Collomb H (1977) La mis à mort de la famille. Psychopathol Enfant 20:245–299 *(107)*
120. Collomb H, Collignon R (1974) Les conduites suicidaires en Afrique. Psychopathol Afr 10:55–114 *(162)*
121. Constant J (1969) Les bouffées délirantes en Guadeloupe. Thèse, Université de Paris *(94; 101; 103)*
122. Cooney JG (1971) Alcohol and the Irish. J Ir Coll Physicians Surg 1:50–54 *(200)*
123. Cooper JE, Kendell RE, Gurland BJ, Sharpe L, Copeland JRM, Simon R (1972) Psychiatric diagnosis in New York and London. Oxford University Press, London *(18; 63; 67; 71; 130)*
124. Cooper JE, Sartorius N (1975) Cultural and temporal variations in schizophrenia; a speculation on the importance of industrialization. Division of Mental Health, WHO. Geneva (Typescript 11 pp) *(92)*
125. Corin E (1971) Le père comme modèle de différentiation dans une société clannique matrilinéaire (Yansi, Congo-Kinshasa). Psychopathol Afr 7:185–224 *(269)*
126. Corin E, Bibeau G (1980) Psychiatric perspectives in Africa. Part II: The traditional viewpoint. Transcult Psychiatr Res Rev 17:204–232 *(260)*
127. Corin E, Murphy HBM (1979) Psychiatric perspectives in Africa. Part I: The western viewpoint. Transcult Psychiatr Res Rev 16:147–178 *(63)*
128. Correa P, Arias-Stella J, Perez Tamayo R, Carbonell LM (1975) Texto de pathologia, 2nd edn. Prensa Medica, Mexico City, p 247 *(210)*
129. Cosminsky S (1971) Sex differences in illnesses of emotional origin in a Guatamalan community. Amer Anthrop Assn annual meeting, New York, 1971 *(254)*
130. Counts DR (1980) Why have you killed my child? Alternative strategies of death in Kaliai. Can Ethnol Assn annual meeting, Montreal, 1980 *(164)*

131. Cox JL (1979) Amakiro: A Ugandan puerperal psychosis? Soc Psychiatr 14:49–52 *(107)*
132. Crocetti GM, Kulkar Z, Kesic B, Lemkau PV (1964) Differential rates of schizophrenia in Croatia. Amer J Public Health 54:196–206 *(68)*
133. Cromley R (1967) Mental illness is low among GIs in Vietnam Ann Arbor News, Oct 31st *(250)*
134. Czaplicka MA (1914) Aboriginal Siberia: A study in social anthropology. Oxford University Press, Oxford *(256)*
135. Czernak J (1858) Ein Beitrag zur Statistik der Psychosen. Allg Z Psychiatr 15:251–271 *(120)*
136. Dalgaard JB (1962) On international comparison of suicide frequencies (in Danish). Sociol Meddelelser 7:53–60 *(156)*
137. Daly MB, Tyroler HA (1972) Cornell medical index response as a predictor of mortality. Br J Prev Soc Med 26:159–164 *(35)*
138. Damaye H (1917) Considérations cliniques sur les commotions de la guerre. Prog Méd 32: 332–334 *(247)*
139. Daneshmand L (1974) Incidence of phobias in Iranian psychiatric patients. In: Leigh D, Noorbakhsh J, Izadi C (eds) Proceedings of international symposium on epidemiological studies in psychiatry. World Psychiatric Association. Teheran, pp 325–329 *(262)*
140. Davis RB (1949) A study of war psychoses in troops of the Indian army. Ind J Neurol Psychiatry 1:160–173 *(113)*
141. De Bonis M (1974) Content analysis of 27 anxiety inventories and rating scales. Mod Probl Pharmacopsychiatry 7:221–237 *(283)*
142. De Lint J, Schmidt W (1971) Consumption averages and alcoholism prevalence; a brief review of epidemiological investigations. Br J Addict 66:97–107 *(183)*
143. Denber HCB, Collard J (1962) Différences de bioréactivité au halopéridol entre deux groupes de psychotiques, américain et européen. Acte Neurol Belg 62:577–588 *(85)*
144. Denber HCB, Bente D, Rajotte P (1962) Comparative analysis of the action of butyrylperazine at Manhattan Hospital and the University Psychiatric Clinic at Erlangen. Am J Psychiatry 119:203–206 *(85)*
145. De Ridder JC (1961) The personality of the urban African in South Africa. Routledge & Kegan Paul, London *(229)*
146. Deussen J (1944) Die Blasenneurose unter besonderer Berücksichtigung der sogenannten Kriegs-Pollakisurie. Arch Psychiatr Nervenkr 117:424–442 *(248; 255)*
147. De Vos GA (1973) Socialization for achievement; Essays on the cultural psychology of the Japanese. University of California Press, Berkeley *(241; 263)*
148. Diaz-Guerrero R (1955) Neurosis and the Mexican family structure. Am J Psychiatry 112: 411–417 *(142)*
149. Dilling H, Weyerer S, Enders I (1978) Patienten mit psychischen Störungen in der Allgemeinpraxis und ihre psychiatrische Überweisungsbedürftigkeit. In: Häfner H (ed) Psychiatrische Epidemiologie. Springer, Berlin Heidelberg New York, pp 135–160 *(45; 61)*
150. Djamour J (1955) The Malay family in Singapore. Thesis, London School of Economics *(142)*
151. Djamour J (1959) Malay kinship and marriage in Singapore. Athlone, London *(142; 182)*
152. Djamour J (1966) The family structure of the Singapore Malay. Colonial Office, London *(111)*
153. Doi T (1973) The anatomy of dependence (translation by J. Bester). Kodansha, Tokyo *(15; 44; 223; 263; 265)*
154. Dollard J, Doob LW, Miller NE, Mowrer OH, Sears RF (1929) Frustration and aggression. Yale University Press, New Haven *(154)*
155. Dube KC (1968) Mental disorder in Agra. Soc Psychiatry 3:139–143 *(49)*
156. Dube KC, Kumar N (1974) An epidemiological study of hysteria. J Biosoc Sci 6:401–405 *(255)*
157. Dublin LI (1963) Suicide: A sociological and statistical study. Ronald, New York *(152)*
158. DuBois C (1961) The people of Alor (paperback edn). Harper, New York *(176)*

159. Durand-Comiot M-L (1977) La psychose puerpérale? Etude en milieu sénégalais. Psychopathol Afr 13:269–336 *(107; 108)*
160. Durkheim E (1951) Suicide: A study in sociology (English translation by S.A. Spaulding, G. Simpson). Macmillan, New York *(149; 151)*
161. Eaton JW, Weil RJ (1955) Culture and mental disorders. Free Press, New York *(48; 71)*
162. Ebie JC (1972) Psychiatric illness in the puerperium among Nigerians. Trop Geogr Med 24:253–256 *(106)*
163. Edgerton RB (1971) The individual in cultural adaptation; a study of four East African peoples. University of California Press, Berkeley *(230)*
164. Eleftheriou BE (ed) (1975) Pharmacogenetics. Plenum, London *(85; 179)*
165. El-Islam MF (1969) Depression and guilt; a study at an Arab psychiatric clinic. Soc Psychiatry 4:56–58 *(136)*
166. Ellenberger HF (1950) Die Putzwut. Der Psychologe 2:91, 138 *(15)*
167. Ellenberger HF (1970) The discovery of the unconscious. Basic Books, New York *(256)*
168. Elnagar MN, Maitra P, Rao MN (1971) Mental health in an Indian rural community. Br J Psychiatry 118:499–503 *(49; 71)*
169. Elwin V (1943) Maria murder and suicide. Oxford University Press, Bombay *(154)*
170. Enke P (1900) Casuistische Beiträge zur männlichen Hysterie. Thesis, Jena University [Quoted in Decker HS (1977) Freud in Germany; Revolution and reaction in science, 1893–1907. International University Press, New York] *(9)*
171. Erikson EH (1968) Identity, youth and crisis. Norton, New York *(253)*
172. Erlich VS (1966) Family in transition; a study of 300 Yugoslav villages. Princeton University Press, Princeton *(69; 100)*
173. Esquirol JED (1938) Des maladies mentales considérées sous les rapport médical, hygiénique et médico-légal. Baillière, Paris *(4; 149)*
174. Essen-Möller E (1956) Individual traits and morbidity in a Swedish rural population. Acta Psychiatr Neurol Scand [Suppl] 100:1–160 *(48)*
175. Ey H (1954) Etudes psychiatriques, vol 3. Structure des psychoses aigues et déstructuration de la conscience. Brouwer, Paris *(92; 94; 102)*
176. Ey H (1958) Les problèmes cliniques des schizophrénies. Evol Psychiatr 2:149–212 *(94; 101)*
177. Ey H, Igert C, Rappard P (1957) Psychoses aigues et évolution schizophréniques dans un service de 1930 à 1956. Ann Méd Psychol 2:231–240 *(94)*
178. Fabrega H (1974) Disease and social behavior. M.I.T. Press, Cambridge, MA *(208)*
179. Fabrega H, Rubel AJ, Wallace CA (1967) Working class Mexican psychiatric out-patients. Arch Gen Psychiatry 16:704–712 *(142)*
180. Faergeman PM (1963) Psychogenic Psychoses. Butterworth, London *(94)*
181. Falret JP (1822) De l'hypochondrie et du suicide. Croullebois, Paris *(147)*
182. Farber ML (1968) Theory of suicide. Funk & Wagnalls, New York *(158; 162)*
183. Fenichel O (1946) The psychoanalytic theory of neurosis. Kegan Paul, French, Trubner & Co London *(162; 242)*
184. Fenna D, Mix L, Schaefer O, Gilbert JAL (1971) Ethanol metabolism in various racial groups. Can Med Assoc J 105:472–475 *(179)*
185. Ferenczi S, Abraham K, Simmel E, Jones E (1921) Psychoanalysis and the war neuroses. Internat Psychoanal Press, London *(248; 253)*
186. Feuerlin W (1967) Klinisch-statistische Untersuchungen über die Entstehungsbedingungen und die Prognosis des Alkoholdelirs. Nervenarzt 38:206–212 *(196)*
187. Field MJ (1960) Search for security. Faber & Faber, London *(14; 103; 104; 136)*
188. Field PB (1962) A new cross-cultural study of drunkenness. In: Pittman DJ, Snyder ST (eds) Society, culture and drinking patterns. Wiley, New York, pp 48–74 *(185)*
189. Fiessinger N (1915) Emotional shock from bursting of big shell. Med Press Circ 99:563–565 *(246)*
190. Fine NL (1960) Coca chewing: A social versus a nutritional interpretation (Mimeograph). Columbia University Dept Anthropol, New York *(183)*
191. Finney R (1972) And what about culture-change syndromes? Conference on Culture and Mental Health in Asia and the Pacific, 1972. Honolulu *(56)*

192. Firth R (1936) We the Tikopia. Allen & Unwin, London *(169)*
193. Firth R (1967) Tikopia ritual and belief. Allen & Unwin, London *(169)*
194. Fishberg M (1901) Comparative pathology of the Jews. NY Med J, pp 538–543, 576–581 *(120)*
195. Fitzgerald RD (1924) A thesis on two tropical neuroses peculiar to the Malays. Trans 5th Cong Far-Eastern Assoc Trop Med. Bate and Davidson, London, pp 148–161 *(256)*
196. Florey C du V, Cuadrado RR (1968) Blood pressure in native Cape Verdeans and in Cape Verde immigrants and their descendants living in New England. Hum Biol 40:189–211 *(226)*
197. Flügel JC (1930) The psychology of clothes. Hogarth, London *(213)*
198. Follin S (1963) Les états oniroides. C R Congr Psychiatr Neurol Lang Français 1:79–216 *(102)*
199. Fortes M (1936) Culture contact as a dynamic process. Africa 9:24–55 *(76)*
200. Fortes M, Mayer D (1966) Psychoses and social change among the Tallensi of Northern Ghana. Cah Etudes Afr 6:5–40 *(76)*
201. Fossen A, Boeke HE (1939) Frequency of acute appendicitis in the Netherland East Indies (in Dutch). Geneesk Tijdschr Ned-Indie 79:2857–2867 *(209)*
202. Foulks E (1972) The arctic hysterias of the North Alaskan Eskimo. Am Anthropol Assoc Anthropol Studies No. 10 *(254)*
203. Freedman AM, Kaplan HI, Sadock BJ (1972) Modern synopsis of the comprehensive textbook of psychiatry. Wilkins & Wilkins, Baltimore *(63)*
204. Fremming KH (1951) The expectation of mental infirmity in a sample of the Danish population. Cassell, London *(50; 51)*
205. Freud S (1936) The problem of anxiety. Psychoanal Quarterly Press, Albany *(270)*
206. Fried J (1959) Acculturation and mental health among Indian migrants in Peru. In: Opler MK (ed) Culture and mental health. Macmillan, New York, pp 119:137 *(120)*
207. Fromm E, Maccoby M (1970) Social character in a Mexican village. Prentice Hall, Englewood *(143)*
208. Fürstner C (1875) Über Schwangerschafts- und Puerperal-Psychosen. Arch Psychiatr Nervenkr 5:505–543 *(93; 105)*
209. Gans A (1922) Ein Beitrag zur Rassenpsychiatrie. Münch Med Wochenschr 69:1503–1506 *(141)*
210. Geertz H (1961) The Javanese family; a study in kinship and socialization. Free Press, New York *(111)*
211. Gerard A (1803) Des perforations spontanées de l'estomac. Gillé fils, Paris. [Cited in: Jennings D (1940) Perforated peptic ulcer. Lancet 1:395–398, 444–447] *(210)*
212. Gharagozlu H, Foulks E, Sherif M, Roknie R (1980) Zar healing in South Iran, Transcult Psychiatr Res Rev 17:178–181 *(260)*
213. Gibbs JP (1958) Status integration and suicide. Am Sociol Rev 23:140–146 *(151)*
214. Giel R, LeNobel CPJ (1971) Psychic disturbances in a Dutch village (in Dutch). Ned Tijdschr Geneesk 115:949–954 *(45; 291)*
215. Giffen PJ (1965) Rates of crime and delinquency. In: McGrath WT (ed) Crime and its treatment in Canada. Macmillan, Toronto, pp 59–90 *(39)*
216. Gilat T, Rozen P (1979) Epidemiology of Crohn's disease and ulcerative colitis; etiological implications. Isr J Med Sci 15:305–308 *(209)*
217. Gilles de la Tourette H (1894) L'ulcère rond de l'estomac dans les hôpitaux de Paris; pathogénie et statistique. Bull Mém Soc Méd Hôp (Paris) 393–408 *(210)*
218. Gillespie RD (1942) Psychological effects of war on citizen and soldier. Norton, New York *(243)*
219. Gillion KL (1962) Fiji's Indian migrants. Oxford University Press, Melbourne *(134)*
220. Gillis LS, Lewis JB, Slabbert M (1968) Psychiatric disorder among the coloured people of the Cape peninsula. Br J Psychiatry 114:1575–1587 *(132)*
221. Glad DD (1947) Attitudes and experiences of American-Jewish and American-Irish male youth as related to difference in adult rates of inebriety. Q J Stud Alcohol 8:406–472 *(200)*
222. Gladwin T, Sarason SB (1953) Truk; Man in paradise, Wenner-Gren Foundation, New York *(166)*

223. Glass DC (1977) Behavior patterns, stress, and coronary disease. Erlbaum, Hillsdale *(240)*
224. Goldberg SC, Schooler NR, Davidson EM, Kayce MM (1966) Sex and race differences in response to drug treatment among schizophrenics. Psychopharmacologia (Berlin) 9:31–47 *(86)*
225. Goldfarb A (1960) Evaluation of children's behavior by teachers and psychiatrists. Thesis, John Hopkins School of Public Health, Baltimore *(57)*
226. Goldhamer H, Marshall A (1949) Psychosis and civilization. Free Press, Glencoe *(74)*
227. Goldstein K (1939) The Organism. American Book Publishers, New York *(253)*
228. Gordon S, Cocks TGB (1952) A people's conscience. Cape, London *(24)*
229. Gorer G, Rickman J (1949) The people of Greater Russia. Cresset Press, London *(17)*
230. Gould J, Kolb WL (eds) (1964) A Dictionary of the Social Sciences. Free Press, New York *(10)*
231. Greely AM (1972) That most distressful nation; the taming of the American Irish. Aldine, Chicago *(125)*
232. Grewel F (1967) Psychiatric differences in Ashkenazim and Sephardim. Psychiatr Neurol Neurochir 70:339–347 *(122)*
233. Grinker RR (1973) Changing styles in psychoses and boderline states. Am J Psychiatry 130:151–152 *(81)*
234. Grinsard (Paper carries no initial) (1939) Etats délirants observés à l'asile d'aliénés de Voi. C.R. 10th congress of the Far East Assn Trop Med, Hanoi. Imprimérie d'Extrême-Orient, Hanoi, pp 211–256 *(95)*
235. Grollman A (1978) A conjecture about the prevalence of essential hypertension and its high incidence in the Black. Tex Rep Biol Med 36:25–32 *(224)*
236. Gross MM, Rosenblatt SM, Lewis E, Chartoff S, Malinowski B (1972) Acute alcoholic psychoses and related syndromes; psychosocial and clinical characteristics. Br J Addict 67:15–31 *(196)*
237. Gurin G, Veroff J, Feld S (1960) Americans view their mental health. Basic Books, New York *(279)*
238. Gussow Z (1963) A preliminary report of Kayak-angst among the Eskimo of West Greenland; a study in sensory deprivation. Int J Soc Psychiatr 9:18–26 *(267)*
239. Gwee AL (1968) Koro: its origin and nature as a disease entity. Singapore Med J 9:3–6 *(247)*
240. Häfner H, Reimann H (1970) Spacial distribution of mental disorders in Mannheim, 1965. In: Hare EH, Wing JK (eds) Psychiatric epidemiology. Oxford University Press, London, pp 341–354 *(46)*
241. Hagnell O (1966) A prospective study of the incidence of mental disorder. Svenska Bokforlaget, Lund *(48)*
242. Halbwachs M (1930) Les causes du suicide. Alcan, Paris *(151)*
243. Halliday A (1828) A general view of the present state of lunatics and lunatic asylums in Great Britain and Ireland, and some other kingdoms. Underwood, London *(4)*
244. Hallowell AI (1938) Fear and anxiety as cultural and individual variables in a primitive society. J Soc Psychol 9:25–47 *(262)*
245. Hamer JH (1965) Acculturation stress and the functions of alcohol among the forest Potawatomi. Q J Stud Alcohol 26:285–302 *(193)*
246. Hamilton JA (1962) Postpartum psychiatric problems. Mosby, St. Louis *(105)*
247. Haroon AS (1979) Attitudes towards sex and sexual problems among university students (Typescript 6 pp). Jinnah Postgraduate Medical Center, Karachi *(271)*
248. Harvey EB, Gazay L, Samuels B (1976) Utilization of a psychiatric-social work team in an Alaskan native secondary boarding school. J Am Acad Child Psychiatry 15:558–574 *(174)*
249. Hassan R, Lian TK (1970) Suicide in Singapore; a sociological analysis. Southeast Asian J Sociol 3:13–36 *(139)*
250. Hatano S (1974) Hypertension in Japan; a review. In: Paul O (ed) Epidemiology and control of hypertension. Stratton, New York pp 63–100 *(224; 225; 232)*
251. Hayem G, Lion G (1913) Maladies de l'estomac. Baillière, Paris, pp 531–535 *(213)*

252. Helgason T (1961) The frequency of depressive states in Iceland as compared with the other Scandinavian countries. Acta Psychiatr Scand [Suppl] 162:81–90 *(158)*
253. Helgason T (1964) Epidemiology of mental disorders in Iceland. Acta Psychiatr Scand [Suppl] 173:1–258 *(51; 190)*
254. Hemphill RE (1952) Incidence and nature of puerperal psychiatric illness. Br Med J 2: 1232–1235 *(105)*
255. Henderson D, Gillespie RD (1950) A textbook of psychiatry for students and practitioners, 7th edn. Oxford University Press, London *(243)*
256. Hendin H (1964) Suicide and Scandinavia. Grune & Stratton, New York *(17; 157)*
257. Hezel TX (1977) Micronesia's hanging spree (Mimeograph 11 pp). Truk, Micronesia *(166)*
258. Hickling FW (1975) Psychiatric care in a general hospital unit in Jamaica. West Indian Med J 24:67–75 *(173)*
259. Hinkle LE, Redmont R, Plummer N, Wolff HG (1950) An examination of the relationship between symptoms, disability and serious illness in two homogeneous groups of men and women. Am J Public Health 50:1327–1336 *(128)*
260. Hippler AE (1973) Some possibly culturally based causes of paradoxical responses to tranquilizing drugs among Alaska Athabaskans (Typescript 7 pp). Anchorage, Alaska *(86)*
261. Hippler AE (1975) Transcultural psychiatric and related research in the North American arctic and sub-arctic. Transcult Psychiatr Res Rev 12:103–115 *(267)*
262. Hobson S (1978) Family web; A story of India. Murray, London *(126)*
263. Hofman O, Kolar M, Reisenhauer R, Matousek V (1973) Significance of the differences in the personal history between normotensive and hypertensive subjects. Univ Carol (Prague) Ser Med 19:583–599 *(224)*
264. Hofstede G (1979) Value systems in forty countries: interpretation, validation and consequences for theory. In: Eckensberger LH, Lonner WJ, Poortinga YH (eds) Cross-cultural contributions to psychology. Swets & Zeitlinger, Lisse, pp 389–408 *(159)*
265. Holding TA, Buglass D, Duffy JC, Kreitman N (1977) Parsuicide in Edinburgh – a seven-year review, 1968–1974. Br J Psychiatry 130:534–543 *(174)*
266. Hollender MH, Hirsch SJ (1964) Hysterical psychosis. Am J Psychiatry 120:1066–1074 *(94)*
267. Horn W (1941) Untersuchungen und Beobachtungen an geisteskranken Juden. Allg Z Psychiatr 117:167–180 *(122)*
268. Horton D (1943) The functions of alcohol in primitive societies; a cross-cultural study. Q J Stud Alcohol 4:199–320 *(184)*
269. Hoskin JO, Friedman MI, Cawte JE (1969) A high incidence of suicide in a preliterate – primitive society. Psychiatry 32:200–210 *(164)*
270. Hoskin JO, Kiloh LG, Cawte JE (1969) Epilepsy and *guria*; the shaking syndromes of New Guinea. Soc Sci Med 3:39–48 *(260)*
271. Hunter R, Macalpine I (1963) Three hundred years of psychiatry: 1535–1860. Oxford University Press, London *(116; 118)*
272. Inkeles A, Smith DH (1970) The fate of personal adjustment in the process of modernization. Int J Comp Sociol 2:81–114 *(55)*
273. Instytut Psychoneurologiczny (1973) Statistical Bulletin, Psychiatry, 1960–1969 (in Polish). Zaklad Organizacji Ochrony Zdrowia, Warsaw *(125)*
274. Itil TM (1975) Transcultural psychopharmacology from the EEG point of view. In: Itil TM (ed) Transcultural Neuropharmacology. Bozak, Instanbul, pp 39–54 *(85)*
275. Jaco EG (1960) The social epidemiology of mental disorders. Russell Sage, New York *(42)*
276. Jacobs J (1894) Family and village life in Greater Achin, 2 vols (in Dutch). Brill, Leiden *(75)*
277. Jahoda M (1958) Current concepts of positive mental health. Basic Books, New York *(294)*
278. Jarvis E (1852) On the supposed increase in insanity. Am J Insanity 8:333–364 *(5; 23)*
279. Jeffreys MDW (1952) Samsonic suicide or suicide of revenge among Africans. Afr Stud 11: 118–122 *(163; 164)*
280. Jellinek EM (1960) The disease concept of alcoholism. Hillhouse, New Haven *(178)*
281. Jennings D (1940) Perforated peptic ulcer. Lancet 1:395–398, 444–447 *(210; 214)*

282. Jessor R, Young HB, Young EB, Tesi G (1970) Perceived opportunity, alienation and drinking behavior among Italian and American youths. J Pers Soc Psychol 15:215–222 *(180; 200)*

283. Jilek-Aall L (1978) Alcohol and the Indian-White relationship; a study of the function of Alcoholics Anonymous among the Coast Salish Indians. Confin Psychiatr 21:195–233 *(204)*

284. Johnson R (1976) Culture and crisis in confinement. Heath, Lexington, DC *(173)*

285. Joseph A, Murray VF (1951) Chamorros and Carolinians of Saipan. Harvard University Press, Cambridge, MA *(227)*

286. Kagan A, Popper J, Rhoads GG, Takeya Y, Kato H, Goode GB, Marmot M (1976) Epidemiological studies of coronary heart disease and stroke in Japanese men living in Japan, Hawaii and California: Prevalence of stroke. In: Scheinberg P (ed) Cerebrovascular diseases; Tenth Princeton conference. Raven Press, New York, pp 267–278 *(222; 240)*

287. Kaila M (1942) Über die Durchschnittshäufigkeit der Geisteskrankheiten und des Schwachsinns in Finnland. Acta Psychiatr Neurol Scand 17:47–67 *(288)*

288. Kakar S (1978) The inner world. A psychoanalytic study of childhood and society in India. Oxford University Press, New Delhi *(252)*

289. Kapur RL (1975) Factors affecting the reporting of mental disorders in others. Soc Psychiatry 10:87–96 *(58)*

290. Karim I, Price J (1973) Suicide in Fiji. Fiji Med J 1:49–55 *(133)*

291. Karnosh LJ, Hope JM (1937) Puerperal psychoses and their sequelae. Am J Psychiatry 94:537–550 *(105)*

292. Karppanen H, Pennanen R, Passinen L (1978) Minerals, coronary heart disease and sudden coronary death. Adv Cardiol 25:9–24 *(234)*

293. Karvonen MJ, Blomqvist G, Kallio V, Orma E, Punsar S, Rautaharju P, Takkunen J, Keys A (1966) Men in rural east and west Finland. In: Epidemiological studies relating to coronary heart disease: Characteristics of men aged 40–59 in seven countries. Acta Med Scand [Suppl] 460:169–190 *(236)*

294. Kasahara Y (1974) Fear of eye-to-eye confrontation among neurotic patients in Japan. In: Lebra TS, Lebra WP (eds) Japanese culture and behavior; Selected readings. University Press Hawaii, Honolulu, pp 396–406 *(262; 263)*

295. Kato M (1969) Self-destruction in Japan; a cross-cultural epidemiological analysis of suicide. Folia Psychiatr Neurol Jap 23:291–307 *(14)*

296. Kedward H (1969) The outcome of neurotic illness in the community. Soc Psychiatry 4: 1–4 *(61)*

297. Kelleher MJ (1972) Cross-national (Anglo-Irish) differences in obsessional symptoms and traits of personality. Psychol Med 2:33–41 *(288)*

298. Kelleher MJ, Copeland JRM (1973) Psychiatric diagnosis in Cork and London; results of a cross-national pilot study. J Irish Med Assoc 66:553–557 *(67)*

299. Kendell RE (1968) The classification of depressive illness. Oxford University Press, London *(115)*

300 Keniston K (1968) Heads and seekers; drugs on campus, counter-cultures and American society. Am Scholar 38:97–113 *(180)*

301. Kennedy J (1967) Nubian Zar ceremonies as psychotherapy. Human Organization 26: 185–194 *(259)*

302. Kesic B, Kulcar Z, Lemkau PV (1972) Differential rates of psychoses in Croatia; Final report. Andrija Stampar School of Public Health, Zagreb *(69; 291)*

303. Keys A (1980) Seven countries: A multivariate analysis of death and coronary heart disease. Harvard University Press, Cambridge, MA *(233; 236)*

304. Keys A, Karvonen MJ, Fidanza F (1958) Serum cholesterol studies in Finland. Lancet 2:175–178 *(235)*

305. Khan VS (1979) Migration and social stress; Mirpuris in Bradford. In: Khan VS (ed) Minority families in Britain; support and stress. Macmillan, London, pp 37–58 *(126)*

306. Khoo OT (1975) Of drugs, alcohol and venereal disease. Ann Acad Med (Singapore) 4:444–457 *(181)*

307. Kimura B (1965) Vergleichende Untersuchungen über depressive Erkrankungen in Japan und Deutschland. Fortschr Neurol Psychiatr 33:202–215 *(44; 136)*

308. Kimura B (1971) Struktur des Selbstbewusstseins beim Japaner im Spiegel der sogenannten "Anthropophobien" (English Abstract). Transcult Psychiatr Res Rev 8:129–130 *(263)*

309. Kino FF (1951) Alien's paranoid reaction. J Ment Sci 97:589–594 *(94; 98)*

310. Kiste RC (1974) The Bikinians: A study of forced migration. Cummings, Menlo Park California *(170)*

311. Kitamura T, Ito K (1976) Acute gastric changes in patients with acute stroke. Stroke 7: 460–468 *(221)*

312 Kits van Heijningen H Treurniet N (1966) Psychodynamic factors in acute myocardial infarction. Int J Psychoanal 47:370–374 *(236)*

313. Kleinman A, Kunstadter P, Alexander ER, Gale J (eds) (1975) Medicine in Chinese cultures. U.S. Gov't Printing Office Washington, DC *(19)*

314. Knight R (1936) The psychodynamics of chronic alcoholism. J Nerv Ment Dis 37:538–548 *(186)*

315. Kohn R, White KL (1976) Health care; an international studv. Oxford University Press London *(288)*

316. Kohut H (1971) The analysis of the self. International Universities Press, New York *(111; 167)*

317. Kraepelin E (1904) Vergleichende Psychiatrie. Zentralbl Nervenheilk Psychiatr 27:433–437 *(1; 3)*

318. Kraepelin E (1906) Psychiatrie: Ein Lehrbuch für Studierende und Ärzte. Barth, Leipzig *(1)*

319. Kraepelin E (1921) Manic depressive insanity and paranoia (Translated by R.M. Barclay). Livingstone, Edinburgh *(134)*

320. Kranz H (1955) Das Thema des Wahns im Wandel der Zeit. Fortschr Neurol 23:58–72 *(82)*

321. Kraus G (1933) Mental disorders in Holland (in Dutch). Wolters, Groningen *(122)*

322 Kraus RF (1972) Changing patterns of suicidal behavior in North Alaskan Eskimos (abstract) Transcult Psychiatr Res Rev 9:69–71 *(172; 173)*

323. Krauss HH, Krauss BJ (1968) Cross-cultural study of the thwarting-disorientation theory of suicide. J Abnorm Psychol 73:353–357 *(155)*

324. Kretchmer E (1956) Hysterie, Reflex und Instinkt. Thieme, Stuttgart *(259)*

325. Kröber E (1946) Der praktische Arzt und die Beurteilung der Kriegsschäden. Dtsch Gesundheitswes 1:347–352 *(255)*

326. Krupinski J, Stoller A, Wallace L (1973) Psychiatric disorders in East European refugees now in Australia. Soc Sci Med 7:31–49 *(290)*

327. Kulcar Z, Crocetti GM, Lemkau PV, Kesic B (1971) Selected aspects of the epidemiology of psychoses in Croatia, Yugoslavia. Am J Epidemiol 94:118–125 *(69)*

328. Kuljzenko A (1933) Stenjevac hospital in the last five years in the light of medical statistics (in Croatian). Glasnik Centralnog Higijenskog Zavoda, Belgrade *(68)*

329. Kunitz SJ, Levy JE, Odoroff CL, Bollinger J (1971) The epidemiology of alcoholic cirrhosis in two southwestern Indian tribes. Q J Stud Alcohol 32:706–720 *(190; 191)*

330. Laing RD, Sterson A (1964) Sanity, madness and the family. Basic Books, New York *(243)*

331. Lamont AM (1948) A study of racial and socio-economic influences on mental disease in a South African mental hospital. M D Thesis, Glasgow University *(130)*

332. Lamont AM (1951) Affective types of psychotic reaction in Cape coloured persons. S Afr Med J 25:40–42 *(130)*

333. Lange J (1921) Über manisch-depressives Irresein bei Juden. Münch Med Wochenschr, pp 1357–1359 *(122)*

334. Langelüddecke A (1941) Über Lebenserwartung und Rückfallshäufigkeit bei Manisch-Depressiven. Z Psych Hyg 14:1–14 *(161)*

335. Langner TS (1965) Psychophysiological symptoms and the status of women in two Mexican communities. In: Murphy JM, Leighton AH (eds) Approaches to cross-cultural psychiatry. Cornell University Press, Ithaca, NY *(139)*

336. Langner TS, Michael ST (1963) Life stress and mental health: The midtown Manhattan study. Free Press, New York *(52)*
337. Langner TS, Gersten JC, Eisenberg JG, Greene EL, Herson JH (No date) Children under stress; Factors in the behavior of urban children and adolescents (Mimeograph 144 pp). Final Report, USPHS Project Grants No MH 11545 and 18260 *(57)*
338. Langness L (1976) Hysterical psychoses and possessions. In: Lebra WP (ed) Culture-bound syndromes, ethnopsychiatry and alternative therapies. University Press Hawaii, Honolulu, pp 56–57 *(259)*
339. Lanham BB (1956) Aspects of child care in Japan; preliminary report. In: Haring DG (ed) Personal character and cultural milieu, 3rd edn. Syracuse University Press, Syracuse NY, pp 565–583 *(263)*
340. Lannois M, Chavanne F (1915) Le pronostic des surdités de guerre; d'après 1,000 cas. Bull Acad Méd 74:781–786 *(246)*
341. Lebra WP (1974) Youth, socialization and mental health. University Press of Hawaii, Honolulu *(290)*
342. Lebra TS (1976) Japanese patterns of behavior. University Press of Hawaii, Honolulu *(239)*
343. Leighton AH, Hughes CC (1955) Notes on Eskimo patterns of suicide. Southwest J Anthropol 11:327–338 *(172)*
344. Leighton AH, Lambo TA, Hughes CC, Leighton DC, Murphy JM, Macklin DB (1963) Psychiatric disorder among the Yoruba. Cornell University Press, Ithaca, NY *(52; 53; 281; 284)*
345. Leighton DC, Harding JS, Macklin DB, MacMillan AM, Leighton AH (1963) The character of danger: Psychiatric symptoms in selected communities. Basic Books, New York *(51; 53)*
346. Leighton DC, Hagnell O, Leighton AH, Harding JS, Kellert SR, Danley RA (1971) Psychiatric disorder in a Swedish and a Canadian community. Soc Sci Med 5:189–210 *(290)*
347. Lemkau PV, Kulcar Z, Crocetti GM, Kesic B (1971) Selected aspects of the epidemiology of the psychoses in Croatia, Yugoslavia, Parts I, II and III. Am J Epidemiol 94:112–117, 118–125, 126–134 *(68; 69)*
348. Leong JHK (1974) Cross-cultural influences on ideas about drugs. Bull Narc 26(4):1–8 *(181)*
349. Levy JE, Kunitz SJ (1974) Indian drinking: Navaho practices and Anglo-American theories. Wiley, New York *(201; 203)*
350. Levy L, Rowitz L (1971) The ecology of mental disorder. Behavioral Publications, New York *(284)*
351. Lewis HB (1971) Shame and guilt in neurosis. International Universities Press, New York *(222)*
352. Lewis HB (1978) Sex differences in supergo mode as related to sex differences in psychiatric illness. Soc Sci Med 12:199–206 *(129)*
353. Lewis IM (1971) Ecstatic religion; An anthropological study of spirit possession and shamanism. Penguin Books, London *(260)*
354. Lin TY (1953) A study of the incidence of mental disorder in Chinese and other cultures. Psychiatry 16:313–336 *(48; 50; 58; 284)*
355. Lin TY, Rin H, Yeh EK, Hsu CC, Chu HM (1969) Mental disorders in Taiwan fifteen years later; a preliminary report. In: Caudill W, Lin TY (eds) Mental health research in Asia and the Pacific. East-West Center Press, Honolulu, pp 66–91 *(6)*
356. Lingens E (1972) Suicide in extreme situations. In: Waldenström J, Larsson T, Ljungstedt N (eds) Suicide and attempted suicide. Nordiska, Stockholm, pp 114–121 *(152)*
357. Littlewood R, Lipsedge M (1981) Acute psychotic reactions in Caribbean-born patients. Psychol Med 11:303–318 *(129)*
358. Llewellyn-Thomas E (1960) The prevalence of psychiatric symptoms within an island fishing village. Can Med Assoc J 83:197–204 *(44)*
359. Logan WPD, Cushion AA (1958) Morbidity statistics from general practice: Volume I (General). Studies on medical and population subjects. HMSO, London, publication no 14 *(45)*

360. Lorry A-C (1765) De melancholia et morbis melancholicus, 2 vol. Lutetiae parisiorum, Paris *(119)*
361. Ludwig AO (1947) Neuroses occurring in soldiers after prolonged combat exposure. Bull Menninger Clin 11:15–23 *(249)*
362. Lynn R (1971) Personality and national character. Pergamon, Oxford *(285; 288)*
363. Lynn R, Hampson SL (1975) National differences in extraversion and neuroticism. Br J Soc Clin Psychol 14:223–240 *(285)*
364. MacAndrew C, Edgerton RB (1969) Drunken comportment. Aldine, Chicago *(110; 182; 193)*
365. Maccoby M (1967) El caracter nacional mexicano. Rev Psicoanal Psiquiatr Psicol 7:41–52 *(142)*
366. Maclaurin BP, Wardill TEM, Faaiuaso ST, McKinnon M (1979) Geographic distribution of peptic ulcer disease in Western Samoa. New Zeal Med J 89:341–344 *(209)*
367. MacPherson WG, Herringham WP, Elliott TR, Balfour A (1923) Medical services; Diseases of the war, vol II. HMSO, London *(246; 247; 253)*
368. Magnan V, Legrain V (1895) Les Dégénérés. Rueff, Paris *(93)*
369 Mahoney FB (1973) Social and cultural factors relating to the cause and control of alcohol abuse among Micronesian youth. Leonard, Washington DC *(193)*
370. Malhotra SL (1964) Peptic ulcer in India and its aetiology. Gut 5:412–416 *(209)*
371. Malhotra HK, Wig NN (1975) Dhat syndrome; a culture-bound sex neurosis of the Orient. Arch Sex Behav 4:519–528 *(271)*
372. Malzberg B (1931) Mental disease among Jews. Ment Hyg 15:766–774 *(122)*
373. Malzberg B (1940) Social and biological aspects of mental disease. State Hospital Press, Utica NY *(17; 65; 195)*
374. Malzberg B (1959) Mental disease among Jews in New York State, (Mimeograph 229 pp) Research Foundation for Mental Hygiene. Inc. Albany, NY *(122; 195)*
375. Malzberg B (1963) Mental disease among Jews in Canada (Mimeograph 88 pp) Research Foundation for Mental Hygiene, Inc. Albany, NY *(122)*
376. Malzberg B (1964) Mental disease among native Whites in New York State, 1949–1951; classified according to parentage. Ment Hyg 48:478–499 *(66)*
377. Mares J, Barre R (1962) Quelques aspects des accidents psychiatriques de la puerpéralité en milieu musulman algérien. Ann Méd Psychol 1:31–49 *(107)*
378. Marks IM (1969) Fears and phobias. Academic Press, London *(263)*
379. Marks IM, Herst ER (1970) A survey of 1,200 agorophobics in Britain; features associated with treatment and ability to work. Soc Psychiatry 5:16–24 *(262)*
380. Marmot MG, Syme SL (1979) Acculturation and coronary heart disease in Japanese-Americans. Am J Epidemiol 104:225–247 *(237)*
381. Mars L (1958) La schizophrénie en Haiti. Bull Bur Ehtnol (Port-au-Prince) 15:3–21 *(103)*
382. Marshall DS, Suggs RC (eds) (1971) Human sexual behavior. Basic Books, New York *(270)*
383. Masaryk TG (1970) Suicide and the meaning of civilization. Chicago University Press, Chicago [English translation of 1881 edition] *(148; 149; 151)*
384. Maslow AH (1954) Motivation and personality. Harper & Row, New York *(5; 295)*
385. Matsumoto YS (1970) Social stress and coronary heart disease in Japan; a hypothesis. Milbank Mem Fund Q 48:9–36 *(236)*
386. Mayer-Gross W, Cross KW, Harrington JA, Sreenivasan U (1958) The chronic mental patient in India and in England. Lancet 1:1265–1267 *(48)*
387. Mayer-Gross W, Slater E, Roth M (1969) Clinical psychiatry, 3rd edn. Baillière, London *(63)*
388. Mayo WJ (1908) A study of gastric and duodenal ulcers, with special reference to their surgical cure. Ann Surg Philad 47:884–898 *(210)*
389. Mazer M (1965) The human predicament of an island population. Sci Psychoanal 8:159–170 *(46)*
390. Mazer M (1967) Psychiatric disorders in general practice: the experience of an island community. Am J Psychiatry 124:63–69 *(45)*
391. McCandless FD (1968) Suicide and the communication of rage; a cross-cultural case study. Am J Psychiatry 125:197–205 *(168)*

392. McCarthy PD, Walsh D (1975) Suicide in Dublin: I – The under-reporting of suicide and the consequences for national statistics. Br J Psychiatry 126:301–308 *(36)*

393. McClelland DC (1961) The achieving society. Van Nostrand, Princeton NJ *(155; 219)*

394. McClelland DC, Davis WN, Kalin R, Wanner E (1972) The drinking man. Free Press, New York *(180; 181; 186; 199; 201)*

395. McCord W, McCord J (1960) Origins of alcoholism. Stanford University Press, Stanford *(186; 198; 200)*

396. McDonough JR, Garrison JE, Haines CG (1964) Blood pressure and hypertensive disease among Negroes and Whites; a study in Evans County, Georgia. Ann Int Med 61:208–228 *(225)*

397. McNeill I (director of film) (1959) Four families (with Margaret Mead as narrator and consultant). National Film Board of Canada, Ottawa *(217; 267)*

398. Mead M (1928) Coming of age in Samoa. Morrow, New York *(72)*

399. Meadow A, Stoker D (1965) Symptomatic behavior of hospitalized patients: a study of Mexican-American and Anglo-American patients. Arch Gen Psychiatry 12:267–277 *(142)*

400. Meakins JC, Eakin WW (1932) Coronary thrombosis; a clinical and pathological study. Can Med Assoc J 26:18–26 *(233)*

401. Medalie JH, Neufeld HN, Goldbourt U, Kahn HA, Riss E, Oron D (1970) Association between blood pressure and peptic ulcer incidence. Lancet 2:1225–1226 *(224)*

402. Medicus FC (1764) Geschichte periodischer Krankheiten. Macklot, Karlsruhe *(119)*

403. Megaw J (1933) An enquiry into certain public health aspects of village life in India. India Office, Simla *(42)*

404. Megaw J (1939) Medicine and public health. In: Blunt E (ed) Social service in India. HMSO London, pp 27–39 *(75)*

405. Mellor WF (ed) (1972) History of the second world war: Casualties and medical statistics. HMSO, London *(250; 251)*

406. Mercer GW, Smart RG (1974) The epidemiology of psychoactive and hallucinogenic drug use. In: Gibbins RJ (ed) Research advances in alcohol and drug problems, vol 1. Wiley, New York, pp 303–354 *(194)*

407 Messenger JC (1969) Innis Beag. Holt Rhinehart, New York *(68; 125; 200)*

408. Meyer E (1914) Psychosen und Neurosen in der Armee während des Krieges. D Med Wochenschr 40:2085–2088 *(245)*

409. Miall WE, Oldham PD, Khosla T, Lovell HG, Moore F (1967) Factors influencing the degree of resemblance in arterial pressure of close relatives. Clin Sci 33:271–283 *(224)*

410. Milew W, Lirow K (1967) Über einige Erscheinungen und Besonderheiten der zyklophrenen Melancholie in Bulgarien. Aktuel Fragen Psychiatr Neurol 6:22–37 *(146)*

411. Mitchell TJ, Smith GM (1931) Medical services: Casualties and medical statistics of the great war. HMSO, London *(246; 247)*

412. Morel B-A (1845) Pathologie mentale en Belgique, en Hollande et en Allemagne. Ann Méd Psychol 6:196–222, 350–358 *(8)*

413. Mulford HA, Wilson RW (1966) Identifying problem drinkers in a household health survey. United States Public Health Service. Washington DC, Publications Series 1000 no 16 *(57)*

414. Mulhall MG (1880) The progress of the world in arts, agriculture, commerce, manufactures, instruction, railways and public health since the beginning of the nineteenth century. Stanford, London *(148)*

415. Mullins WS, Glass AJ (eds) (1973) Neuropsychiatry in world war II, vol 2. US Government Printing Office, Washington DC *(248; 249)*

416. Murasaki, Lady (1935) The tale of Genji (translated by A. Waley). Allen & Unwin, London (5 books in one volume) *(265)*

417. Murphy HBM (1954) The mental health of Singapore; Part I – Suicide. Med J Malaya 9: 1–45 *(139; 171)*

418. Murphy HBM (ed) (1955) Flight and resettlement. UNESCO, Paris *(77; 144; 282)*

419. Murphy HBM (1958) Culture, society and mental disorder in South East Asia. MD Thesis, Edinburgh University *(144)*

420. Murphy HBM (1959) Culture and mental disorder in Singapore. In: Opler MK (ed) Culture and mental health. Macmillan New York, pp 291–316 *(97; 139)*

421. Murphy HBM (1959) Cultural factors in the mental health of Malayan Students. In: Funkenstein D (ed) The student and mental health: An international view. WFMH, Cambridge MA, pp 164–222 *(97)*
422. Murphy HBM (1963) Juvenile delinquency in Singapore. J Soc Psychol 61:201–231 *(37; 97; 168)*
423. Murphy HBM (1971) The beginning of psychiatric treatment in the Peninsula. In: Wagner MN, Tan ES (eds) Psychological problems and treatment in Malaysia. University of Malaya Press, Kuala Lumpur, pp 13–18 *(92)*
424. Murphy HBM (1972) The evocative role of complex social tasks. In: Kaplan AR (ed) Genetic factors in schizophrenia. Thomas, Springfield, pp 407–422 *(70)*
425. Murphy HBM (1972) Psychopharmacologie et variations ethno-culturelles. Confront Psychiatr 9:163–185 *(42; 86; 138)*
426. Murphy HBM (1973) Chronicité, communauté et culture. In: Chiland C, Béquart P (eds) Traitement au Long Cours des Etats Psychotiques. Editions Privat, Toulouse, pp 371–384 *(79; 87)*
427. Murphy HBM (1973) History and the evolution of syndromes: The striking case of *Latah* and *Amok*. In: Hammer M, Salzinger K, Sutton S (eds) Psychopathology. Wiley, New York, pp 33–55 *(108; 111; 256)*
428. Murphy HBM (1974) Differences between mental disorders of French Canadians and British Canadians. Can Psychiatr Assoc J 19:247–257 *(84)*
429. Murphy HBM (1975) Alcoholism and schizophrenia in the Irish: a review. Transcult Psychiatr Res Rev 12:116–139 *(65; 68; 200)*
430. Murphy HBM (1976) Notes for a theory on Latah. In: Lebra WP (ed) Culture-bound syndromes, ethnopsychiatry and alternate therapies. University Press of Hawaii, Honolulu, pp 3–21 *(258)*
431. Murphy HBM (1976) Two stress measures in three cultures: Their prognostic efficiency, significance and incongruities. In: Leigh D, Noorbakhsh J (eds) Proceedings of international symposium on epidemiological studies in psychiatry, Teheran 1974. Iran Psychiatr Soc, Teheran, pp 248–260 *(6; 61)*
432. Murphy HBM (1977) Migration, culture and mental health. Psychol Med 7:677–684 *(76)*
433. Murphy HBM (1978) The meaning of symptom-check-list scores in mental health surveys: a testing of multiple hypotheses. Soc Sci Med 12:67–75 *(56; 295)*
434. Murphy HBM (1978) The advent of guilt feelings as a common depressive symptom: a historical comparison on two continents. Psychiatry 41:229–242 *(118)*
435. Murphy HBM (1978) European cultural offshoots in the new world: differences in their mental hospitalization patterns. Part I: British, French and Italian influences. Soc Psychiatry 13:1–9 *(65; 68; 125; 294)*
436. Murphy HBM (1978) Mental health trends in the Pacific Islands. Report on a tour of Pacific territories, September 1977–March 1978. South Pacific Commission, Noumea, New Caledonia *(73; 196; 292)*
437. Murphy HBM (1978) Historic changes in the sex ratio for different disorders. Soc Sci Med 12B:143–149 *(13; 211; 233)*
438. Murphy HBM (1979) Depression, witchcraft beliefs and supergo development in preliterate societies. Can J Psychiatry 24:437–449 *(136)*
439. Murphy HBM (1980) [Review of] Schizophrenia: An international follow-up study. Transcult Psychiatr Res Rev 17:158–161 *(78)*
440. Murphy HBM (1980) European cultural offshoots in the new world: differences in their mental hospitalization patterns. Part II: German, Dutch and Scandinavian influences. Arch Psychiatr Nervenkr 228:161–174 *(65; 125; 292)*
441. Murphy HBM, Lemieux M (1967) Quelques considérations sur le taux élevé de schizophrénie dans un type de communauté canadienne-française. Can Psychiatr Assoc J (Numéro Spécial) 12:572–581 *(60; 284)*
442. Murphy HBM, Narayan R (1979) Mental hospitalisation in Fiji. Fiji Med J 7:4–11 *(133)*
443. Murphy HBM, Negrete JC (1967) Psychological deficit in chewers of coca leaf. Bull Narc 19 (4):11–17 *(196)*

444. Murphy HBM, Raman AC (1971) The chronicity of schizophrenia in indigenous tropical peoples. Br J Psychiatry 118:489–497 *(34; 79)*
445. Murphy HBM, Taumoepeau BM (1980) Traditionalism and mental health in the South Pacific: a re-examination of an old hypothesis. Psychol Med 10:471–482 *(72; 292)*
446. Murphy HBM, Wittkower ED, Fried J, Ellenberger HF (1963) A cross-cultural survey of schizophrenic symptomatology. Int J Soc Psychiatry 9:237–249 *(42; 81)*
447. Murphy HBM, Wittkower ED, Chance NA (1967) Cross-cultural inquiry into the symptomatology of depression: a preliminary report. Int J Psychiatry 3:6–15 *(42; 134; 137)*
448. Murphy HBM, Engelsmann F, Tcheng-Laroche F (1976) The influence of fosterhome care on psychiatric patients. Arch Gen Psychiatry 33:179–183 *(89)*
449. Murphy HBM, Negrete JC, Tousignant M (1979) Exploring a new type of alcoholism survey. Int J Epidemiol 8:119–126 *(58)*
450. Murthy RS, Kala K, Wig NN (1978) Mentally ill in a rural community: some initial experiences in case identification and management. Ind J Psychiatry 20:137–142 *(49)*
451. Nalin DR (1973) Epidemic of suicide by Malathion poisoning in Guyana; report of 264 cases. Trop Geogr Med 25:8–14 *(168)*
452 Nandi DN, Ajmany S, Ganguli H, Banerjee G, Boral GC, Ghosh A, Sarkar S (1976) The incidence of mental disorders in one year in a rural community in West Bengal. Ind J Psychiatry 18:79–87 *(48; 49)*
453. Nandi DN, Mukherjee SP, Banerjee G, Boral GC, Ghosh A, Sarkar S, Das S, Banerjee K, Ajmany S (1978) Psychiatric morbidity in an uprooted community in rural West Bengal. Ind J Psychiatry 20:137–142 *(49)*
454. Naroll R (1962) Data quality control – A new research technique. Free Press, New York *(7)*
455. Naroll R (1965) Thwarting disorientation and suicide: a cross-cultural survey (Abstract). Transcult Psychiatr Res Rev 2:89–92 *(154)*
456. National Center for Health Statistics (1968) Vital statistics rates for the United States, 1940–1960. U.S. Gov't Printer, Washington DC *(214)*
457. National Institute of Mental Health (1973) Suicide, Homicide and Alcoholism among American Indians. U.S. Government Printer, Washington DC *(201)*
458. Neel S (1973) Medical Support of the U.S. Army in Vietnam, 1965–1970. U.S. Government Printer, Washington DC *(250)*
459. Negrete JC (1970) Les attitudes envers le comportement des alcooliques; étude comparative dans trois sous-cultures québecoises. Toxicoman 3:193–212 *(191)*
460. Negrete JC (1973) Cultural influences on social performance of chronic alcoholics: a comparative study. Q J Stud Alcohol 34:905–916 *(191)*
461. Neki JS (1976) An examination of the cultural relativism of dependence as a dynamic of social and therapeutic relationships. Br J Med Psychol 49:1–22 *(217; 264)*
462. Neuringer C (1976) Current developments in the study of suicidal thinking. In: Schneidman ES (ed) Suicidology: Contemporary developments. Grune & Stratton, New York, pp 234–252 *(165)*
463. New Zealand Department of Health (1962) Maori patients in mental hospitals. Government Printer, Wellington, Special Report Series no 8 *(132)*
464. Ngui PG (1969) The koro epidemic in Singapore. Aust NZ J Psychiatry 3:263–266 *(274)*
465 Norman-Taylor W, Rees WH (1963) Blood pressures in three New Hebrides communities. Br J Prev Soc Med 17:141–145 *(225)*
465a. Obeyesekere G (1976) The impact of Ayurvedic ideas on the culture and the individual in Sri Lanka. In: Leslie C (ed) Asian Medical Systems; A Comparative Study. University of California Press, Berkeley, pp 201–226 *(270)*
466. Ødegaard Ø(1932) Emigration and insanity. Acta Psychiatr Neurol [Suppl] 5 *(70)*
467. Ødegaard Ø (1952) The incidence of mental diseases as measured by census investigations versus admission statistics. Psychiatr Q 26:212–218 *(23)*
468. O'Flaherty WD (1973) Asceticism and eroticism in the mythology of Siva. Oxford University Press, London *(271)*
469. O'Hare A, Walsh D (1965–1976) Activities of Irish psychiatric hospitals and units. Medico-Social Research Board, Dublin (Annual volumes) *(66)*

470. Opler ME (1957) Anxiety, spirit possession and culture in a rural area of North India. Am Anthropol Assoc annual meeting, 1957, Chicago *(255)*
471. Opler MK, Singer JL (1956) Ethnic differences in behavior and psychopathology: Italian and Irish. Int J Soc Psychiatry 2:11–23 *(18; 44; 82)*
472. Oppenheim H (1908) Zur Psychopathologie und Nosologie der russisch-jüdischen Bevölkerung. J Psychol Neurol 13:1–7 *(122)*
473. Oppenheim H (1915) Der Krieg und die traumatischen Neurosen. Berl Klin Wochenschr 52:257–261 *(246)*
474. Orth-Gomer K (1979) Ischemic heart disease and psychological stress in Stockholm and New York. J Psychosom Res 23:165–173 *(234)*
475. Ortigues MC, Martino P, Collomb H (1967) L'utilisation des données culturelles dans un cas de bouffée délirante. Psychopathol Afr 3:121–147 *(102)*
476. Ortigues MC, Ortigues E (1973) Oedipe Africain. Plon, Paris *(18; 105)*
477. Osgood CE, May WH, Miron MS (1975) Cross-cultural universals of affective meaning. University of Illinois Press, Urbana *(12)*
478. Overbeck-Wright AW (1921) Lunacy in India. Chapman, London *(93)*
479. Paffenberger RS (1961) The picture puzzle of the postpartum psychoses. J Chron Dis 13:161–173 *(106)*
480. Painter NS (1967) Diverticular disease of the colon: a disease of this century. Am J Dig Dis 12:222–227 *(207)*
481. Palmer S (1965) Murder and suicide in forty non-literate societies. J Crim Law Criminol Police Sci 56:320–324 *(155)*
482. Parin P (1948) Die Kriegsneurose der Yugoslawen. Schweiz Arch Neurol Psychiatr 61: 303–324 *(100)*
483. Parin P (1978) Der Widerspruch im Subjekt: ethno-psychoanalytische Studien. Syndikat, Frankfurt/M *(136)*
484. Parin P, Parin-Matthey G (1978) The Swiss and Southern German lower-middle class; an ethno-psychoanalytic study. J Psychol Anthropol 1:101–119 *(17; 44)*
485. Parker S, Kleiner RJ (1966) Mental health in an urban negro community. Free Press, Glencoe, IL *(88)*
486. Parsons A (1964) Is the Oedipus complex universal; the Jones-Malinowski debate revisited. Psychoanal Stud Soc 3:278–328 *(269)*
487. Parsons A (1969) Belief, magic and anomie; Essays in psychosocial anthropology. Free Press, New York *(82; 293)*
488. Peck WM (1978) Interim report on hypertension program in Saipan, Palau, Ponape, Truk and Yap, P.O. Box 602, Saipan. Commonwealth of the Northern Mariana Islands. (Typescript 15 pp) *(227)*
489. Peters DWC (1863) Remarks on the evils of youthful enlistments and nostalgia. Am Med Times 6:75–76 *(244)*
490. Pfeiffer WM (1974) Psychosen in einer traditionsbestimmten Kultur (Nias/Indonesien). Confin Psychiatr 17:15–41 *(141)*
491. Pfeiffer WM, Gebelein H (1969) Zur klinischen Wirkung des Fluphenazindecanoat bei einer deutschen und einer indonesischen Patientengruppe. Arzneim-Forsch 19:500–502 *(85; 86)*
492. Philip AE (1972) Social and psychological pathology of attempted suicide in Edinburgh. In: Diekstra RWF, VanderLoo KJM (eds) The cost of crisis. Gorcum, Assen pp 76–99 *(175)*
493. Piault C (ed) (1975) Prophétisme et Thérapeutique. Hermann, Paris *(104; 136; 144)*
494. Piedmont EB (1962) An investigation of ethnic grouping differences in the development of schizophrenia. Ph D Thesis, University of Buffalo *(82)*
495. Pilcz A (1902) Sur les psychoses chez les juifs. Ann Med Psychol (8th Series) 15:5–20 *(120; 121)*
496. Pilcz A (1919/1920) Beitrag zur vergleichenden Rassenpsychiatrie. Psychiatr Neurol Wochenschr 23:157–162; 24:179–182 *(98; 99; 247)*
497. Pitts FN, Winokur G (1964) Affective disorder: III – diagnostic correlates and incidence of suicide. J Nerv Ment Dis 139:176–181 *(161)*
498. Pollock HM (1913) A statistical study of the foreign-born insane in New York state hospitals. State Hosp Bull 5 (special number) 10–27 *(65; 195)*

499. Pollock HM (1928) Frequency of schizophrenia in relation to sex, age, environment, nativity and race. In: Schizophrenia. (NY Nerv Ment Dis Monogr vol 5) *(65)*
500. Porterfield AL (1949) Indices of suicide and homicide by states and cities. Am Sociol Rev 14:481–489 *(155)*
501. Primrose EJR (1962) Psychological illness; A community study. Tavistock, London *(44; 45)*
502. Prior IAM, Evans JG, Harvey HPB, Davidson F, Lindsey M (1968) Sodium intake and blood pressure in two Polynesian populations. New Engl J Med 279:515–520 *(226)*
503. Prokupek J (1968) Programs and research in Czechoslovakia. In: Williams RH, Ozarin L (eds) Community mental health. An international perspective. Jossey-Bass, San Francisco *(290)*
504. Pulvertaft CN (1968) Comments on the incidence and natural history of gastric and duodenal ulcer. Postgrad Med J 44:597–601 *(215)*
505. Rahe RH, Hervig L, Romo M, Siltanen P, Punsar S, Karvonen MJ, Rissanen V (1978) Coronary behavior in three regions of Finland. J Psychosom Med 22:453–460 *(235; 236)*
506. Raman AC, Murphy HBM (1972) Failure of traditional prognostic indicators in Afro-Asian psychotics. J Nerv Ment Dis 154:238–247 *(81; 127)*
507. Reay M (1977) Ritual madness observed; a discarded pattern of fate in Papua New Guinea. J Pacific Hist 12:55–79 *(260)*
508. Ree GH (1971) Suicide in Macuata province, Fiji. Practitioner 207:669–671 *(168)*
509. Regeringscommissaris voor de Emigratie (1958) The Man who leaves (in Dutch). Staatsdrukkerij, The Hague *(146)*
510. Régis E (1916) Psychic and neuropsychic affections in war (English-language abstract of report prepared for the French War Ministry in November 1914). Boston Med Surg J 175: 784–792 *(246)*
511. Rin H (1957) The alcoholism problem in the Nan Shi Ami people. Studia Taiwanica 2:7–16 *(193)*
512. Rin H, Lin TY (1962) Mental illness among Formosan aborigines as compared with the Chinese in Taiwan. J Ment Sci 108:134–146 *(48; 50; 72; 284)*
513. Ripley H, Wolf S (1947) Mental illness among Negro troops overseas. Am J Psychiatry 103:499–512 *(250)*
514. Robbs JV, Moshal MG (1979) Duodenal ulceration in Indians and Blacks in Durban. S Afr Med J 55:39–42 *(209; 215)*
515. Robins LN (1974) The Vietnam drug user returns: Final report. Special Action Monograph Series A. U.S. Government Printer, Washington DC *(181; 190; 251)*
516. Robins E, Murphy GE, Wilkinson RH, Gassner S, Kayes J (1959) Some clinical considerations in the prevention of suicide based on a study of 134 successful suicides. Am J Public Health 49:888–898 *(160)*
517. Robins LN, Bates WM, O'Neal P (1962) Adult drinking patterns of former problem children. In: Pittman DJ, Snyder CR (eds) Society, culture and drinking patterns. Wiley, New York, pp 395–412 *(198)*
518. Romo M, Siltanen P, Theorell T, Rahe RH (1974) Work behavior, time urgency and life dissatisfactions in subjects with myocardial infarction: a cross-cultural study. J Psychosom Res 18:1–8 *(235)*
519. Rosanoff AJ (1917) Survey of mental disorders in Nassau County, New York, July – October 1916. Psychiatr Bull 2:109–178 *(48)*
520. Rosen G (1968) Madness in society: Chapters in the historical sociology of mental illness. Harper & Row, New York *(23)*
521. Ross DC, Thomas CB (1965) Precursors of hypertension and coronary disease among healthy medical students: discriminant function analysis III: Using ethnic origin as the criterion. Bull Johns Hopkins Hosp 117:37–57 *(291)*
522. Roth GK (1953) The Fijian way of life. Oxford University Press, London *(133)*
523. Roussy G, Lhermitte J (1917) Psychonévroses de guerre. Masson, Paris *(247)*
524. Rubel AJ (1964) The epidemiology of a folk illness; susto in Hispanic America. Ethnology 3:268–284 *(255)*

MIX
Papier aus verantwortungsvollen Quellen
Paper from responsible sources
FSC® C105338

If you have any concerns about our products,
you can contact us on
ProductSafety@springernature.com

In case Publisher is established outside the EU,
the EU authorized representative is:
Springer Nature Customer Service Center GmbH
Europaplatz 3, 69115 Heidelberg, Germany

Printed by Libri Plureos GmbH
in Hamburg, Germany